RECENT ADVANCES IN SCOLIOSIS

Edited by **Theodoros B. Grivas**

Recent Advances in Scoliosis
Edited by Theodoros B. Grivas

Published by InTech
Janeza Trdine 9, 51000 Rijeka, Croatia

Publishing Process Manager Ana Skalamera

Technical Editor Teodora Smiljanic

Cover Designer InTech Design Team

Additional hard copies can be obtained from orders@intechopen.com

Recent Advances in Scoliosis, Edited by Theodoros B. Grivas
p. cm.
ISBN 978-953-51-0595-4

For EU product safety concerns:
IN TECH d.o.o., Prolaz Marije Krucifikse Kozulić 3, 51000 Rijeka, Croatia,
info@intechopen.com or visit our website at intechopen.com.

Meet the editor

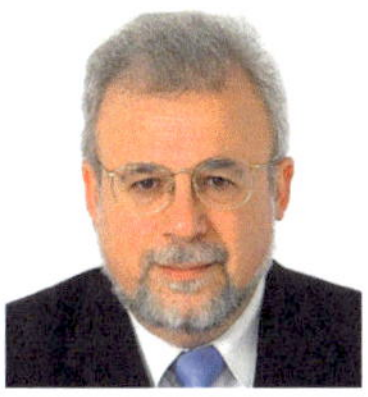

Dr Theodoros B. Grivas (MD, PhD Orthopaedic and Spinal Surgeon) graduated from the Medical School at "Aristotle" University of Thessaloniki, Central Macedonia, Greece. He completed his training in General Surgery, Paediatric and Adult Orthopaedics and Traumatology in Greece and received his MD Diploma and his PhD degree. He worked at the "University Hospital", Queen's Medical Centre in Nottingham, "Harlow Wood" Orthopaedic Hospital in Mansfield, UK under Mr JK Webb and Professor RG Burwell, as well as at "Evangelismos" and "Thriasio" Hospital in Athens, Greece. He is a member and Traveling Fellow of both AAOS and SRS, a member of the Hellenic Association of Orthopaedic Surgery and Traumatology and a member of numerous other scientific societies. He served as an IRSSD and SOSORT elected president. He completed several research projects, studied and implemented the School Screening program, published numerous peer-review articles and chapters in books and was invited to lecture on various general orthopaedic and spinal topics. He wrote or was the editor of eight books. He is the Chief Editor of "Scoliosis" and a member of editorial board or reviewer for several peer-review journals. Currently he is the Director of the Trauma and Orthopaedic Department at "Tzanio" General Hospital of Piraeus, Greece.

Contents

Preface

Idiopathic scoliosis (IS) is of yet unknown aetiology and its treatment is symptomatic and not aetiological. Every effort must be undertaken to reverse this treatment into aetiological. Professor RG Burwell, a recognised authority in the study of IS aetiology, states that "although considerable progress had been made in the past two decades in understanding the etiopathogenesis of adolescent idiopathic scoliosis (AIS), it still lacks an agreed theory of etiopathogenesis. One problem may be that AIS results not from one cause, but several that interact with various genetic predisposing factors". Epigenetic concepts, which may relate to AIS pathogenesis, were also recently introduced and reported.

The first two chapters of this book focus on concepts related to the pathogenesis of IS and provide suggestions for improving scoliosis research. A related chapter tapping the aetiological aspects of IS reports on the Ritscher-Schinzel syndrome. The chapter on Sensorimotor Integration in AIS Patients provides some evidence of a relation between IS and dysfunction of neurological mechanisms. In the chapter "Virtual Anatomy of Spinal Disorders by 3-D MRI/CT Fusion Imaging" the methods used in the authors' hospital for obtaining, evaluating and displaying 3-D MRI/CT fusion imaging are discussed, focusing on their application in the field of spinal surgery.

The chapter entitled "Quantitative MRI for Scoliosis Follow-Up" introduces the MRI parameters and presents how they are acquired in vivo. The studies on MRI parameters of bone are presented, in order to show how these parameters may be involved in bone health research related to scoliosis. The same chapter describes the studies on the relation between MRI parameters and biochemical or mechanical properties of the intervertebral disc. It focuses on the relationships between MRI parameters and muscle properties, as well as the possible applications to scoliosis. Finally, the potential of quantitative MRI to become a very important diagnostic and treatment assessment tool in scoliosis is discussed.

The chapter "Moiré Topography: From Takasaki Till Present Day" presents a literature review on the main characteristics of the Moirι phenomenon, and its use as a topographical method for the clinical diagnosis of postural deviations. The chapter entitled "Three-Dimensional Assessment of the Scoliosis" reports on spine assessment in 3D through reconstruction models, and discusses their importance for the diagnosis, the follow-up and the treatment of scoliosis. The chapter entitled "Emerging Technology and Analytical Techniques for the Clinical Assessment of Scoliosis" provides an overview of current clinical models for the assessment of scoliosis, and brings to attention new approaches that may allow enhancing fundamental knowledge and complementing clinical models of assessment. In the same chapter, the theoretical construct of posture is also reviewed and the clinical terms and frames of reference are identified which are commonly adopted to describe the posture of children and youth with IS. The chapter also identifies and discusses the potential of emerging techniques that may enhance current clinical models of assessment. The chapter "Predicting Curve Progression in Adolescent Idiopathic Scoliosis - An Outline of Different Indicators of Growth" provides a concise outline of several indicators of growth and curve progression, thus offering a clear overview of which indicators can be helpful in predicting the timing of pubertal growth spurt and therefore the timing of possible scoliosis progression. In "The Impact of Spinal Deformity on Gait in Subjects with Idiopathic Scoliosis" the authors describe various walking disorders in subjects with different types of scoliosis, which were measured by appropriate systems and instruments. The chapter "Characteristics of Body Posture in Children and Youth with Hearing Disorders" aims to assess the body posture of children and youth with hearing impairment, with an emphasis on the frequency of the occurrence of abnormalities. The percentage of abnormalities in the body posture is defined, which allows for corrective work to be planned.

In the chapter "Scoliosis Idiopathic? The Etiologic Factors in Scoliosis Will Affect Preventive and Conservative Therapeutic Strategies" the author presents a novel conservative therapeutic model. In "Long-Term Outcome of Surgical Treatment in Adolescent Idiopathic Scoliosis" the authors present their long-term results of posterior instrumentation and spondylodesis in patients with AIS, and critically review original papers, compiled in a chronological manner, that present long-term results. In "Complications in Scoliosis Surgery" the authors review the published literature on complications related to surgical treatment of scoliosis.

"Health Related Quality of Life in Adolescents with Idiopathic Scoliosis" attempts to deepen the concept of HRQOL and to understand how it is used, as well as its strong and weak points. The authors intend to complement the medical model with the psychological one, in a bio-psycho-social framework. The chapter "Psychological Aspects of Scoliosis Treatment in Children" emphasises the fact that the patients with scoliosis and their families need to be provided with psychological support through the whole period of the treatment, and discusses related issues.

The patient's perspective is described in "Untreated Early Onset Scoliosis - The Natural Progression of a Debilitating and Ultimately Deadly Disease". A case of an adult patient with untreated early onset IS is presented; evidence-based facts and data regarding health related issues, natural progression and surgical management of untreated early onset and AIS that results in severe adult deformity is summarized.

In "Congenital Kyphoscoliosis due to Hemivertebra" the treatment options and results for this congenital disease are reviewed.

Closing this short introduction to this open access book, I would like to express my gratitude to all authors for their enthusiasm and willingness to document their knowledge and share it with all peers interested in scoliosis. I would also like to thank Mrs Ana Skalamera, the Publishing Process Manager, and InTech Open Access Publisher for inviting me to do the editorship of this book.

Dr Theodoros B. Grivas, MD, PhD
Orthopaedic and Spinal Surgeon
Director of the Trauma and Orthopaedic Department
"Tzanio" General Hospital of Piraeus,
Greece

Section 1

Aetiology – Pathogenesis of Idiopathic Scoliosis

1

Hypothesis on the Pathogenesis of Idiopathic Scoliosis

F.H. Wapstra and A.G. Veldhuizen
University Medical Center of Groningen
The Netherlands

1. Introduction

Idiopathic scoliosis is a deformity of the torso, characterized by lateral deviation and axial rotation of the spine. Although good anatomic descriptions of the structural changes seen in scoliosis were first made by the ancient Greeks, we have not as yet elucidated its pathogenesis. The deformity always develops from a straight spine into a curved spine, usually accompanied by a rib cage deformity, during the growth period in general and in particular in the rapid growth period. In the growing scoliotic spine, the loss of mechanical stability results in deformation of the vertebral bodies and ribs. The eventual magnitude of an idiopathic scoliotic curve varies and is unpredictable. The extent of the alterations in the shape of the vertebrae and ribs is strongly related to the severity of the scoliotic curve. Pain is a rare symptom, and the patient seems unaware of his or her condition. The idiopathic scoliotic curves follow a geometric pattern: (1) primary thoracic; (2) thoraco-lumbar; (3) primary lumbar (4) double primary. The primary curve invariably has associated secondary curves which follow similar geometric pattern. The axial rotation of the vertebrae is towards the convexity of the curve (Boos & Aebi, 2008). The most important problem related to scoliosis is progression of the deformity, i.e. worsening of the scoliotic curve. The amount of progression is different in each individual patient, some progress very fast, others don't progress at all (Charles et al, 2006; Cheung et al, 2005 & 2006; Dimeglio, 2001; Escalada et al, 2005; Sanders et al, 2007; Wever et al, 2000; Yronen & Ylikoski, 2006). Earlier when the growth velocity of the spine is 20 mm/year or more, the idiopathic scoliosis is nearly always progressive (Cheung et al, 2004). When growth is completed progression generally stops, although research has shown that the risk of curve progression is primarily related to periods of rapid skeletal growth of the patient, most often during the pubertal growth spurt. It was shown that curves of more than 40 degrees Cobb angle are able to progress even after skeletal maturity, because of degeneration of the disk and the fibro-cartilage at load transfer points on the concave side of the curve, although this progression will be at a very low rate of 1° or 2° a year (Duval-Beaupere et al, 1970; Duval-Beaupere & Lamireau, 1985). The prevalence of scoliosis is approximately 4% of the children between 10 and 16 years of age. However, adolescent idiopathic scoliosis does not necessarily progress, and the prevalence of children having a Cobb angle larger than 45 degrees, and therefore needing operative treatment, is approximately 0.1%. Spontaneous improvement is however rare and almost never seen in moderate to large curves. Although many types or causes of scoliosis are known, the idiopathic variety comprises the largest group (80%) and its aetiology remains unknown. A strong familiar history is usual and a hereditary transmission suggesting an autosomal dominant or multifactorial defect is described (Duthie, 1959; Duval-Beaupere et al, 1970). The effect of industrial environmental factors been investigated, but those factors probably do not significantly influence the prevalence of AIS (Grivas et al, 2008). Some workers favour a neuromuscular basis for the condition, others believe that asymmetrical growth is the primary etiological factor (Deacon et al, 1984 & 1987; Dickson et al, 1984; Duthie, 1959; Millner & Dickson, 1996). Some workers have attributed the initial spinal

deformity of AIS to changes in ribs (Pal, 1991; Burwell et al, 1992; Grivas et al, 1991, 1992, 2002, 2007 & 2008; Sevastik, 2000; Sevastik et al, 2003; Erkula et al, 2003). Many workers hold the view that the rib deformities of progressive AIS are adaptations to forces imposed by the scoliotic spine (Wever et al, 1999; Burwell et al, 2003) with the sternum, held nearly stationary by abdominal ties and providing the opposing forces needed to deform the ribs (Closkey & Schultz, 1993).Whatever factors underlie the aetiology, they ultimately express themselves in the biomechanical changes that define scoliotic curve progression. This paper proposes a possible model for the pathomechanics of idiopathic scoliosis.

2. Neuromuscular factors

Awareness of the position of the body in space is a highly developed sense in humans. It is the result of input from the vestibular, visual and proprioceptive neural pathways. In recent years, strong evidence has been found for the idea that, for visuomotor co-ordination and exploration of space, the brain uses abstract, neural representations of space interposed between sensory input and motor output. These neural representations seem to be organised in nonretinal, body-centred and/or world-centred coordinates (Andersen et al, 1993; Snijder et al, 1993). Spatial information in non-retinal coordinates allows the subject to determine the body position with respect to visual space, which is a necessary prerequisite for accurate behaviour in space. To obtain such a frame of reference, the information coded in coordinates related to the peripheral sensory organs must be transformed and integrated. Defective postural equilibrium has been proposed as a contributing factor in the development of scoliosis (Guyton, 1976). In this regard, defects in visual and vestibular input have been studied extensively as a possible genesis of idiopathic scoliosis (Herman & McEwen, 1979; Herman et al, 1982 & 1985; Sahlstrand et al, 1979; Sahlstrand & Petruson, 1979; Sahlstrand & Lindstrom, 1980; Sahlstrand, 1980; Kapetanos et al, 2002). The occurrence of vestibular-related deficits in AIS patients is well established but it is unclear whether a vestibular pathology is the common cause for the scoliotic syndrome and the gaze/posture deficits or if the latter behavioral deficits are a consequence of the scoliotic deformations. A possible vestibular origin was tested in the frog Xenopus laevis by unilateral removal of the labyrinthine end organs at larval stages. After metamorphosis into young adult frogs, X-ray images and three-dimensional reconstructed micro-computer tomographic scans of the skeleton showed deformations similar to those of scoliotic patients. The skeletal distortions consisted of a curvature of the spine in the frontal and sagittal plane, a transverse rotation along the body axis and substantial deformations of all vertebrae (Lambert et al, 2009). A clinical study from Wiener-Vacher (Wiener-Vacher & Mazda, 1998) supports the hypothesis that central otolith vestibular system disorders lead to a vestibule-spinal system imbalance, and may be a factor in the cause of AIS. In a pilot study on scoliotic patients we used Vestibular Evoked Myogenic Potentials (VEMP) (Hain et al, 2006). The purpose of the VEMP test is to determine if the saccule, one portion of the otoliths, as well the inferior vestibular nerve and central connections, are intact and working normally. The saccule, which is the lower of the two otolithic organs, has a slight sound sensitivity and this can be measured. This sensitivity is thought to be a remnant from the saccule's use as an organ of hearing in lower animals. We found an asymmetry in Idiopathic scoliosis patients and not in other types of scoliosis (unpublished data). Vestibulo-ocular reflex changes may be viewed as a function of asymmetrical control of reflex gain, which is disturbed further during any postural task requiring control of body motion in the presence of visual fixation. Hence, postural instability is ascribed to the conflict between visual and vestibular information within the higher central nervous system (CNS) centres, which can integrate and calibrate converging sensory data for perception and control of postural movement (Herman & McEwen, 1979; Herman et al, 1979 & 1985). Proprioceptive input from joints, ligaments and tendons has been recognised as an integral contribution to the body's postural equilibrium Guyton, 1976). Defects in the muscle spindle system and tone in the spinal muscles have been implicated in scoliosis (Barrack et al, 1984; Hoogmartens & Basmajian, 1976; Low et al, 1978; Matthews, 1969; Matthews, 1969, Whitecloud et al, 1984; Yekutiel et al, 1981). Neural pathways involving visual, vestibular and proprioceptive afferents all have discrete interconnections in the brainstem. A lesion in this anatomical location could affect all three pathways. Congenital lesions in this area are associated with scoliosis (Tezuka, 1971), and scoliosis has been successfully induced by damaging this area (Dubousset et al, 1982).

Experimentally created defects in the vestibular system of a rat resulted in delayed posture and motor development (Geisler, 1997). Previous studies of CNS function in AIS have suggested that altered cerebral cortical/subcortical function (Herman & McEwen, 1979; Mixon & Steel, 1982; Petersen et al, 1979; Sahlstrand et al, 1979) or hemispherical dominance (Enslein & Chan, 1987) may be related to the aetiology of AIS. Patients with scoliosis and primary alteration of the motor system, so-called neuromuscular scoliosis, are known to have a curve morphology and natural history very different from that of the "typical" idiopathic curve. Magnetic resonance imaging studies of the brain stem in adolescent idiopathic scoliosis by Geissele et al. showed an asymmetry in the ventral pons or medulla in a number of patients (Geissele et al, 1991). Abnormalities in the paraspinal muscles have been implicated by several investigators as a possible causative factor in the production and progression of adolescent idiopathic scoliosis (Fidler et al, 1974; Fidler & Jowett, 1976; Ford et al, 1984; Spenser & Eccles, 1976; Yarom & Robin, 1979). An increased myoelectric response on the convex side of the curve, near its apex, was the main finding reported by various authors (Alexander & Season, 1978; Alexander et al, 1978; Butterworth & James, 1969; Guth & Abbink, 1980; Henssge, 1962; Redford et al, 1969; Spenser & Eccles, 1976; Wong et al, 1980; Yarom & Robin, 1979; Zetterberg et al, 1984), but not all agreed on the meaning of these findings. In early reports a fatigue mechanism was suggested (Riddle & Roaf, 1955), while others explained the difference as an effect of the stretching of the erector spinae muscles on the convex side (Butterworth & James, 1969).

This view was supported by the finding of a stretch reflex (H-reflex) that was more sensitive to vibration and hammer tapping on the spinous processes in larger curves (Hoogmartens & Basmajian, 1976). Others believed that the increased myoelectric activities on the convex side were only a secondary effect of the muscles adapting to a higher load demand in larger curves (Zetterberg et al, 1984). This would be consistent with the reported findings of differences in the morphology of the paravertebral muscles between the left and right sides (Saltin et al, 1977; Spenser & Eccles, 1976; Wong et al, 1980; Yarom & Robin, 1979). However, the increase of type 1 muscle fibres on the convex side can be explained on the basis of muscle denervation (Ford et al, 1984; Webb, 1973 & 1981; Zetterberg et al, 1984), produced by an alteration of the motor drive arising at the spinal cord level, either from altered sensory input at the same level (Pincott, 1980; Pincott & Taffs, 1982; Taffs et al, 1979) or from a central mechanism (Barrack et al, 1984; Dubousset et al, 1982; Michelsson, 1965; Sahlstrand et al, 1979; Whitecloud et al, 1984). The ocular and postural control systems reach maturation in early adult life (Forssberg & Nasher, 1982; Nasher, 1982; Sharp et al, 1979).

Children with idiopathic scoliosis in the age range of 9–16 years exhibit delay in the complete development of smooth pursuit and optokinetic nystagmus; moreover, they demonstrate a delay in tasks that couple the vestibular and visual systems, particularly those requiring voluntary suppression of the vestibulo-ocular reflex (Herman & McEwen, 1979). This behaviour is required to ensure optimal visual acuity in phase with head motion. Incomplete maturation of visual and visuo-vestibular functioning is ascribed to inefficient extraretinal processing of perceptual information by cortical structures within the CNS, e.g. to delayed development of perception of the position of visual images in space (Herman & McEwen, 1979; Sharp & Rabinovitch, 1979; Yasui & Young, 1976; Young, 1977). The maturation of the ocular and postural control systems coincides with the secondary rapid growth period. Some workers believe that not only the somatic nervous system is involved but the autonomic nervous system as well (Burwell, 2003; Grivas et al, 2009; Burwell et al, 2009). AIS in girls may then be the result from developmental disharmony expressed in spine and trunk between autonomic and somatic nervous systems. The autonomic component involves *selectively increased sensitivity* of the hypothalamus to circulating leptin (genetically-determined up-regulation possibly involving inhibitory or sensitizing intracellular molecules, such as SOC3, PTP-1B and SH2B1 respectively), with asymmetry as an adverse response (hormesis); this asymmetry is routed bilaterally via the sympathetic nervous system to the growing axial skeleton where it may initiate the scoliosis deformity.

We propose, therefore, that the most likely cause of idiopathic scoliosis includes a neuromuscular condition and an asymmetry of the transversospinalis muscles, produced by alteration of the motor drive at the spinal cord level, either from altered sensory input at the same level or from a central mechanism, which may produce enough lateral deviation and axial rotation to disturb the delicate balance of forces in the region, thereby producing an idiopathic scoliosis. Growth disturbance may not be a primary cause of idiopathic scoliosis, but it certainly plays a prominent part in the progression of this deformity, although it is not very clear how.

2.1 Spinal growth factor

Researchers of spinal deformity have always been interested in spinal growth and its relationship to spinal curvature. Normal longitudinal growth does not proceed in a uniform, linear pattern (Tanner, 1962 & 1978; Tanner & Davies, 1985; Tanner et al, 1965). There are two periods of rapid growth, the first from birth to three years of age, and the second during the adolescent growth spurt. The intervening period is a period of quiet but steady growth. For over 100 years the association between idiopathic scoliosis and vertebral growth has been debated (Anderson et al, 1965; Burwell & Dangerfield, 1974; Calvo, 1957; Duthie, 1959; Duval-Beaupere et al, 1970; Duval-Beaupere & Lamireau, 1985). A large number of studies on growth differences between normal and scoliotic girls have been conducted.

Unfortunately, the results of these studies were not consistent. Willner observed a taller mean standing height in girls with scoliosis compared to healthy controls (Willner, 1974 & 1975 & 1975). These findings were supported by other cross-sectional studies (Buric & Momcilovic, 1982; Hagglund et al, 1992; Leong et al, 1982; Low et al, 1978; Nordwall & Willner, 1975; Normelli et al, 1985; Shohat et al, 1988). Loncar-Dusek et al. demonstrated a higher peak velocity for scoliotic children (Loncar-Dusek, 1991). Moreover, Goldberg et al. and Ylikowski et al. reported that girls with adolescent idiopathic scoliosis (AIS) have an earlier growth spurt and earlier attainment of adult height compared to healthy nonscoliotic controls (Goldberg et al, 1993; Ylikowski, 1993). This is in marked contrast to many other reports, which found no difference in growth pattern or height between AIS patients and nonscoliotic controls (Drummond & Rogala, 1980; Taylor, 1983; Veldhuizen, 1985; Veldhuizen et al, 1986). However, one should keep in mind that most of the studies on growth differences between scoliotic and nonscoliotic girls mentioned above were based either on length measurements of the sitting height, without correction for the error introduced by the scoliotic deformity itself, or were corrected using the method described by Bjure (Bjure et al, 1968) This method overestimates the real length of the spine, and may not be valid for curves of 30° or less Cobb angle, since they had no patients with such mild curves in their material (Skogland & Miller, 1981). The advocates of a deviating growth pattern explain the initiation of idiopathic scoliosis as the result of a greater tendency of taller and more slender spines to buckle out of the sagittal plane under loading (Dickson et al, 1984 & 1987; Millner & Dickson, 1996; Smith & Dickson, 1987).

Roaf (Roaf, 1960 & 1966) and Dickson (Dickson et al, 1984 & 1987) explain the pathogenesis of idiopathic scoliosis as a result of biplane asymmetry. Increased anterior vertebral height at the apex of the curve with posterior end-plate irregularity characterises the median plane asymmetry. This lordosis at bony level was an important basis for their theory that thoracic lordosis, which is caused by a relative overgrowth of the anterior part of the vertebral body, triggers the initiation of scoliosis by buckling. In a three-dimensionally rendered CT scan study we have previously described the vertebral and rib deformities in idiopathic scoliosis (Wever et al, 1999). The observed vertebral deformities suggest that these are caused by bone remodelling due to an imbalance between forces in the anterior and posterior spinal column (Meyer, 1866; Wever et al, 1999). In our study, we also noted a minimal wedge deformation in the local sagittal plane in certain apical vertebrae, as mentioned by Deacon and Dickson, but it is questionable whether this deformation in the sagittal plane is a primary aetiological phenomenon, as they suggest, or whether it is rather a secondary phenomenon, comparable to the other vertebral deformations. They do not offer an explanation for this growth disturbance. Deane and Duthie (Deane & Duthie, 1973; Duthie, 1959) found in a cadaveric study that the anterior body lengths either singly, or as total length were almost normal in the scoliotic patients, but the posterior lengths were considerably reduced due to a strong inhibitory force to growth of the posterior vertebral structures. Furthermore, no proof of the "Euler theory", that idiopathic scoliosis is the result of buckling under load, has ever been given. The mechanical behaviour of such a complex and highly non-linear structure as the human vertebral column is very difficult to analyse. Using a new finite element model of the spine, we have previously examined this buckling theory (van de Plaats, 1997; van de Plaats et al, 2007). Judging from the results of this finite element study, buckling can not initiate idiopathic scoliosis, because the characteristic coupling of lateral deviation and axial rotation is absent. Furthermore, no difference in spinal flexibility can be established between patients with idiopathic scoliosis and controls (Mattson et al, 1983; Veldhuizen, 1985; Veldhuizen & Scholten, 1990). Mechanical and computer models of the spine are frequently used to analyse the mechanisms by which scoliosis is initiated and aggravated. In a relatively simple stable physical model of the trunk, progression of the scoliosis due to growth can be shown (Murray & Bulstrode, 1996; Nijenbanning, 1998), but there is little evidence that growth initiate idiopathic scoliosis.

The question is what growth is.

2.2 Human growth

Growth is inextricable associated with life. It is defined as a quantitative increase in size or mass, and it is a consequence of hyperplasia and hypertrophy; i.e. the size of the cells increases, as well as the number of cells. The term 'growth' is generally used for an increase in height or weight. Several body length dimensions can be measured, like total body height, sitting height, arm span, foot length, head circumference etc. Leg length is calculated by protraction of sitting height from total height. The increase in length is calculated per year, this is called the growth velocity. Unfortunately, in literature several terms are used alternatively, like growth, growth velocity, height velocity, or growth rate. Often timing or the magnitude of the growth spurt is simply indicated as peak growth velocity (PGV). Furthermore, many authors just refer to peak growth velocity of total body height as peak height velocity. It is often confusing whether the magnitude of the growth velocity is meant, or the age at which the maximum growth velocity takes place. In this article the term 'growth' is used for the increase in a certain length dimension in centimetres. The term 'growth velocity' is used for the increase of a certain length dimension per year, expressed in cm/year. The term 'peak growth velocity (PGV)' of a certain length dimension is used for the maximum growth velocity during adolescence. For example, PGV of total body height, or PGV of foot length. Growth is a volumetric revolution. From birth onwards, total body height increases 350% and weight increases 20-fold. Growth involves changes in proportion. At birth, the lower limbs make up 30% of the total body height in contrast to 48% at skeletal maturity. The infant head makes up 25% of the total body height and only 13% at skeletal maturity. All the changes in body length dimensions are gradual and each dimension has its own period of rapid growth (Busscher et al, 2010 & 2011; Dimeglio, 2001). Tanner (Tanner, 1962 & 1978) was the first to describe the distal-to-proximal growth gradient theory. This theory states that humans grow "from the outside to the inside", in other words, distal body parts will have their growth spurt earlier in adolescence in comparison to more proximal body parts. Four main characteristics dominate puberty: an increase in total body height, change of upper and lower body segment proportions, change in overall morphology, and the development of secondary sexual characteristics. Wide individual variations exist in onset and duration of puberty, and many factors play a role in the timing of the pubertal growth spurt. Beyond the age of 10 years, the growth patterns of boys and girls diverge. This is mainly due to the fact that boys have their pubertal growth spurt later in adolescence. The average age for the pubertal growth spurt, or the peak growth velocity of total body height, to occur is between ages 10 and 14 in 95% of the girls and between ages 12 and 16 in 95% of the boys (Gerver & de Bruin, 2001 & 2003; Tanner & Davies, 1985), see Figure 1A.

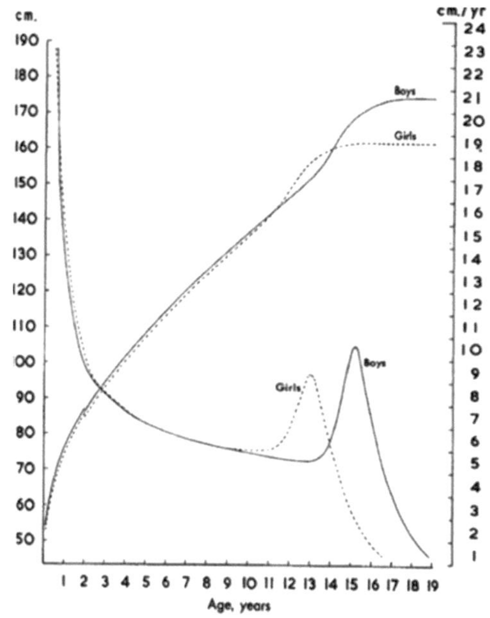

Fig. 1A. Average growth curves and growth velocity curves of boys and girls.

Furthermore, it is known that the magnitude of the peak growth velocity is significantly larger for those individuals with an early pubertal growth spurt as compared to those with a late growth spurt (Figure 1B). However, the growth period before the peak is longer and therefore the ultimate total body height will be similar or higher compared to children with an early growth spurt (Gerver & de Bruin, 2003; Tanner & Davies, 1985)

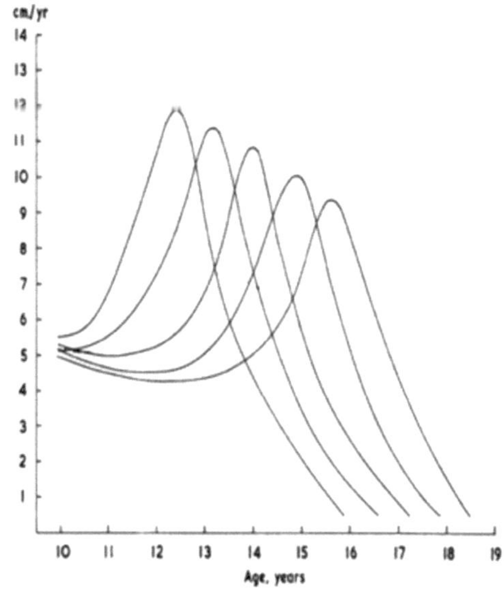

Fig. 1B. Examples of growth velocity curves of children having their peak growth velocity at a different age.

Generally, the increase in height of the vertebral bodies is the result of enchondral growth at the upper and lower growth plate (Bick, 1961; Gooding & Neuhauser, 1965; Knuttson, 1961), whereas the increase in width is a result of periosteal growth (Bick, 1961). It has been suggested (Neugebauer, 1976) that the regulating(hormonal) mechanism is different for the two types of bone growth, but there is in fact little definite evidence for the endocrine pathways by which any particular hormone influences skeletal growth (Sisson, 1971). The growth of the posterior elements (lamina, pedicles) comes in part from enchondral ossification initiated in the articular cartilages of the articular processes (Enneking & Harrington, 1969). Growth can also be described as a mechanical process.

2.3 Growth as a mechanical processi

In his classic "On Growth and Form "D' Arcy Thompson (D' Arcy Wentworth Thompson, 1961) analyses biological processes in their mathematical and physical aspects. In his opinion the form and change of any object in its movement and its growth may be described as due to the action of forces. In the Newtonian language of elementary physics, force is recognised by its action in producing or changing motion or in preventing change of motion or in maintaining rest. In accordance with D'Arcy Thompson's view we describe growth as a mechanical process; a process that elapses in time and can be described by mechanical input and output variables. All parts of the skeleton show visco-elastic behaviour, meaning that a change in form is the sum of the changes in elastic and viscous transformations. The main difference between elastic and viscous transformation is time response. Elastic transformation can be understood as the action of a spring: by putting a weight on a spring, the length of that spring will increase immediately and after removing this weight, it regains its original length (Figure 2A). Viscous transformation can be understood as the action of a damper: by putting a weight on a damper, at first nothing will happen, but after a while the damper will move. After removing this weight, the damper will remain in its new position. (Figure 2B)

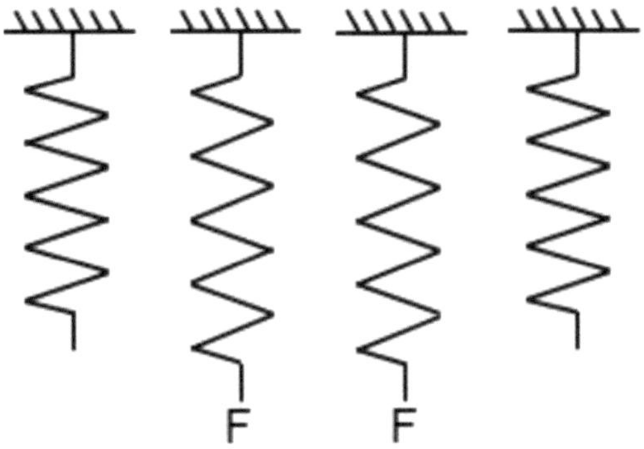

Fig. 2A. Elastic Element.

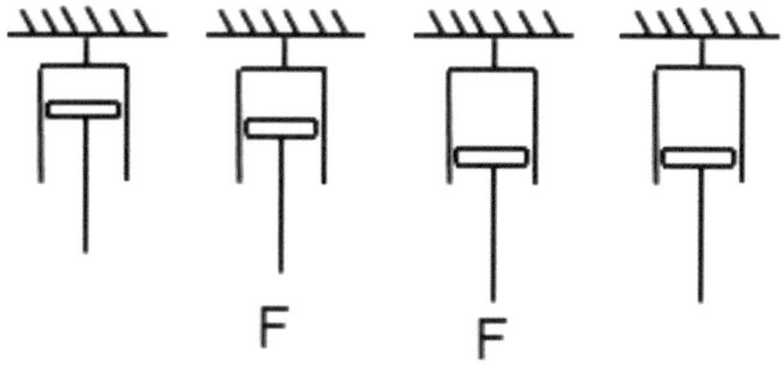

Fig. 2B. Viscous Element.

The growth in bone takes place in the growth-plate. As shown in figure 3 the genesis of growth can be thought of as a hydraulic system: the barrel left in the drawing contains liquid under pressure, representing the nursery-room of new cells. The liquid flows through tubes in which switch-back valves are incorporated to form a piston-cylinder combination. The liquid pressure will move the piston. Every piston-cylinder combination represents a growing cell and will produce an internal force on the growth-plate. The pistons are mechanically coupled resulting in a total force on the growth-plate, called the force of growth. The displacement of the coupling beam models the increase in length. Unequal distribution of force on the coupling beam results in an inclination of the coupling beam, simulating asymmetric growth. The switch-back valve supports the permanent character of the transformation by growth.

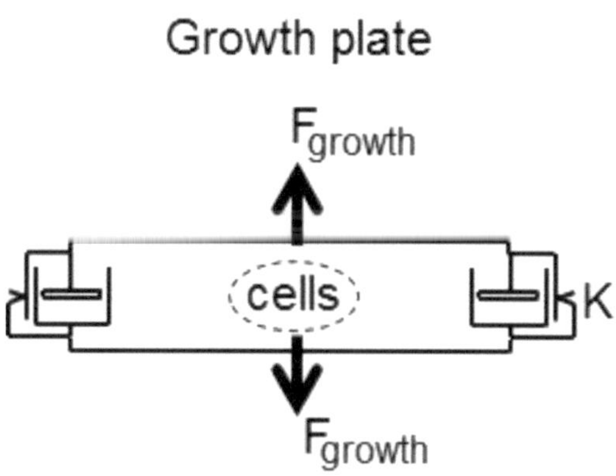

Fig. 3. Genesis of growth, represented as a hydraulic system. The switch-back valve (K) supports the permanent character of the transformation by growth.

If bone grows the soft tissues like muscles and ligaments have to follow and increase their length as well against their own tractive powers. This force is referred to as Soft tissue Complex Force and opposes growth. As shown in figure 4 this Soft Tissue Complex Force will induce a suction tension through traction on the piston. If the suction force is larger than the spring-force on the switch-back valve, liquid will flow into the cylinder. The lengthening will be permanent through the action of the switch-back valve. Only one piston-cylinder combination has been drawn, representing the total of growing cells.

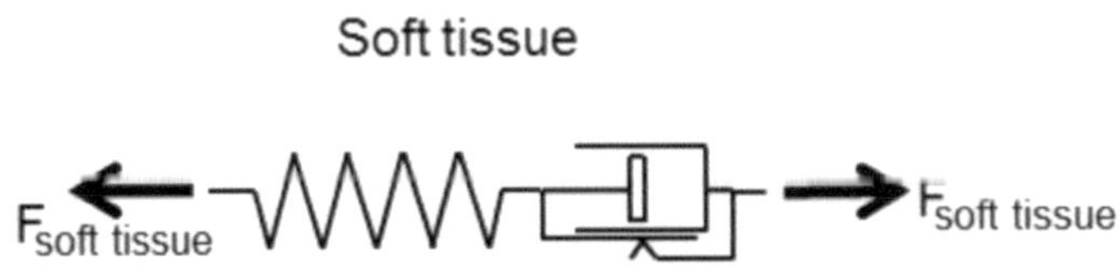

Fig. 4. Hydraulic representation of traction Force: $F_{Soft\ Tissue\ Complex}$.

In figure 5 a scheme of the growth-process of bone-soft tissue combination is presented. The in the growth-plate generated Force of Growth will induce growth in bone but will be inhibited by the Force of Soft Tissue Complex, required for lengthening of soft tissue.

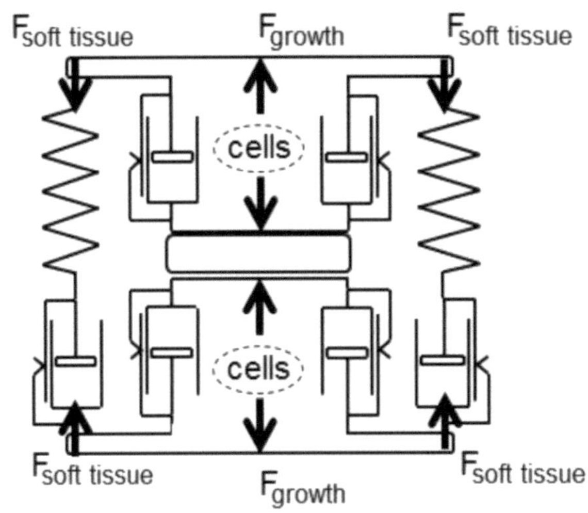

Fig. 5. A scheme of growth process of bone and soft tissue is presented.

The difference between these two forces creates a growth-velocity in bone resulting in growth only if there is a positive force difference. This mechanical concept of growth explains easily the greater length of bony elements in Marfan Disease: the force of soft tissue complex will be smaller and will have a less opposing effect on the force of growth.

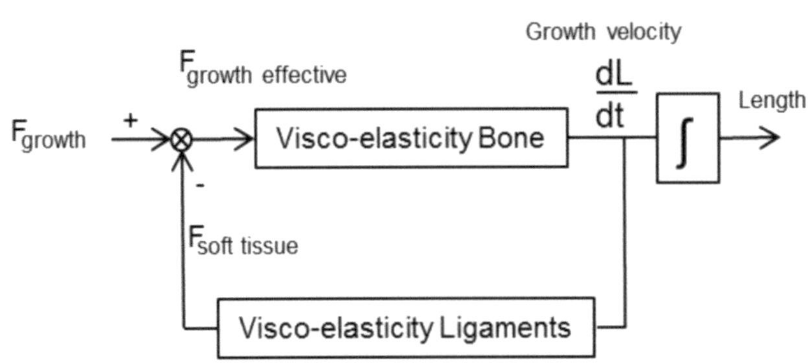

Fig. 6. Growth-process.

In table 1 a summary of forces acting on the spine are given. For the growth process only the Force of Growth and the Force of Soft Tissue Complex are important. The other forces, mentioned in table 1, act relatively too shortly to influence the slow reacting viscous elements.

Forces	Duration of Action	Effect
Gravity	Long	
Ligaments/muscles passive	Short	Viscous
Muscles active	Short	
External load	Short	
Growth	Long	Viscous

Table 1. Summary of forces, acting on the spine.

Our basic model of growth shows a one- dimensional situation: bone-growth equals soft tissue lengthening. In practice the soft tissue will show a non-linear and dynamic behaviour. The introduction of a joint makes the system multi-dimensional and enables small rotation of skeletal parts as a result of growth. Sometimes these small rotations are part of nature's plan, e.g. when considering the formation of the s-shape in the sagittal plane during the first years of life.

3. Curve progression

The initiation of idiopathic scoliosis can be explained on the basis of a neuromuscular condition. However, the proposed neurological defects are not correlated with the degree of subsequent progression for the curve. According to Perdriolle (Perdriolle et al, 1993) the progression of idiopathic scoliosis is the result of a mechanical phenomenon. It has been demonstrated that the expected spinal growth at the moment that the initial curve is diagnosed is of crucial importance for the further development of scoliosis (Lonstein & Carlson, 1984). In a recent study, we demonstrated that progression of an idiopathic scoliotic curve correlates with periods of moderate and rapid growth, measured on successive radiographs (Wever et al, 2000).The variations in growth speed across individuals, as seen in our study, may explain the variations in expression of AIS, together with other factors such as the type of curve. Different biomechanical mechanisms are given to explain scoliosis progression during spinal growth (Kamman, 2003; Pincott & Taffs, 1982; van de Plaats, 1997; van de Plaats et al, 2007; Raso, 1998). It has been suggested that asymmetrical growth of the apical vertebral bodies due to chronic axial asymmetrical loading on the physes, according to the Hueter- Volkmann law, may result in scoliosis progression (Agadir et al, 1988; Perdriolle et al, 1993). Stokes et al. quantified the relationship between the degree of a symmetrical loading and the degree of asymmetrical growth in a rat-tail model and confirmed that vertebral wedging results from asymmetric growth in the physes (Stokes et al, 1996). In our study, there was a strong correlation between the degrees of apical vertebral deformation (wedging) and the degree of lateral deviation (Cobb angle), meaning that more vertebral deformation was found in more severe curves (Wever et al, 1999 & 2000). However, we have not found a direct relation between curve progression and an increase in wedging in progressive scoliosis. Others have stressed the importance of the posterior musculo-ligamentous structures of the spinal column, which have a strong tendency to shorten. It was postulated that the tethering tendency of the musculo-ligamentous structures of the posterior compared to the rapid growth of the anterior spinal column will result in curve progression and the complex geometry of scoliosis (Murray & Bulstrode, 1996, Roaf, 1960 & 1966, Somerville, 1952). Several major sensory systems, the general proprioceptors and the special receptors of the vestibular, visual, auditory and olfactory systems, are believed to be the principal sensors. Lack of feedback, inappropriate feedback, or faulty programming within the CNS, due to pathology, results in varying degrees of abnormal muscle tone, movement, and / or problems associated with gravity and orientation in space. The postural tone depends largely on the stretch reflex in the extensor muscles (Matthews, 1969; Michelsson, 1965). This reflex acts so that any external factor that brings the body out of equilibrium will stretch the appropriate extensor muscles and their muscle spindles, thereby activating the primary afferents, which monosynaptically excite homonymous alpha afferents. The latter will induce a contraction in the stretched muscles and restore the body to its position of equilibrium. The sensitivity of muscle spindle afferents is known to be under control of supraspinal centres, which act through the supraspinal gamma route and through the gamma motor neurons at the spinal level. The gamma motor neurons innervate the muscle spindles, which are sensitive to stretch in a minor or major degree, according to whether they are more or less biased by the gamma motor neurons. The central parts of the muscle spindle are surrounded by primary and secondary afferent fibres, transmitting stretch information to the alpha motor neurons in the anterior horns and to higher centres. The sensory input from the muscle spindle depends on the amount of stretch and the amount of gamma bias. Recently, it has been shown that in human intervertebral discs and longitudinal ligaments mechanoreceptors are present and it is more than likely that this will be also the case in the other ligaments of the spine. As mentioned in previous paragraph growth (Force of Growth) will stretch the soft tissues (Force of Soft Tissue Complex) and this will lead through a dysfunction of the muscle spindle system to asymmetric muscle contraction resulting in an increase of the scoliosis, meaning the higher Force of Growth (i.e. more growth) and the more dysfunction of the mechanoreceptors the greater the scoliosis. Only a dysfunction of the mechanoreceptors and no growth will not lead to a serious scoliosis. The various degrees of scoliosis seen clinically depend on the growth velocity and the degree of malfunctioning of the mechanoreceptors. A failure of the supportive musculo-ligamentous structures and/or their neuromuscular control system for stabilizing the spine may explain the occurrence of progression in AIS. Lack of feedback, inappropriate feedback, or faulty programming within the CNS, due to pathology, may be an important contributing factor in curve progression (Dobosiewicz, 1997).

4. Summary

The natural history of AIS involves an initial stage in which a small curve develops due to a small defect in the neuromuscular control system and a second stage, during adolescent growth, in which the scoliotic curve is exacerbated by biomechanical factors, whereas neurological dysfunction may play a role in the extent of progression during normal growth (Dobosiewicz, 1997). We propose that the most likely cause of idiopathic scoliosis is neuromuscular. Asymmetry of the transversospinalis muscles may produce enough lateral deviation and axial rotation to disturb the delicate balance of forces in the region, thus producing a scoliotic deformity. This asymmetry of the transversospinalis muscles may be produced by alteration of the motor drive arising at the spinal cord level, either from altered sensory input at the same level or from a central mechanism, and "the altered muscle pull" is the final common pathway for the production of a scoliotic curve. Growth (Force of Growth) will stretch the soft tissues (Force of Soft Tissue Complex) and this will lead through a dysfunction of the muscle spindle system to asymmetric muscle contraction resulting in an increase of the scoliosis, meaning the higher Force of Growth(i.e. more growth) and the more dysfunction of the mechanoreceptors the greater the scoliosis. Only a dysfunction of the mechanoreceptors and no growth will not lead to a serious scoliosis. The various degrees of scoliosis seen clinically depend on the growth velocity and the degree of malfunctioning of the mechanoreceptors.Secondary to the scoliosis, a force system arises which may be held responsible for the geometrical and morphological characteristics of adolescent idiopathic scoliosis (Pincott & Taffs, 1980; Wever et al, 1999).

5. References

Agadir, M; Sevastik, J; Persson, A & Isberg, B (1988) Induction of scoliosis in growing rabbits by unilateral growth stimulation. Spine 13: 1065- 1969

Alexander, MA & Season, EH (1978) Idiopathic scoliosis. Arch Phys Med Rehabil 59:314-315

Alexander, MA; Bunch, WH & Ebbersson, SOE (1978) Can experimental dorsal rhizotomy produce scoliosis? J Bone Joint Surg Am 54:1509-1513

Andersen, RA; Snijder, LH; Li, CS & Stricane B (1993) Coordinate transformations in the representation of spatial information. Curr Opin Neurobiol 3: 171-176

Anderson, M; Shih-Chen Hwang, AM & Green WT (1965) Growth of the normal trunk in boys and girls during the second decade of life, related to age, maturity, and ossification of the iliac epiphysis. J. Bone Joint Surg. Am 47: 1554-1564

Arkin, AM (1949)The mechanism of the structural changes in scoliosis. J Bone Joint Surg Am 31: 519-528

Barrack, RL; Whitecloud, TS; Burke, SW; Cook, SD& Harding, AF (1984) Proprioception in idiopathic scoliosis. Spine 9:681-685

Bick, E (1961) Vertebral growth. Its relation to spinal abnormalities in children. Clin.orthop 21. 43-48

Bjure, J; Grimby, G & Nachemson, A (1968) Correction of the body height in predicting spirometric values in scoliotic patients. Scand J Clin Lab Invest 21:189-192

Boos, N & Aebi, M (2008) *Spinal disorders: fundamentals of diagnosis and treatment.*

Buric, M & Momcilovic, B (1982) Growth pattern and skeletal age in school girls with idiopathic scoliosis. Clin Orthop 170:238-242

Burwell, RG & Dangerfield PH (1974) In: Zorab PA (ed) Scoliosis. Proceedings of the Fifth Symposium. Academic Press, pp 123-163

Burwell, RG & Dangerfield, P H (1992). Pathogenesis and assessment of scoliosis. In: G. Findlay and R. Owen (editors) Surgery of the Spine. A Combined Orthopaedic and Neurosurgical Approach, Volume 1 (Oxford: Blackwell Scientific Publications), Chapter 19, pp. 365-408

Burwell, RG; Cole, AA & Grivas, TB (1992) Screening, aetiology and the Nottingham theory for idiopathic scoliosis. In: A. Alberti, B. Drerup and E. Hierholzer (editors) Sixth International Symposium on Surface Topography and Spinal Deformity (Stuttgart: Gustav Fischer), pp. 136-161

Burwell, RG; Cole, AA; Cook, TA; Grivas, TB;Kiel, AW; Moulton, A; Thirlwall, AS; Upadhyay, SS, Webb, JK; & Wemyss-Holden, SA (1992). Pathogenesis of idiopathic scoliosis. The Nottingham Concept. Acta Orthop Belg.58 Suppl 1:33-58

Burwell, RG; Aujla, R K & Cole, AA (2003) Relation of ribs to the spine in the transverse plane at the curve apex in preoperative adolescent idiopathic scoliosis (AIS): evaluation using an ultrasound method and radiographs. In: Proceedings of the British Scoliosis Society, Leeds, 9–11 April. J of Bone & Joint Surg., vol. 86-B. pp 112

Burwell, RG (2003) Aetiology of idiopathic scoliosis: current concepts. Pediatr Rehabil.Jul-Dec; 6 (3-4):137-70

Burwell, RG; Aujla, RK; Grevitt, MP; Dangerfield, PH; Moulton, A; Randell, TL & Anderson, SI (2009) Pathogenesis of adolescent idiopathic scoliosis in girls - a double neuro-osseous theory involving disharmony between two nervous systems, somatic and autonomic expressed in the spine and trunk: possible dependency on sympathetic nervous system and hormones with implications for medical therapy. Scoliosis. Oct 31; 4:24

Busscher, I; Wapstra, FH & Veldhuizen, AG(2010) Predicting growth and curve progression in the individual patient with adolescent idiopathic scoliosis: design of a prospective longitudinal cohort study. BMC Musculoskeletal Disease 11:93 11-93, 1-21

Busscher, I; Gerver, WJM; Kingma, I; Wapstra, FH; Verkerke, GJ & Veldhuizen, AG (2011) The growth of different body length dimensions is not predictive for the peak growth velocity of sitting height in the individual child Eur Spine J 20:791–797

Busscher, I; Kingma, I; Wapstra, FH; Bulstra, SK; Verkerke, GJ & Veldhuizen, AG (2011) The value of shoe size for prediction of the timing of the pubertal growth spurt. Scoliosis 2011, 6:1, 1-7

Busscher, I; Kingma, I; Wapstra, FH; de Bruin, R; Verkerke, GJ & Veldhuizen, AG (2011) Predicting the peak growth velocity in the individual child: validation of a new growth model Eur Spine J DOI 10.1007/s00586-011-1845-z

Butterworth, TR & James, C (1969) Electromyographic studies in idiopathic scoliosis. South Med J 62: 1008–1010

Calvo, IJ (1957) Observations on the growth of the female adolescent spine and its relation to scoliosis. Clin Orthop. 10:40–46

Charles, YP; Daures, JP & de Rosa, V (2006) Progression risk of idiopathic juvenile scoliosis during pubertal growth. *Spine*; 31:1933-42.

Cheung, J; Veldhuizen, AG; Halbertsma, JP; Maurits, NM; Cool, JC & van Horn, JR (2004) The relation between electromyography and growth velocity of the spine in the evaluation of curve progression in idiopathic scoliosis. *Spine*; 29:1011-6.

Cheung J; Veldhuizen, AG; Halbertsma, JP; Maurits, NM; Cool, JC & van Horn, JR (2005) A preliminary study on electromyographic analysis of the paraspinal muscalure in idiopathic scoliosis. Euro Spine J: 14, 130-137

Cheung, J; Veldhuizen, AG; Halbertsma, JPK; Sluiter, WJ & van Horn, JR (2006) Geometric and Electromyographic Assessment in the Evaluation of Curve Progression In Idiopathic Scolioisis. Spine: vol.31, 322-329

Closkey, R F & Schultz, AB (1993). Ribcage deformities in scoliosis: spine morphology, rib cage stiffness, and tomography imaging. J of Orthopedic Research, 11: 730–737

D'Arcy Wentworth Thompson (1961) On Growth and Form. Cambridge University Press ISBN 0521 437768

Deacon, P; Flood, BM & Dickson, RA (1984) Idiopathic scoliosis in three dimensions. A radiographic and morphometric analysis. J Bone Joint Surg Br 66:509-512

Deacon, P; Archer, IA & Dickson, RA (1987) The anatomy of spinal deformity: a biomechanical analysis. Clin Orthop 10:897-903

Deane, G & Duthie, RB (1973) A new projectional look at articulated scoliotic spines. Acta Orthop Scand 44: 351-365

Dickson, RA; Lawton, JO; Archer, IA & Butt, WP (1984). The pathogenesis of idiopathic scoliosis. Biplanar spinal asymmetry. J Bone Joint Surg Br 66: 8-15

Dickson, RA & Deacon, P (1987) Spinal growth. J Bone Joint Surg Br 69: 690- 692

Dimeglio, A (2001) Growth in pediatric orthopaedics. J.Pediatr.Orthop: 21: 549-55

Dobosiewicz, K (1997) Neurophysiological mechanism of the unloading reflex as a prognostic factor in the early stages of idiopathic scoliosis. Eur Spine J 6:93-97

Drummond, DS & Rogala, EJ (1980) Growth and maturation of adolescents with idiopathic scoliosis. Spine 5: 507-511

Dubousset, J; Queneau, P & Thillard, MM (1982) Experimental scolisis induced by pineal and diencephalic lesions in young chickens: its relation with clinical findings in idiopathic scoliosis. Proceedings of the 17th Annual Scoliosis Research Society Meeting, Denver,Colorado

Duthie, RB (1959) The significance of growth in orthopaedic surgery. Clin Orthop 14:7-19

Duval-Beaupere, G; Dubousset, J; Queneau, P & Grossiord, S (1970) Pour une théorie unique de l'évolution des scolioses. Press Med 78:1141-1146

Duval-Beaupere, G & Lamireau, T (1985) Properties at less than 30 degrees. Properties of the Evolutivity (risk of progression). Spine 5:421- 424

Enneking, WF & Harrington, P (1969) Pathological changes in scoliosis. J Bone & Joint Surg. Br 51: 165-184

Enslein, K & Chan, DP (1987) Multiparameter pilot study of adolescent idiopathic scoliosis. Spine 12:978-982

Erkula, G; Sponseller, PD & Kiter, AE (2003) Rib deformity in scoliosis. European Spine Journal, 12: 281-287

Escalada, F; Marco, E & Duarte, E (2005) Growth and curve stabilization in girls with adolescent idiopathic scoliosis. Spine 30: 411-417

Fidler, MW; Jowett, RL & Troup, JDG. (1974) Histochemical study of the function of multividus in scoliosis. In:Zorab PA (ed) Scoliosis and muscle. William Heinemann, London, 184-192

Fidler, MW & Jowett, RL (1976) Muscle imbalance in the etiology of scoliosis. J Bone Joint Surg Br 58:200-201

Ford, DM; Bagnall, KM; McFadden, KD; Greenhill, BJ & Rasco, VJ (1984) Paraspinal muscle imbalance in adolescent idiopathic scoliosis. Spine 9: 373-376

Forssberg, H & Nasher, LM (1982) Ontogenetic development of postural control in man. Adaptation to altered support in visual conditions during stance. J Neurosci 2:545-552

Geisler, HC (1997) The influence of the vestibular system on the development of posture in the rat. Thesis, University of Groningen

Geissele, AE; Mark, LTC; Kransdorf, J; Geyer, CA; Jelinek, JS; Bruce, LTC & Van Dam E (1991) Magnetic resonance imaging of the brain stem in adolescent idiopathic scoliosis. Spine 16:761-763

Gerver, WJ & de Bruin, R (2001) Paediatric morphometrics: a reference manual. Second extended edition ed. UPM Maastricht

Gerver, WJ & de Bruin, R (2003) Growth velocity: a presentation of reference values in Dutch children. Horm Res; 60:181-184

Gooding, CA & Neuhauser, EBD (1965) Growth and development of the vertebral body in the presence and absence of normal stress. Am J Roentgenol: 93, 338-394

Goldberg, CJ; Dowling, FE & Fogarty, EE (1993) Adolescent idiopathic scoliosis: early menarche, normal growth. Spine 18:529–535

Grivas, TB ; Burwell, RG & Purdue, M (1991) A segmental analysis of thoracic shape in chest radiographs of children. Changes related to spinal level, age, sex, side and significance for lung growth and scoliosis. Journal of Anatomy, 178: 21–38,

Grivas, TB ; Burwell, RG & Purdue, M (1992) Segmental patterns of rib-vertebra angles in chest radiographs of children: changes related to rib level, age, sex, side and significance for scoliosis. Clinical Anatomy, 5: 272–288

Grivas, TB; Burwell, RG & Purdue, M (1992). The rib cage deformity in infantile idiopathic scoliosis—the funnel-shaped upper chest in relation to specific rotation as a prognostic factor.An evaluation of thoracic shape in progressive scoliosis and control children during growth. In: A. Alberti, B. Drerup and E. Hierholzer (editors) Sixth International Symposium on Surface Topography and Spinal Deformity (Stuttgart: Gustav Fischer), pp. 93–109

Grivas, TB; Samelis P; Polyzois, BD; Giourelis, B & Polyzois, D (2002). School screening in the heavily industrialized area--Is there any role of industrial environmental factors in idiopathic scoliosis prevalence?. Stud Health Technol Inform; 91: 76-80.

Grivas, TB,; Dangas, S; Polyzois, BD & Samelis, P (2002) The Double Rib Contour Sign (DRCS) in lateral spinal radiographs: aetiologic implications for scoliosis. Stud Health Technol Inform; 88: pp 38-43

Grivas, TB; Vasiliadis, ES; Mihas, C, & Savvidou, O (2007). The effect of growth on the correlation between the spinal and rib cage deformity: implications on idiopathic scoliosis pathogenesis.. Scoliosis: 14; 2: 11.

Grivas, TB; Vasiliadis, ES; Mihas,C ; , Triantafyllopoulos,G & Kaspiris, A (2008).Trunk asymmetry in juveniles. Scoliosis: 23; 3: 13.

Grivas, TB; Vasiliadis, E; Savvidou, OD & Triantafyllopoulos, G(2008). What a school screening program could contribute in clinical research of idiopathic scoliosis aetiology. Disabil Rehabil; 30(10): 752-62

Grivas, TB; Burwell, RG; Mihas, C; Vasiliadis, ES; Triantafyllopoulos, G & Kaspiris, A(2009) Relatively lower body mass index is associated with an excess of severe truncal asymmetry in healthy adolescents: Do white adipose tissue, leptin, hypothalamus and sympathetic nervous system influence truncal growth asymmetry?. Scoliosis: 30; 4:13

Guth, V & Abbink, F (1980) Vergleichende electromyographische und kinesiologische Skoliosen. Z Orthop 118:165–172

Guyton, AC (1976) Textbook of medical physiology, 5th edn. WB Saunders, Philadelphia, pp 640–708

Hain, TC; Yoo, H; Rudisill, H & Tanaka-Cameron, A (2006) Vemp testing in bilateral vestibular loss. Poster at ANA annual meeting, Chicago Oct 9

Hagglund, G; Karlberg, J & Willner, S (1992) Growth in girls with adolescent idiopathic scoliosis. Spine 17: 108–111

Henssge, J (1962) Electromyographischen Befunde der Rückenmusculatur nach Poliomyelitis und bei idiopatischen Scoliosen. Z Orthop 96:324–334
Herman, R & McEwen, D (1979) Idiopathic scoliosis: a visio-vestibular disorder of the central nervous system. In: Zorab PA (ed) Scoliosis. Proceedings of the Sixth Symposium. Academic Press, pp 61–69
Herman, R; Stuyck, J & Maulucci, R (1982) Development and plasticity of visual and vestibular generated eye movements. Exp Brain Res 47:69–78
Herman, R; Mixton, J; Fisher, A; Maulucci, R & Stuyck, J (1985) Idiopathic scoliosis and the central nervous system: a motor control problem. Spine 10:1–14
Hoogmartens, MJ & Basmajian, JV (1976) Postural tone in the deep spinal muscles of idiopathic scoliosis patients and their siblings. Electromyogr Clin Neurophysiol 16:93–114
Kamman, LLJ (2003) Siability of the Spinw. An Application to Scoliosis Progression. Thesis, University of Twente. ISBN 90-365-1857-1
Kapetanos, G; Potoupnis, M; Dangilas, A; Markou, K & Pournaras,J(2002). Is the labyrinthine dysfunction a causative factor in idiopathic scoliosis? Stud Health Technol Inform.; 91:7-9.
Knuttson F (1961) Growth and differentiation of the postnatal vertebra. Acta Radiol 55, 401-408
Lambert, FM; Malinvaud, D; Glaune`s, J; Bergot, C; Straka, H & Vidal, PP (2009) Vestibular asymmetry as the cause of idiopathic scoliosis, A possible answer from Xenopus J Neuroscience, October 7, 29(40): 12477-12483
Leong, JC; Low, WD; Mok, CK; Kung, LS & Yau, AC (1982) Linear growth in southern Chinese female patients with adolescent idiopathic scoliosis. Spine 7: 471–475
Loncar-Dusek, M; Pecina, M & Preberg, Z (1991) A longitudinal study of growth velocity and development of secondary gender characteristics versus onset of idiopathic scoliosis. Clin Orthop 270:278–282
Lonstein, JE & Carlson, JM (1984) The prediction of curve progression in untreated idiopathic scoliosis during growth. J Bone Joint Surg Am 66: 1061–1071
Low, WD; Mok, CK; Leong, JC; Yau, AC & Lisowski, FP (1978) The development of southern Chinese girls with adolescent idiopathic scoliosis. Spine 3:152–156
Low, WD; Chew, EC; Kung, HTC; Hisli, LCS & Leong, JCY (1983) Ultrastructures of nerve fibres and muscle spindles in adolescent idiopathic scoliosis. Clin Orthop 174: 217-221
Matthews, PBC (1969) Muscle spindles and their motor control. Physiol Rev 44:219–288
Matthews, PBC (1969) Evidence that the secondary as well as primary endings of the muscle spindles may be responsible for the tonic stretch reflex of the decerebrate cat. J Physiol 204: 365–393
Mattson, G; Haderspeck-Grib, K; Schultz, AB & Nachemson, A (1983) Joint flexibility in structural normal girls and girls with idiopathic scoliosis. J Orthop Res 1:57–62
Meyer, GH (1866) Die Mechanik der Skoliose. Archiv für pathologische Anatomie und Physiologie und für klinische Medicin 35:15–253
Michelsson, JE (1965) The development of spinal deformity in experimental scoliosis. Acta Orthop Scand Suppl 81:1–91
Millner, PA & Dickson, RA (1996) Idiopathic scoliosis. Biomechanics and biology. Eur Spine J 5:362–373

Mixon, R & Steel, H (1982) Oculomotor control in children with idiopathic scoliosis. Presented at the Seventeenth Annual Scoliosis Research Society Meeting, Denver, Colorado

Murray, DW & Bulstrode, CJ (1996) the development of adolescent idiopathic scoliosis. Eur Spine J 5:251–257

Nasher, LM (1982) Adaptation of human movement to altered environments. Trends Neurosci 5:358–361

Neugebauer, H (1976) Skoliose, Stoffwechsel und Wirbelsäulenwachstum. Arch Orthop Unfallchir 85; 87-99

Nijenbanning, G (1998) Scoliosis redress.Design of a force controlled orthosis. Thesis, University of Twente, ISBN 90-36511925

Nordwall, A & Willner, SA (1975) A study of skeletal age and height in girls with idiopathic scoliosis. Clin Orthop 110:6–10

Normelli, A; Sevastik, J; Ljung, G; Aaro, S & Jonsson-Soderstrom, AM (1985) Anthropometric data relating to normal and scoliotic Scandinavian girls. Spine 10:123–126

Pal, GP (1991) Mechanism of production of scoliosis: a hypothesis. Spine, 16: 288–292, 1991.

Perdriolle, R; Becchetti, S; Vidal, J & Lopez, P (1993) Mechanical process and growth. Essential factors in the progression of scoliosis. Spine 18: 343–349

Petersen, I; Sahlstrand, T & Sellden, U (1979) Electroencephalographic investigation of patients with adolescent idiopathic scoliosis. Acta Orthop Scand 50:283–293

Pincott, JR (1980) Observations on the afferent nervous system in idiopathic scoliosis. In: Zorab PA, Siegler D (eds) Scoliosis. Academic Press, London New York, 45–49

Pincott, JR & Taffs, LF (1982) Experimental scoliosis in primates: a neurological cause. J.Bone Joint Surg Br 64:503–507

Plaats, A van de (1997) Numerical analysis of idiopathic scoliosis using the finite element method. Internal report: BW-91. Technical University of Twente

Plaats, A van de; Veldhuizen, AG, & Verkerke, GJ (2007) Numerical simulation of asymmetrically altered growth as initiation mechanism of scoliosis. Ann Biomed Eng: 35(7):1206-1215..

Raso, VJ (1998) Review of biomechanics in the aetiology of idiopathic scoliosis Presented at the Tenth International Philip Zorab Symposium, Oxford

Redford, JB; Butterworth, TR & Clements, EL (1969) Use of electromyography as a prognostic aid in the management of idiopathic scoliosis. Arch Phys Med Rehabil58:433–438

Riddle, HFV & Roaf, R (1955) muscle imbalance in the causation of scoliosis. Lancet: 1245–1247

Roaf, R (1960) Vertebral growth and its mechanical control. J Bone Joint Surg Br 42:40–59Roaf, R (1966) The basic anatomy of scoliosis. J Bone Joint Surg Br 48:786–792

Sahlstrand, T; Petruson, B & Ortengren, R (1979) Vestibulospinal reflex activity in patients with adolescent idiopathic scoliosis. Acta Orthop Scand 50:275–281

Sahlstrand, T & Petruson, B (1979) A study of labyrinthine function in patients with adolescent idiopathic scoliosis. Acta Orthop Scand 50:759–769

Sahlstrand, T & Petruson, B (1979) Postural effects on nystagmus response during caloric labyrinthine stimulation in patients with adolescent idiopathic scoliosis. Acta Orthop Scand 50:771–775

Sahlstrand, T & Lindstrom, J (1980) Equilibrium factors as predictor of the prognosis in adolescent idiopathic scoliosis. Clin Orthop 152:232-236

Sahlstrand, T (1980) An analysis of lateral predominance in adolescent idiopathic scoliosis with special reference to convexity of the curve. Spine 5:512-517

Saltin, B; Henriksson, J; Nijgaard, E & Andersen, P(1977) Fibre-types and metabolic potentials of skeletal muscles in sedentary man and endurance runners. 1. Metabolism in prolongedm exercise. Ann N Y Acad Sci 301:3-29

Sanders, JO; Browne, RH & McConnell, SJ(2007) Maturity assessment and curve progression in girls with idiopathic scoliosis. J.Bone Joint Surg.Am; 89:64-73.

Sevastik, JA (2000).The thoracospinal concept of the etiopathogenesis of idiopathic scoliosis. Spine: State of the Art Reviews, 14: 391-400

Sevastik, JA; Burwell, RG & Dangerfield, PH (2003) A new concept for the etiopathogenesis of the thoracospinal deformity of idiopathic scoliosis: summary of an electronic focus group debate of the IBSE. European Spine Journal, 12: 440-450

Sharp, JA; Lo, AW & Rabinovitch, HE (1979) Control of saccadic and smooth pursuit systems after cerebral hemidecortication. Brain 102:387- 403

Shohat, M; Shohat,T & Nitzan, M(1988) Growth and ethnicity in scoliosis. Acta Orthop Scand 59:310-313

Skogland, LB & Miller, JAA (1981) The length and proportions of the thoracolumbar spine in children with idiopathic scoliosis. Acta Orthop Scand 52:177-185

Smith, RM & Dickson, RA (1987) Experimental structural scoliosis. J Bone Joint Surg Br 69:576-581

Snijder, LH; Brotchie, P & Andersen, RA (1993) World-centred encoding of location in posterior parietal cortex of monkey. Soc Neurosci Abstr 19:770

Somerville, EW (1952) Rotational lordosis. The development of the single curve. J Bone Joint Surg Br 34:421- 427

Spencer, GSG & Eccles, MJ (1976) Spinal muscle in scoliosis. 2. The proportion and size of Type 1 and Type 2 skeletal muscles fibres measured using computer- controlled microscope. J Neurol Sci 30:143-156

Sisson, HA (1971) The biochemistry and physiology of bone. Deveopment and Growth (Ed.GH Bourne) vol 111, page 116, Academic Press, New York

Stokes, IAF; Spense, H; Aronsson, DD & Kilmer, N (1996) Mechanical modulation of vertebral body growth. Implication for scoliosis progression. Spine 21:1162-1167

Taffs, LF; Magrath, DI & Lytton, NA (1979) Monkey scoliosis. Lancet 1:1078-1079

Tanner, JM (1962) Growth at Adolescence. 2nd Edition ed.Oxford: Blackwell Scientific Publ Tanner, JM (1978) Foetus into Man. Physical Growth from Conception to Maturity.OBP London

Tanner, JM & Davies, PS (1985) Clinical longitudinal standards for height and height velocity for North American children. J.Pediatr; 107: 317-29.

Tanner, JM; Whitehouse, RH & Takaishi, M (1965) Standards from birth to maturity for height, weight, height velocity, and weight velocity: British children, Arch.Dis.Child 41: 454-71.

Taffs, LF; Magrath, DI & Lytton, NA (1979) Monkey scoliosis. Lancet 1:1078-1079

Taylor, JR (1983) Scoliosis and growth: patterns of asymmetry in normal vertebral growth. Acta Orthop Scand 54:596-602

Tezuka, A (1971) Development of scoliosis in cases with congenital organ abnormalities of the brainstem. Tokushima J Exp Med 18:49-62

Veldhuizen, AG (1985) Idiopathic scoliosis. A biomechanical and functional- anatomical study. Thesis, University of Groningen, van Denderen

Veldhuizen, AG; Baas, P & Webb, PJ (1986) Observations on the growth of the adolescent spine. J Bone Joint Surg Br 68:724–728

Veldhuizen, AG & Scholten, PJM (1990) Flexibility in structural normal young females and in young females with idiopathic scoliosis. Clin Biomech 5:117–119

Webb, PJ (1973) The effect of innervation, denervation and muscle type on the reunion of skeletal muscle. Br J Surg 60: 180–182

Webb, PJ (1981) Electromyographic changes in scoliosis. Presented at the British-Scandinavian Joint Scoliosis Meeting of the British Scoliosis Society, Jersey

Wever, DJ; Veldhuizen,AG; Klein, JP; Webb, PJ; Nijenbanning, G; Cool JC& v Horn, JR (1999) A biomechanical analysis of the vertebral and rib deformities in structural scoliosis. Eur Spine J 8:252–260

Wever, DJ; Tonseth, KA; Veldhuizen, AG; Nijenbanning, G; Cool, JC & v Horn, J (2000) Curve progression and spinal growth in brace treated idiopathic scoliosis. Clin Orthop Res 377, 169-179

Whitecloud, TS; Cook, SD; Burke, SW; Leinhardt, T & Barrack, RL (1984) Upper extremity proprioceptive deficit in idiopathic scoliosis. Presented at the Nineteenth Annual Scoliosis Research Society Meeting, Orlando, Florida

Wiener-Vacher, SR & Mazda, K (1998) Asymmetric otolith vestibulo-ocular responses in children with idiopathic scoliosis. J Pediatr 132: 1028-32

Willner, SA (1974) Study of growth in girls with adolescent structural scoliosis. Clin Orthop 101: 29–135

Willner, SA (1975) Study of height, weight and menarche in girls with idiopathic structural scoliosis. Acta Orthop Scand 46:71–83

Willner, SA (1975) The proportion of legs to trunk in girls with idiopathic scoliosis. Acta Orthop Scand 46:84– 89

Wong, VC; Yak, ACMC; Low, WD; Chin, NK & Lisowsky, FK (1980) Ultrastructural changes of the back muscles in idiopathic scoliosis. Spine 2: 251–260

Yarom, R & Robin, GC (1979) Studies on spinal and peripheral muscles from patients with scoliosis. Spine 4:12–21

Yasui, S & Young, LR (1976) Eye movements during and after image tracking under sinusoidal and random vestibular stimulation. In: Monty RA, Senders JW (eds) Eye movements and psychological process. Erlbaum, New Jersey, 33–37

Yekutiel,M; Robin, GC & Grimby, G (1981) Proprioceptive function in children with adolescent idiopathic scoliosis. Spine 6:560–566

Ylikowski, M (1993) Spinal growth and progression of adolescent idiopathic scoliosis. Eur Spine J 1:236– 239

Young, LR (1977) Pursuit eye movement – what is being pursued? In: Baker R, Berthoz A (eds) Control of gaze by brainstem neurons. Elsevier/ North Holland, Amsterdam, 29–36

Yrjonen, T & Ylikoski, M (2006) Effect of growth velocity on the progression of adolescent idiopathic scoliosis in boys. J.Pediatr.Orthop.B; 15:311-5.

Zetterberg, C; Bjork, R; Ortengren, R & Andersson, GBJ (1984) Electromyography of the paravertebral muscles in idiopathic scoliosis. Acta Orthop Scand 55:304–309

2

How to Improve Progress in Scoliosis Research

Keith M. Bagnall
United Arab Emirates University
United Arab Emirates

1. Introduction

Since the time of Hippocrates, patients with abnormally-curved spines have been observed and their condition well documented. It is recognized that there are several different types of scoliosis identified by the age of initial appearance and the curves can take several different forms including single and double, directed to the left or to the right, spanning different vertebral levels, and with differing degrees of curvature. Whatever the form, the curves are 3-dimensional and involve vertebral rotation as an additional defining characteristic. The most common form of scoliosis is adolescent idiopathic scoliosis (AIS) and refers to the development of abnormal curvature of the vertebral column that becomes evident at the time of puberty. As its name suggests, it also has no apparent cause. AIS represents 80% of the cases of scoliosis and will be the primary focus of this chapter.

Patients with scoliosis form a small but significant portion of the general population. Many of the curves are sufficiently small to be simply of a cosmetic nature but, nevertheless, are very noticeable and upsetting for the patient who is at an important stage of their adolescent development. Understandably, the patients request treatment and elimination of the curve. However, for the unfortunate few, the curves go beyond being cosmetic and are of such magnitude that the rotation causes the ribs to impinge on the heart and lungs and severely affects cardio-respiratory function (Keim, 1979).

The mechanism behind the development of such curves is both fascinating and complex and has been the focus of much research especially in the last 100 years or so. Unfortunately, in spite of this intense activity, very little is known about scoliosis with any degree of certainty and, quite simply, the return on any research investment has been limited. So much so that if a patient could be identified with 100% certainty that they will develop scoliosis in the near future then there is little that can be done other than watch its development (see Figure 1). There are many treatment strategies that might be considered (e.g. bracing and exercise) and applied but none seem able to guarantee prevention of the curve development other than the insertion of long metal rods and fusion of the affected vertebrae. This is drastic, invasive treatment and is not acceptable.

If the curve develops sufficiently (~50 degrees) then the insertion of metal rods is made. While this effectively curtails further curve development it is a drastic procedure that can surely be replaced by something better and less invasive in this day and age. A better understanding of the aetiology of AIS and the underlying mechanics of curve development would lend itself towards the development of improved treatment strategies at earlier stages that would be more effective and far less invasive.

This chapter will focus on the changes that are needed in regards to research into scoliosis so that much greater progress can be made in comparison with the limited progress that has been made so far. Albert Einstein is often quoted as saying that: 'To continue doing the same thing and expecting different results is a sign of madness'. This statement can be used as a platform on which to build.

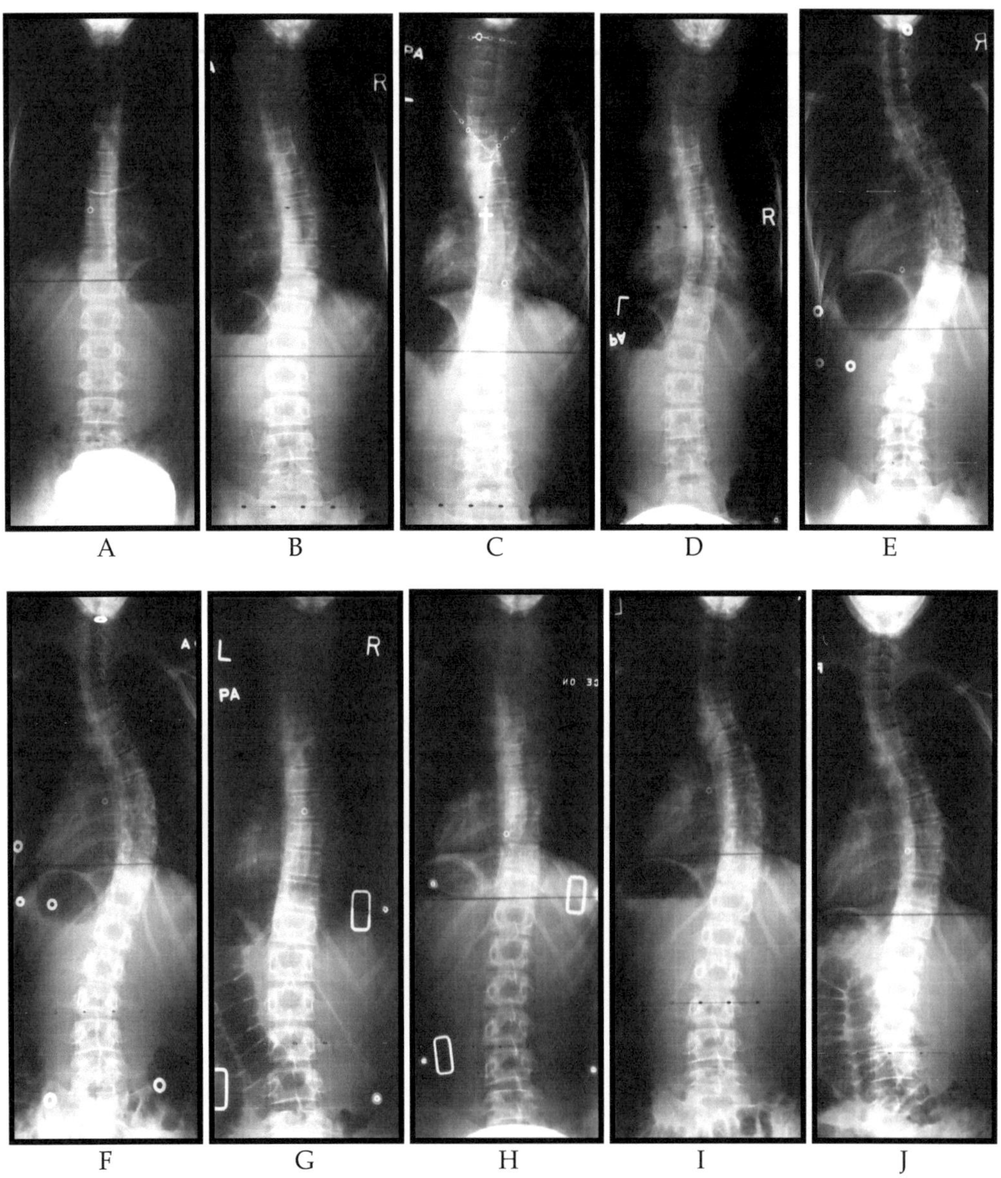

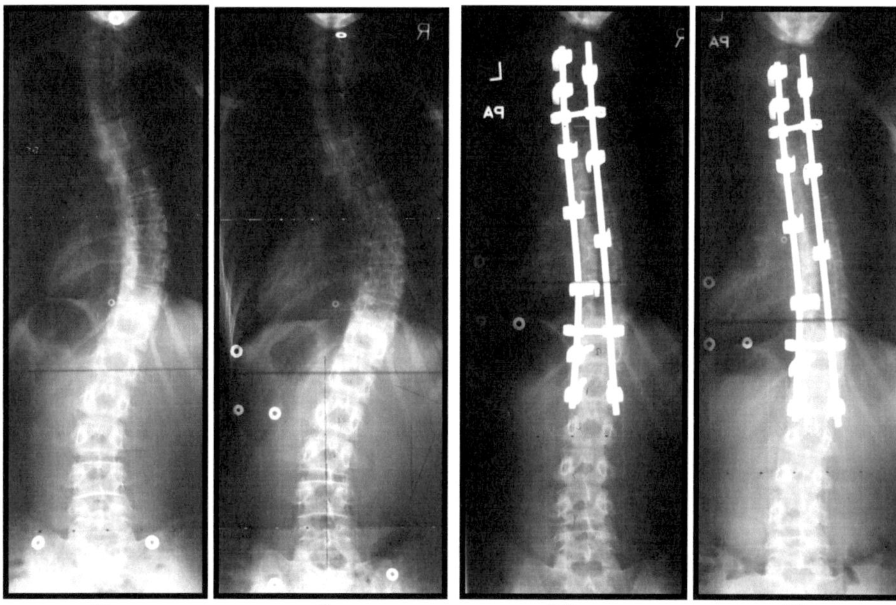

K L M N

Fig. 1. A series of radiographs showing development of AIS in a young girl.

Such a sequence of radiographs is rare because there is a radiograph available of the times when she did not have an abnormal spinal curve and radiographs which show the early curve development are usually not available. A - radiograph before any curve development. B, C, D, E, and F - curve development over the next two years. G and H - reduction of the curve during brace treatment. I, J, K, and L - continued curve development after brace treatment was stopped. M and N - radiographs after surgery for the insertion of metal supporting rods. This sequence of radiographs illustrates the lack of effective treatment strategies currently available to deal effectively with patients who have AIS.

2. What have we learned with certainty from the research conducted into scoliosis in the past 100 years?

The vertebral column is a complicated structure consisting of many interactive and overlapping components. Using many different techniques, research into AIS appears to have explored many, if not all, of the components of the vertebral column in an effort to discover the underlying mechanism of any abnormal development. Unfortunately the results of such research have often been contradictory and confusing with those indicating a positive result being counteracted by results from similar research showing either equivalent negative or neutral conclusions. For example, different research projects measuring the levels of growth hormone during development of AIS have shown negative influence, neutral influence and positive influence all with seemingly similar patients and experimental protocols.

Research into scoliosis has been intense over the last 100 years but really there are only four basic facts that appear to be beyond dispute:

- Development of AIS requires the presence of a growth spurt.
- Most (80%) of the patients are female.
- Many different kinds of curve can develop and be present within the group of patients
- AIS appears to be familial (present in families)

Although there have perhaps been other less significant findings, it is these four facts that summarize the research findings in relation to the aetiology of AIS during the past 100 years. This is disappointing because observation for just 20 minutes in a scoliosis clinic would provide the same information! The patients would be adolescents undergoing significant growth, most of them would be female, there would be a variety of curves among the patients, and there might well be a relative accompanying the patient who also has the same problem. This lack of specific findings is disappointing but perhaps as a whole they provide us with the motivation, impetus and guidance to change the way that we are approaching the research. They emphasise to us the need to change.

3. Where to focus efforts

Figure 2 shows the hypothetical development of a scoliosis curve in a typical patient. When the patient is born there is no obvious curve present and this remains so until approximately the age of 10 years. At this age a curve starts to develop but it is not yet of sufficient magnitude to be noticeable. The curve continues to develop for approximately 18 months, steadily getting more severe. (Because of the nature of the curve development, the length of time for a patient to have a spinal curve before it is noticed is unknown.) It is interesting to note that the patient is unaware of a curve developing with no intrinsic symptoms being manifest. Eventually, 'somebody' notices a curve (usually somebody else – *'stand up straight', 'your shoulders are not level....*) and so the patient visits their family physician for advice. An appointment is made with a specialist with an inevitable further delay because of a surfeit of patients. The diagnosis of scoliosis is subsequently confirmed and the curve at this point can get worse, remain the same or improve.

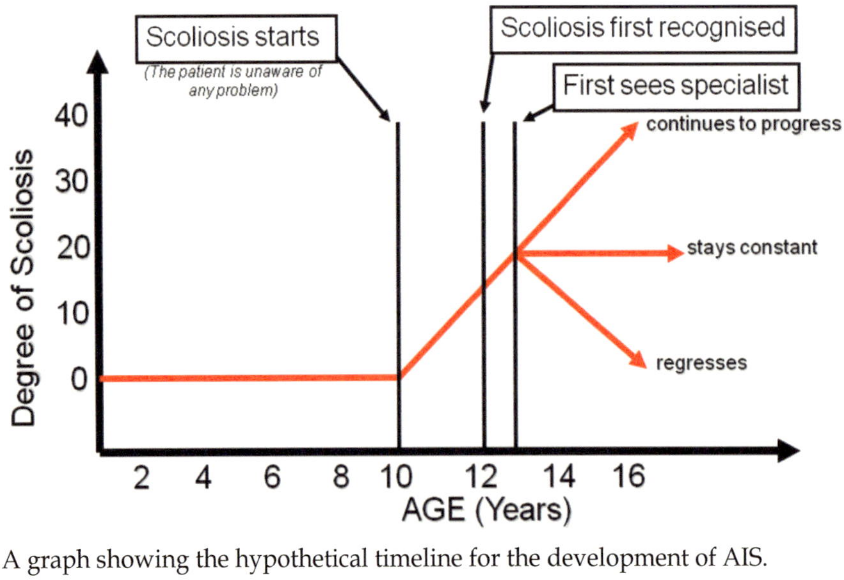

Fig. 2. A graph showing the hypothetical timeline for the development of AIS.

There is no curve development until approximately the age of 10 years old at which time the curve starts to develop steadily. The curve is not noticed until it is sufficiently severe (~15 degrees) which has taken possibly 2 years. After seeing a specialist the curve can either continue to progress, stay constant or even regress.

Following this hypothetical pathway, the initiation of treatment of the spinal curve is delayed perhaps 2 years since the inception of curve development. This in itself presents significant difficulties in research:

- When the patient is first seen in the scoliosis clinic, they have had a curve for perhaps 2 years. During this time the underlying cause might well have resolved and the patient might have nothing wrong with them at the time of examination other than having a scoliosis curve.
- Bone is very malleable and responds to extrinsic forces. The presence of a force producing a spinal curve over a period of time leads to vertebral malformation, especially of the vertebral body. This malformation might be such as to not allow the spine to become straight even if the underlying, deforming cause is able to be removed. With a curved spine that has developed over several months, the underlying cause might not be present any more and the presence of the curve and its potential for increase is now a purely biomechanical one with the foundation being malformed vertebrae.
- The period of time that would be very beneficial for research focus is the time when the curve first starts to form. However, this cannot currently be identified because the curve is small and not noticeable at this time. The initial stages in the study of curve development are inevitably made after the curve has been present for a considerable time and not at the critical period when the curve is first initiated.
- This argument is often amplified when differences between patients with scoliosis and normal subjects are examined because patients with advanced scoliosis are often selected for study and their curves are particularly severe. In such cases, the scoliosis has often been present for many years and the biomechanical influence has had a major influence.

By the time the patient is examined in the scoliosis clinic, the underlying cause might no longer be present. Certainly a curve can be demonstrated and it might well be seen to progress over time but the problem might simply be a biomechanical problem. Gathering samples of tissue at this time might well be futile because the patient could be entirely normal. The underlying cause might no longer be present.

The fact that a patient with AIS has had the spinal curve for at least several months (if not years) also presents another major problem for researchers. The development of the curve and its accompanying mechanics has many effects on the tissues of the spine. Separating the effects that have been created by the development of the curve from those that were present before the development of the curve is very difficult. Nevertheless, when the research involves comparison of tissues collected from patients with AIS with similar tissues collected from normal subjects, then this becomes an important issue which is difficult to resolve and clarify. Research into the study of AIS is fraught with separation of *'cause from effect'*.

Observation and analysis of the initial stages of scoliosis development are critical to an understanding of the aetiology of AIS and yet they have never been studied because patients are identified only after this period. Attempts have been made to identify the early stages of curve development by associating them with ribcage deformity but for this to be visible, the curve has to have been present for a considerable time and any observations are not being made at the critical time when the curve is first initiated.

School-screening studies have shown that the incidence of scoliosis is ~2% and that development of severe scoliosis requiring surgery is only 3% of that population. While these studies have been proved to be very valuable, these figures make very difficult the continued observation of a group of normal subjects to observe early curve development and certainly impractical financially. Consequently, a case can be made to identify a population in which the incidence of scoliosis is higher than in the normal population. Perhaps this population can be developed from the relatives of the patients who attend the scoliosis clinic – their siblings and cousins. As AIS is familial, then such a population would have a higher probability of developing AIS. Maybe if this population was then followed closely, more cases in which the early identification of curve development could be found and invaluable data collected.

From Figure 2. it can be seen that there are three areas where efforts should be focused if significant progress is to be made:

- Development of a marker that can predict the future development of scoliosis would be of enormous benefit. Such a marker could be applied at an early age (~5 years of age) so that preparation can be made for appropriate treatment strategies and initial curve development thwarted.
- In combination or separately, a marker that would predict the severity of future curve development would also be of great benefit. When the scoliosis curve is first detected it is not possible to predict future development with accuracy. Currently, the age of the patient, physical maturity, current curve development and rate of development are all taken into account to predict future development but the addition of a definitive marker would be a tremendous advance for diagnosis application.
- There is a need for appropriate strategies to be developed for the treatment of small curves so that they do not develop into major curves. All major curves started off as small curves and so there is a need for the development of treatment strategies that will curtail any further development.

Figure 2 also offers other areas for consideration as major issues for the focus of attention (for example, the development of better treatment strategies for severe curves which do not involve such invasive surgery) but if the three areas outlined above can be resolved then the other areas of interest would be dramatically reduced as a result. If a better understanding of the aetiology of AIS can be obtained, then better treatment strategies can be developed as a consequence.

4. Changes in experimental design

The underlying cause of AIS is unknown and confirmation of the diagnosis of AIS is by elimination rather than by positive means. When a patient presents with AIS, all the known causes are considered and if they are all excluded then the patient is diagnosed with AIS. An important, fundamental question in this area relates to whether or not there is a single cause for AIS development or whether there are multiple causes each with a similar outcome that have been included under the umbrella of AIS. The answer to this question is of paramount importance because it affects how research experiments are designed.

Patients with scoliosis have been reported and recorded since the time of Hippocrates, 2000 years ago. One might imagine his 'clinic' where there would have been patients with curved spines who would have formed a very visible group. However, identification of an underlying cause would not have been available for any of them and so they would all have been labeled simply as 'idiopathic'. As the number of patients with curved spines increased, Hippocrates would have been able to identify and isolate patients with apparently common causes and relate these causes to the curved spines. Over the years this has been shown to be true with cases of Neurofibromatosis, Friedrich's Ataxia, Poliomyelitis etc. - all such patients develop scoliosis and the underlying cause has been recognized as such. However, this culling of patients from the idiopathic group has only reduced the number of AIS patients by 20% with 80% remaining as idiopathic. It seems arrogant to suggest that there is just one, single underlying cause remaining to be found among these many patients. Perhaps it is just that the remaining causes are more difficult to identify but, nevertheless, still exist. Furthermore, scoliosis curves have tremendous variety with some being single or double, some being to the left or to the right, and some covering different levels of the vertebral column! And yet they are all included in the same category as being cases of AIS. While these differences in form may be the consequence of biomechanical differences rather than any underlying cause, they do support more the idea that there are several, if not many, separate, underlying causes of AIS yet to be discovered.

In spite of this evidence to suggest that there are many different causes of AIS, the usual experimental design found in the literature has relied on an underlying principle that there is just a single cause remaining to be found despite the facts suggesting otherwise.

A theory of scoliosis is tested by experiment. The usual experimental design consists of selecting a group of patients with AIS and a similar group of control subjects and examining the parameter in question. If there is a single cause for AIS then this experimental design might be considered satisfactory. But if there are many causes for scoliosis then this experimental design is seriously flawed because any abnormal results related to scoliosis in the experimental group of patients will be smothered by the large number of patients in whom this particular parameter is normal. For example:

- Imagine, hypothetically, that it is suspected that the underlying cause for the development of AIS is an unequal number of muscle spindles in the muscles on the two sides of the spine. This inequality has led to an unequal input of sensory information to the central nervous system which has subsequently led to a poor distribution of muscle response. This inequality has resulted in a change in force distribution and the development of a spinal curve.
- If this hypothesis were to be tested, then the logical experiment would be to collect samples of muscle tissue from the spines of patients with AIS and compare them with similar samples collected from normal subjects.
- The muscle samples would be sectioned and stained and the number of muscle spindles counted and compared between the left and right sides of the spine and between the two groups.
- If the hypothesis is correct and the imbalance in numbers of muscle spindles is the underlying mechanism responsible for all the cases of AIS, then the results table might

look like those seen in Table 1 below. Subsequent analysis would show that there is a significant difference in the number of muscle spindles in the paraspinal muscles of patients with AIS with a significantly greater number being on the concave side. These results would suggest that there is just one underlying mechanism for the cause of AIS.

Experiment #1				
	Scoliosis Patients		Normal Patients	
	Concave side	Convex side	Left	Right
	15	5	15	14
	13	4	14	13
	14	6	14	12
	16	5	13	15
	14	3	16	16
	12	2	15	14
	15	7	14	14
	16	3	15	14
	17	5	12	13
	14	3	13	15
Mean	14.6	4.3	14.1	14
S.D.	1.51	1.57	1.20	1.15

Table 1. The results from a hypothetical experiment in which the number of muscle spindles in paraspinal muscles on both sides of the vertebral column has been determined in patients with AIS and in controls. The assumption has been made that there is one underlying mechanism for the development of AIS namely, an imbalance of muscle spindle number. If such was the case, then this is the type of result that might be expected. In the scoliosis patients the number of muscle spindles on the convex side of the vertebral column is significantly less than on the concave side. In the normal patients, there is no difference in the number of muscle spindles between the two sides of the vertebral column.

- However, if there is more than one underlying cause for the development of AIS and an imbalance of muscle spindles was just one of several, then the results of a similar, but more realistic, experiment might possibly be those as shown in Table 2. Here there are two AIS patients in whom the number of muscle spindles is significantly different between the two sides of the vertebral column but their results would be masked in any statistical analysis. Such an experiment would conclude that an imbalance in the number of muscle spindles is not an underlying cause of development of AIS - which would probably be incorrect.

This experimental design is not suited for identifying single causes for the development of AIS when there are many potential causes but unfortunately many experiments relating to identification of the underlying causes of AIS have been conducted on this basis e.g. several projects looking at the levels of serum melatonin in patients with and without AIS simply compared levels in blood collected from normal subjects and from patients with AIS. While low levels of melatonin might be a cause of AIS development in some patients it probably is not the only cause. Perhaps this explains the wide variety of results to be found in the literature that are often contradictory.

Experiment #2				
	Scoliosis Patients		Normal Patients	
	Concave side	Convex side	Left	Right
	15	15	15	14
	13	14	14	13
	13	16	14	12
	16	5*	13	15
	14	13	16	16
	12	12	15	14
	15	17	14	14
	16	3*	15	14
	17	15	12	13
	14	13	13	15
Mean	14.5	12.3	14.1	14
S.D.	1.58	4.64	1.20	1.15

Table 2. The results from a hypothetical experiment in which the number of muscle spindles in paraspinal muscles on both sides of the vertebral column has been determined in patients with AIS and in controls. If there is more than one underlying cause for the development of AIS then this is the type of result that might be expected. The assumption has been made that there is more than one underlying mechanism for the development of AIS e.g. muscle imbalance, ligament strength imbalance, unbalanced neural feedback, differences in growth hormone levels etc. In this scenario it is assumed that an imbalance of the number of muscle spindles between the two sides of the vertebral column is a separate cause for the development of AIS but only in some patients, not in all patients. Note that two patients reflect this imbalance (*). However, the analysis of the overall data would overwhelm the data from these two patients and no significant differences in average values would be found. At the end of the statistical analysis, the conclusion would be that differences in the number of muscle spindles between the concave and convex sides of the vertebral column do not contribute to the development of AIS – but this would be incorrect, at least for the two patients as shown in this hypothetical example.

Whenever an experiment is conducted as described above, the authors should be asked to explain why they selected this particular experimental design. The design is only appropriate when there is a belief that there is only one underlying cause for development of AIS and the authors should be asked to explain why they believe this is so.

While most experiments related to the aetiology of AIS are designed on the basis that there is a single underlying cause there is little reason to suspect that this is actually the case.

5. Measurement of scoliosis curves must be made in 3-dimensions

Traditionally, spinal curves have been measured from postero-anterior (PA) radiographs using the Cobb angle. This method has proved to be very successful especially for surgery and is useful for comparison of curve development and to present to patients to show progress. However, a radiograph is a two-dimensional (2-D) representation of a 3-D structure and all the structures in the image are compressed into a 2-D plane. As such, this is a distortion of the 3-D structure and can be easily misrepresented. Figures 3 and 4 provide a good example of the type of 2-D distortion that can occur when a simple, fixed, 3-D curved metal bar is rotated.

Figure 3 represents a piece of equipment in a children's playground. It consists of a single metal bar that is connected to a swivel at both the top and the bottom. The bar is curved and goes through a 360° spiral along its length. The idea is for the children to turn the bar easily by simply by pulling on it and watching the spiral rotate. Apparently, this provides great entertainment. Figure 4 shows the metal bar stopped in 4 different positions (B, C, D, and E) that are each separated by 90° rotation. The four images can be seen to represent the 4 most common types of curve seen in patients with AIS - single curves to the right and left (B and D) and double curves to the right and left (C and E). Therefore, from a single, curved, fixed rod different images of curved spines can be seen simply by rotation.

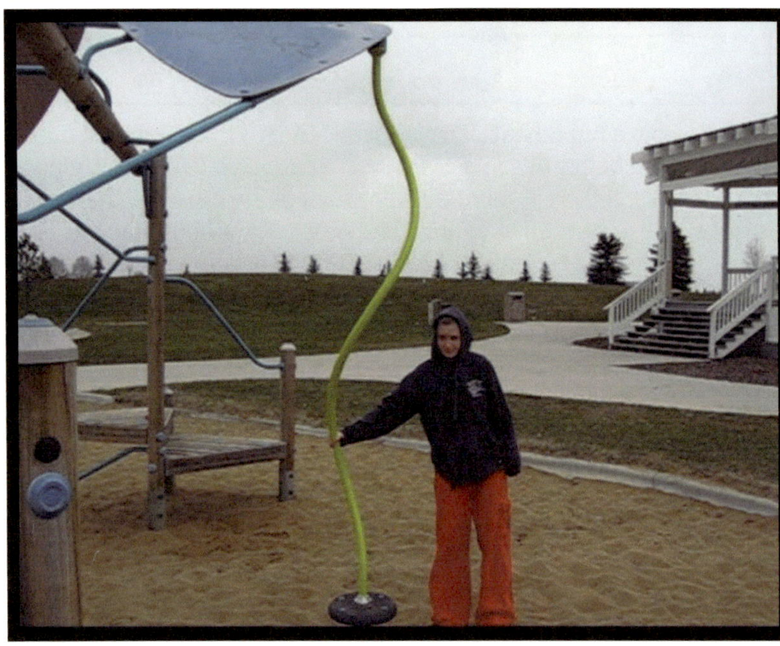

Fig. 3. A 'twirly bar' in a children's playground.

The equipment consists of a single, metal rod that curves through a complete 360°. It is anchored to a swivel at both the top and the bottom and can be rotated continuously simply by turning the bar.

A radiograph compresses three-dimensions into two-dimensions and the Cobb angle is consequently a two-dimensional measurement. Scoliosis curves are far from being two-dimensional as they involve vertebral rotation, rotation of the ribs, and malformed vertebrae, all of which are in three dimensions. While the Cobb angle successfully provides measurement of deformity in two-dimensions, there is a great need to study curve development and improvement in three-dimensions if advances in the understanding of curve structure are to be made. *If you measure in three-dimensions, you will think in two-dimensions; if you measure in three-dimensions, then you will think in three-dimensions* - and that is what is needed to be done.

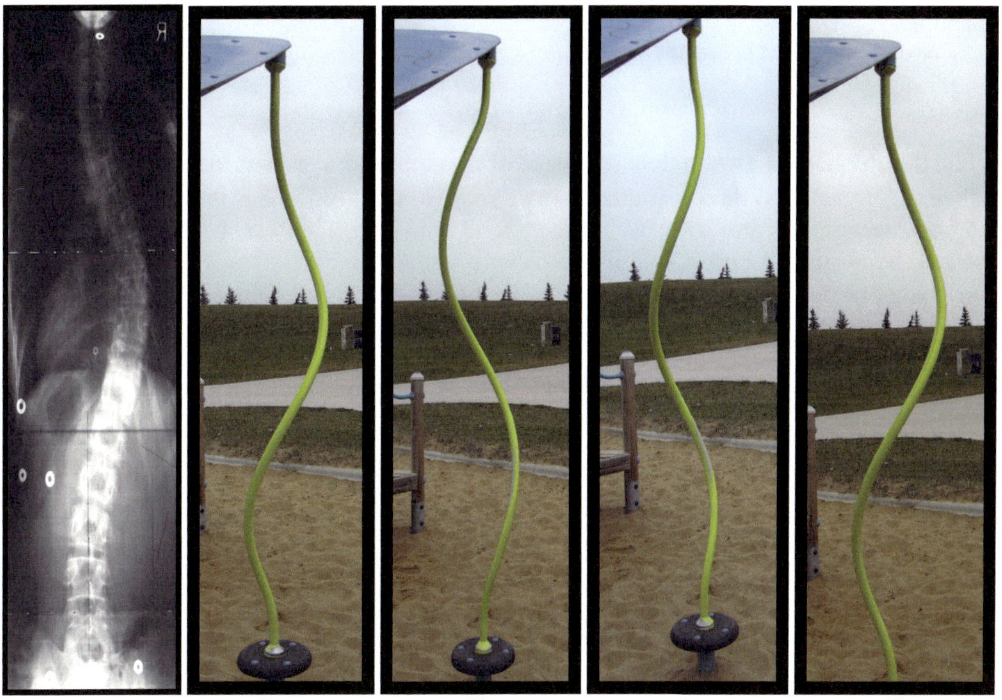

Fig. 4. A – a typical radiograph of a patient with AIS presented to show a resemblance to the position of the fixed, metal bar seen in B. B – the metal bar positioned to represent a single curve similar in shape to that seen in AIS with the curve being to the right. C - the metal bar positioned to represent a double curve in AIS with the thoracic curve being to the left. D - the metal bar positioned to represent a single curve in AIS with the curve being to the left. E - the metal bar positioned to represent a double curve in AIS with the thoracic curve being to the right. Overall, the four major curves commonly seen in AIS can be represented by the same fixed curve viewed in different positions. This sequence highlights the importance of rotation being a major factor in the analysis and evaluation of AIS from 2-D radiographs.

The measurement of a spinal curve in 2-D from a PA radiograph is easy to make and easy to understand, especially for the patients and their relatives: *'Six months ago your curve was 30° and now it is 20°. The treatment is effective and your curve is being reduced.'* There are considerable errors associated with taking radiographs of curved spines and measuring the Cobb angle but these are well-recognised and much effort has been made to overcome them especially those associated with consistent positioning and observer errors. However, as Figures 3 and 4 have shown, a simple rotation of the spine can produce a completely different image. This change in image can easily be mistaken for a change in the structure of the spinal curve (e.g. a decrease/increase in curvature) where none has actually occurred. A spinal curve is a 3-D structure and that fact cannot be ignored. No amount of 2-D measuring can overcome this basic issue.

A 3-D curve is a much more complicated structure to measure than a 2-D curve and the problem now arises as to how to keep such measurements simple for communication purposes. A 3-D curve is perhaps best represented by an equation which can be calculated quite easily using a 3-D coordinate system. A simple example might be:

$$A = 3xy^3z^2 + x^3yz^3 + x^2y^2z \quad (1)$$

While this might depict accurately the shape of the curve in its present form, it is much more difficult to understand than a simple number of degrees (e.g. 30 °) as is presented with the 2-D measurement. It is also difficult to understand how a change in such an equation can be made to be meaningful especially to the patients and to their relatives who simply want to know whether the curve has got better or worse. For example, analysis of the same spinal curve on a subsequent visit might reveal an equation such as:

$$A = 4y^2z^4 + 10x^2yz^3 + 3x^2y^2 \quad (2)$$

and it is difficult to provide a method whereby the subtle changes between the two equations could be expressed clearly to the patient!

Methods for producing 3-D images of scoliosis spines are becoming more readily available. Methods for describing these curves in 3-D should receive high priority because of their usefulness in providing a more accurate description of the spinal curve and any changes that might be involved. While the 2-D measurement provided by the Cobb angle has been useful in the past and remains useful to the clinician, if significant advances are to be made in scoliosis research, there has to be a shift in attitude and 3-D measurement should become routine and used as the gold standard.

6. The promise of genetic studies

The rapid development of genome-sequencing techniques in recent years has reduced the time to sequence the genome of a patient to a matter of just a few days. For the past few years, utilizing this ability has led to much research into many diseases being focused on selecting patients with a common problem and analyzing the genetic make-up of such patients to identify problem genes. In some diseases this has been very successful, especially where a single problem gene has been able to be identified. Such techniques have been applied to patients with AIS but, unfortunately, the picture that has emerged does not seem to be a simple one. Genetic research into AIS has shown many genes possibly to be involved and the picture is most certainly complex even though diagnostic tests are currently being developed (Akoume et al, 2010; Leboeuf et al., 2009; Ogilvie, 2010; Weinstein et al, 2008). This complexity might well reflect the complex nature of AIS (as described above) and the mixed nature of patients with possibly very different underlying causes. Alternatively, it might well describe the multifactorial nature of AIS with many factors being involved even in just a single case. Whatever the outcome, the results from the genetic studies of AIS seem to have the greatest potential for providing a solution and much better understanding of the problem. In addition, the results from such studies would provide much needed guidance to many other areas of research.

One aspect of the complexity of AIS has always been the question of whether all cases have a similar underlying cause (as discussed earlier) or whether the patients represent similar manifestations of a variety of different causes. The lack of resolution of this problem has had repercussions for AIS research. For example, in the past a group of patients with AIS selected for research might have included both males and females, patients with single or double curves, patients with curves to the left or to the right, curves that span just a few vertebrae, curves that span many vertebrae, curves of just a few degrees, much more severe curves, curves that have been present for a long time, curves that have been present for a short time etc. The only common feature in selection of such a group is that they all fall under the umbrella of AIS with all its apparent diversity. Such a selection process leaves much to be desired and it is not difficult to recognize the inherent problems within such a group especially if there are several different underlying causes which are different for each case and even more so if there are multiple factors contained within those different underlying causes. The selection of such groups is not ideal but is often made by necessity with a lack of numbers of patients having to be overcome to make statistical analysis worthwhile.

With genetic research, the opportunity to overcome such difficulties has been presented because of the intricacy of the work. To overcome or simplify the issue of there being many different causes of AIS and consequently reduce the number of potential genes involved, many genetic studies are now looking at Familial Idiopathic Scoliosis (FIS) where only patients from the same family are being investigated. In theory, this should narrow the scope of investigation to a single (albeit multifactorial) underlying cause but even here, from the results so far, there are still many genes that appear to contribute to the abnormal development. However, at least it is a step in the right direction and should be encouraged.

The concept of the underlying cause of AIS being multifactorial is also important to consider in this context, even within the family environment. Interestingly, research has shown that if a patient has AIS there is a ~10% probability that a sibling will also develop AIS. This probability is too high for this second development of AIS to be random and so AIS is referred to as being familial i.e. it can be found in several people within the same family.

In the case of identical (monozygotic - identical DNA) twins, it has been shown that there is only a ~70% probability of both twins developing scoliosis. This is important because it highlights the impact of factors other than genetic make-up in developing scoliosis and has spawned the concept of epigenetics where factors other than genetics are considered to be major contributing factors (Grivas et al., 2002a, 2002b, 2006, 2007, 2008a, 2008b, 2009, 2001). Factors that might be considered must certainly include environmental conditions and their influence on spinal curve development and might present alternative treatment strategies (Hermus et al., 2007). This probability of ~70% also shows the limitations of genetic screening being successful in this search because individuals with identical DNA can have diverse degrees of scoliosis, sometimes ranging from severe in one twin to none in the other. This is a dilemma that needs to be resolved and would be an important key in the solution to the problem.

Most interesting though is the finding that for non-identical twins (dizygotic - with non-identical DNA that merely has sibling similarity) there is a ~35% probability that they will both develop scoliosis. Non-identical twins are nothing more than siblings who have shared a common uterus at the same time. This would suggest that the probability of both twins getting scoliosis should be 10% and not the ~35% as is found. It remains to be seen what complexities exist in relation to the uterine environment that might create this increased probability. Again, this is a dilemma of genetic studies that remains to be resolved and one that requires focus if greater progress is to be made

7. Devolopment of computer-assisted methods of research

The development of scoliosis is a slow process and takes several years in humans. There are very few reliable and successful animal models that approach being able to replicate the development of AIS in humans and even these take several weeks if not months for any curve to become manifest. The use of computer-assisted methods and models to mimic the curve development are essential research tools to be developed because their application would have many advantages:

- The time for development of the scoliosis curves would be greatly reduced and results could be seen in hours rather than weeks and months.
- The development of such methods would eliminate/reduce the need for animal research
- Such methods would allow for many different methods and ideas to be tested quickly and simply. The quick results could also enable alternative ideas and thoughts to be tested immediately.
- The results from such methods would allow for a better understanding of the mechanics and underlying mechanisms for the development of spinal curves
- The methods would allow for the development of better treatment strategies which could be applied before actual treatment to predict results.

However, currently the time required for the development of computer-assisted modeling is long and very time-consuming. Furthermore, many practical results relating to tissue parameters are still required to provide adequate and accurate input data and collection of these data all requires time. However, the benefits of being able to use computer assisted modeling to view curve development quickly are well worthwhile. Moreover, the extended application of developing treatment strategies and viewing their predictive value prior to their actual application would be immense (Driscoll et al., 2010, 2011a, 2011b).

8. Is anybody looking for a cure?

In his recent book (Where are all the leaders?), Lee Iacocca, the former, very successful CEO of Chrysler reported on his retirement activities. Having tried all the usual activities such as playing golf he realized he was bored and so focused on raising funds for research for a health-related charity. Again, he was very successful but after a while he realized something that he thought influenced the research world. He came to the conclusion that research is never-ending and has become an industry all on its own. In effect: *'Researchers get grants to do research so that they can write papers to get more grants to do more research so that they can write more papers to get more grants to do more research .... and on it goes.'* In the book he asks quite simply: *'Is nobody looking for a cure?'* How many people are looking for a cure for AIS?

It would be a great relief if a cure for AIS could be announced tomorrow. If a means by which a spinal curve could be prevented from developing as well as a cure for all those patients who already have a curve were to be announced it would be incredible. If that happened then people involved with research into the aetiology of AIS would be very excited and all the effort that is being put into research of AIS could be channeled elsewhere.

9. Conclusion

An understanding of scoliosis involves an enormous amount of interest and covers many areas of academia. The ideas and thoughts related to AIS in particular are scattered in many different directions. This chapter has attempted to identify those areas of research where most progress towards a better understanding of scoliosis might be made. This is not to say that other areas of research in scoliosis have less value but the chapter has tried to identify those areas where most progress can potentially be made and where focus should be directed. Whether this can be achieved as such remains to be seen.

10. References

Akoume, M, Azeddine, B, Turgeon, I, Franco, A, Labelle, H, Poitras, B, Rivard, C., Grimard, G, Ouellet, J, Parent, S & Moreau, A. (2010) *Spine*. Cell-based screening test for idiopathic scoliosis using cellular dielectric spectroscopy. 35, pp. E601-608.

Driscoll, M, Aubin, C, Moreau, A, & Parent, S. (2011a) Biomechanical comparison of fusionless growth modulation corrective techniques in pediatric scoliosis. *Med Biol Eng Comput* (Epub ahead of print).

Driscoll, M, Aubin, C, Moreau, A, & Parent, S. (2011b) Spinal growth modulation using a novel intravertebral epiphyseal device in an immature porcine model. *Eur Spine J* (Epub ahead of print).

Driscoll, M, Aubin, C, Moreau, A, & Parent, S. (2010) Finite element comparison of different growth sparring instrumentation systems for the early treatment of idiopathic scoliosis. *Stud Health Technol Inform* 158, pp 89-94.

Grivas, TB, Dangas, S, Polyzois, BD, & Samelis, P. (2002a). The Double Rib Contour Sign (DRCS) in lateral spinal radiographs: aetiologic implications for scoliosis. *Stud Health Technol Inform*. 88, pp.38-43.

Grivas TB, Dangas S, Samelis P, Maziotou C, & Kandris K. (2002b) Lateral spinal profile in school-screening referrals with and without late onset idiopathic scoliosis 10 degrees-20 degrees. *Stud Health Technol Inform*. 91, pp.25-31.

Grivas, TB, Vasiliadis, E, Malakasis, M, Mouzakis, V., & Segos, D. (2006) Intervertebral disc biomechanics in the pathogenesis of idiopathic scoliosis. *Stud Health Technol Inform*. 123, pp.80-3.

Grivas TB, Vasiliadis ES, Mihas C, & Savvidou O. (2007) The effect of growth on the correlation between the spinal and rib cage deformity: implications onidiopathic scoliosis pathogenesis. *Scoliosis*. Sep14, pp.2-11.

Grivas, TB, Vasiliadis, ES, Mihas, C, Triantafyllopoulos, G & Kaspiris, A. (2008) Trunk asymmetry in juveniles. *Scoliosis*. Sep 23, pp.3-13.

Grivas TB, Vasiliadis ES, Rodopoulos G, & Bardakos N. (2008a) The role of the intervertebral disc in correction of scoliotic curves. A theoretical model of idiopathic scoliosis pathogenesis. *Stud Health Technol Inform*. 140, pp.33-6.

Grivas TB, Vasiliadis E, Savvidou OD, & Triantafyllopoulos G. (2008b) What a school screening program could contribute in clinical research of idiopathic scoliosis aetiology. *Disabil Rehabil*.;30(10):752-62. Review.

Grivas TB, Burwell RG, Mihas C, Vasiliadis ES, Triantafyllopoulos G, & Kaspiris A. (2009) Relatively lower body mass index is associated with an excess of severe truncal asymmetry in healthy adolescents: Do white adipose tissue, leptin, hypothalamus and sympathetic nervous system influence truncal growth asymmetry? *Scoliosis.* Jun 30, pp.4:13.

Grivas TB, Vasiliadis ES, Kaspiris A, Khaldi L, & Kletsas D. (2011) Expression of matrix metalloproteinase-1 (MMP-1) in Wistar rat's intervertebral disc after experimentally induced scoliotic deformity. *Scoliosis.* May 9, pp.6(1):9.

Hermus, J, Rhijn, L, Ooij, A. (2007). Non-genetic expression of adolescent idiopathic scoliosis: a case report and review of the literature. *Eur Spine J.* 16 (suppl 3) 338-341.

Keim, H. (1979) Scoliosis. CIBA Clinical Symposia. Vol 31, number 2.

Leboeuf, D, Letellier, K., Alos, N, Edery, P, & Moldovan, F. (2009) Do estrogens impact adolescent idiopathic scoliosis? *Cell.* 20, 4, pp147-152.

Ogilvie, J. (2010). Adolescent idiopathic scoliosis and genetic testing. *Curr Opin Pediatr.* 22 (1), 67-70.

Weinstein, S, Dolan, L, Cheng, J, Danielsson, A & Morcuende, J. Adolescent idiopathic scoliosis. (2008) The Lancet. 371, pp. 1527-1537.

3

Ritscher – Schinzel Syndrome – 3C (Cranio-Cerebello-Cardiac) Syndrome: Case Report

Sibila Nankovic, Sanja Hajnsek, Zeljka Petelin,
Andreja Bujan Kovac and Vlatko Sulentic
*University Department of Neurology, School of Medicine,
Zagreb University Hospital Centre,
Referal Centre for Epilepsy of the Ministry of Health
and Social Welfere of the Republic of Croatia
Croatia*

1. Introduction

Ritscher-Schinzel syndrome was first described 1987, in the case of two sisters of healthy parents who have had posterior fossa malformations, congenital heart defects and craniofacial anomalies (5). It is believed that this is an autosomal recessive hereditary disorder. So far, according to ORD data (Office of Rare Disease of the National Institutes of Health), only about 30 cases are reported all over the world, mostly from North America and Europe, mostly in the age of 6 and the oldest patient was 21 years old. In 2001, Leonardi et al. proposed criteria for the diagnosis of 3C ("Cranio-cerebello-cardiac") syndrome in a chromosomally normal sporadic cases - Table 1 (3). Clinically the disorder consists of: 1. various forms of craniofacial anomalies, as well as sceletal malformations of other parts, including cleft palate, ocular coloboma, prominent forehead or occiput, hypertelorism, depressed nasal bridge, micrognathia, down-slanting palpeberal fissurae; 2. cardiac malformations (ventricular or atrial septal defect, tetralogy of Fallot, hipoplastic left heart, aortic or pulmonary stenosis, and other forms of valvular anomalies), 3. anomalies of the central nervous system, including Dandy-Walker malformation, vermis hypoplasia and enlargement or posterior fossa cyst. Criteria to establish certain diagnosis inculde presence of a cardiac malformation, described malformations of posterior cranial fossa, cleft palate or ocular coloboma or 4 of these other forms of craniofacial anomalies previously mentioned.

2. Case report

We report on a patient E.K. born in 1972, who soon after his birth underwent surgery for cleft soft palate, and in 1996 because of ventricular septal defect. At he age of 20 he was diagnosed with thoracic spine scoliosis and received physical therapy, but no surgery was preformed. From year 1989 he has been treated for epilepsy, with clinical fenotype of grand mal seizures and with signs of psychomotor retardation. CT scan of the brain made in 2008 showed a Dandy-Walker malformation. In March 2009 he was hospitalized in University Hospital Centre Zagreb, University Department of Neurology, for frequent seizures despite regular antiepileptic barbiturates therapy (MPB). The clinical examination showed

Craniofacial malformation:	
Low-set ears	58%
Hypertelorism	50%
Down-santing palpebral fissures	40%
Depressed nasal bridge	36%
Prominent occiput	30%
Cleft palate	25%
Micrognathia	22%
Ocular coloboma	21%
Cleft lip and palate	4%
Cardiac malformation:	
Septal defects	82%
Valvular defects	32%
Cono-truncal anomalies	14%
Cerebellar malformation:	
Dandy-Walker	68%
Dandy-Walker Variant	21%
Hydrocephalus	11%
Other malformations noted in less than 10% of the patients:	
Absent ribs	
Adrenal hypoplasia	
Anal atresia	
Congenital glaucoma	
Cutis aplasia	
Hemangioma	
Hemivertebrae	
Hypospadias	
Inguinal hernia	
Malrotation of the gut	
Nail hypoplasia	
Nippler hypoplasia	
Penis hypoplasia	
Polydactyly	
Renal malformations	

Table 1. Summary of possible clinical findings and the frequency in patients with Ritscher-Schinzel (3C) syndrome (3)

craniofacial anomalies in terms of prominent forehead, down-slanting palpeberal fissurae, depressed nasal bridge (Figure 1), with syndactyly of 1st and 2nd finger on his right foot (Figure 2), flexural contractures of distal phalanges of 2nd and 3rd finger of both hands and scoliosis of thoracic spine segment. X-ray imaging study of the whole spine have been performed. Images of the cervical spine show proper bone mineralization. Congenital block of vertebral body and articular processes in C6-C7 segment. Reduced intervertebral space in C2-C3 segment. Alordosis with preserved posterior vertebral line. Uncovertebral arthrosis, and with hypoplasia of 1st rib on the right side. Sinistro-convex scoliosis of the thoracis spine segment. Normal intervertebral space. Imaging of the thoracolumbar transition and lumbosacral spine show normal intervertebral space and normal height and width of vertebral body. Preserved posterior vertebral line.

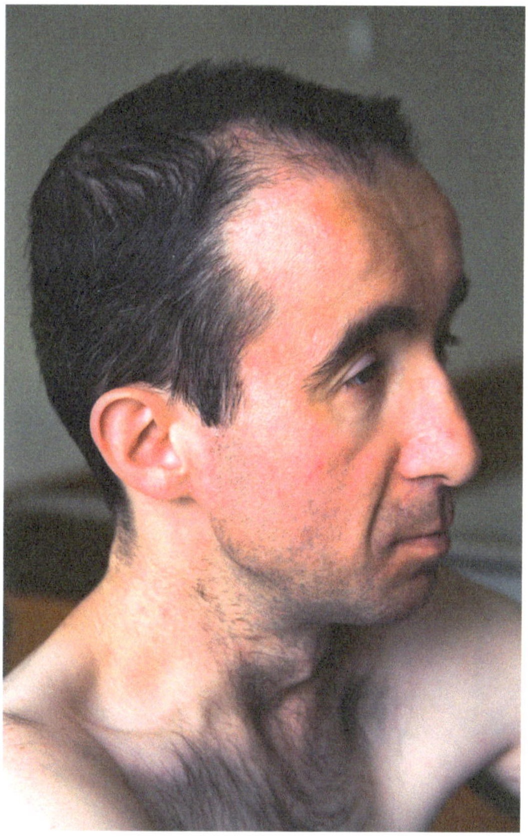

Fig. 1. Craniofacial anomalies. prominent forehead, down-slanting palpeheral fissurae, depressed nasal bridge.

MRI of the brain showed Dandy-Walker malformation, enlargement of the cisterna magna because of the posterior fossa cyst and aplasia of the caudal part of the cerebellar vermis, but also bilateral subependimal heterotopia of grey matter (Figure 3-6). EEG showed diffuse dysrhythmic activity with the focus frontotemporobasal left, and with paroxysmic activity and vulnerability on hyperventilation. Visual and auditory evoked potentials were normal. Cardiac ultrasound showed a dilated right heart, with no signs of residual obstruction after resection of the right ventricular ridge, and minor L-D shunt at membranous part of interventicular septum. Abdominal ultrasound displayed in the VI / VII liver segment hyperechogenic zone, 15x9,6 mm in diameter, corresponding liver hemangioma, with other findings were normal. EMNG verified mild chronic lesions in the muscles of the foot. Laboratory analysis was done in terms of multisystem metabolic diseases (lactate /perchlorate in perchloric acid, ammonia, amino acids quantitatively, organic acids, oligosaccharides, mucopolysaccharides excretion, transferrin phenotypes, chitotriosidase) and all findins were proper. Chromosomal analysis showed normal male karyotype.

During hospitalization we have observed two epileptic seizures of a new clinical phenotype, the type of complex partial seizure of the parietal origin (giratory crisis). Antiepileptic therapy was changed and Oxcarbazepine (OXC) was introduced, on which the epileptic manifestations were completely ckupirale. The patient was presented at neurosurgical-neuroradiologic-neurological meeting which concluded that there is no indication for neurosurgical treatment.

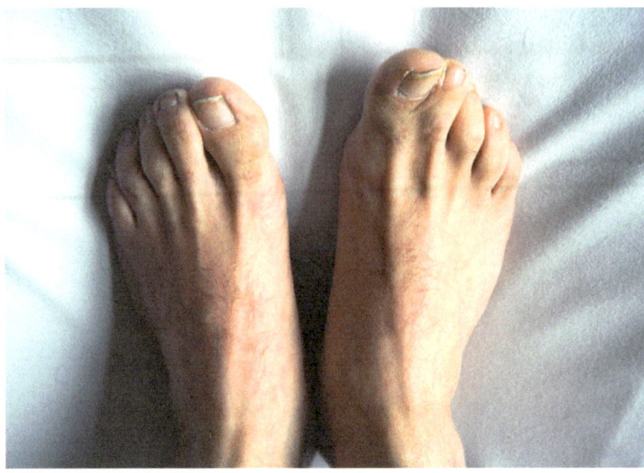

Fig. 2. Complete syndactyly of 1st and 2nd finger of right foot.

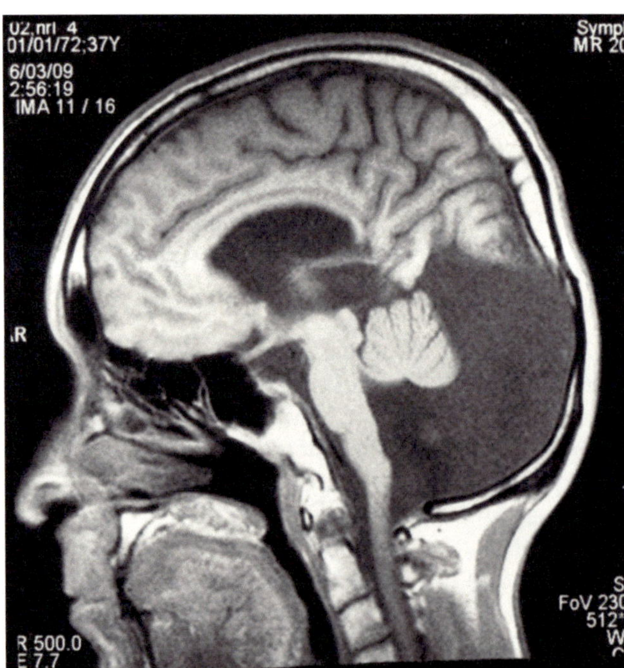

Fig. 3. MRI of the brain: T1-weighted sagittal view showes Dandy-Walker malformation with enlarged posterior fossa because of the cyst, aplasia of the caudal part of the cerebellar vermis, and extensive IV ventricle communication with the cyst.

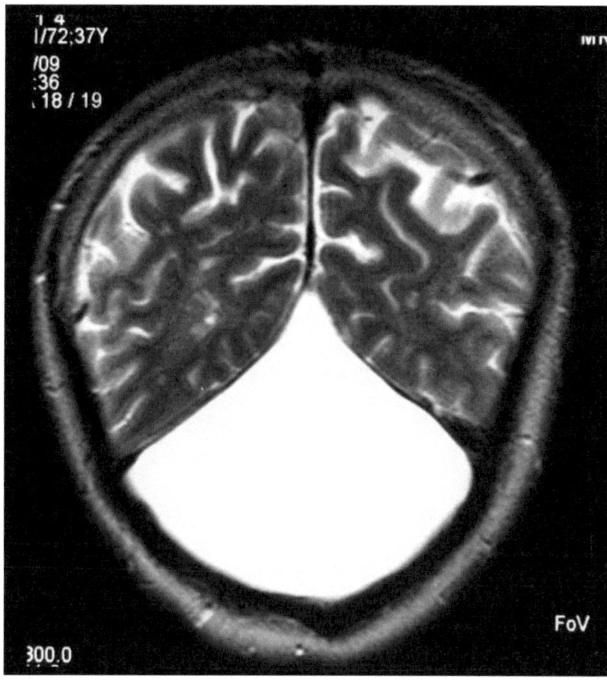

Fig. 4. MRI of the brain: Axial T2-weighted image shows large cystic formation.

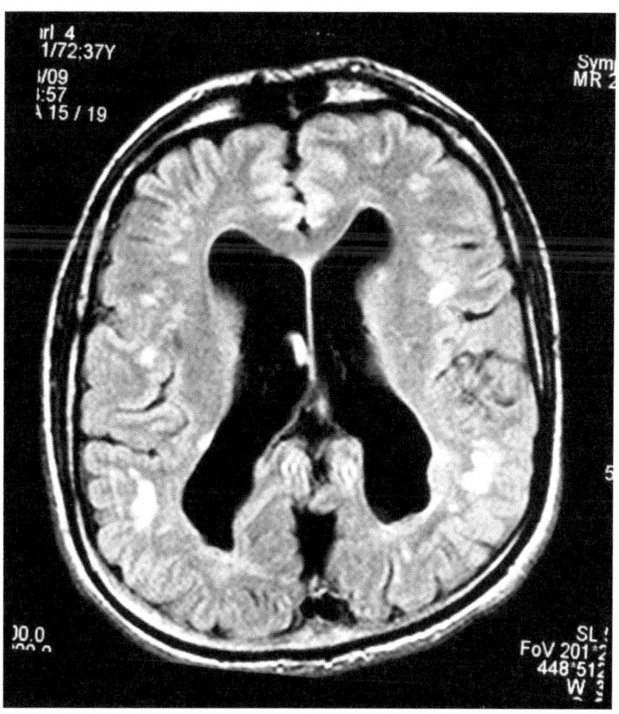

Fig. 5. MRI of the brain: Axial T1-weighted image shows multiple bilateral subependimal heterotopia of grey matter.

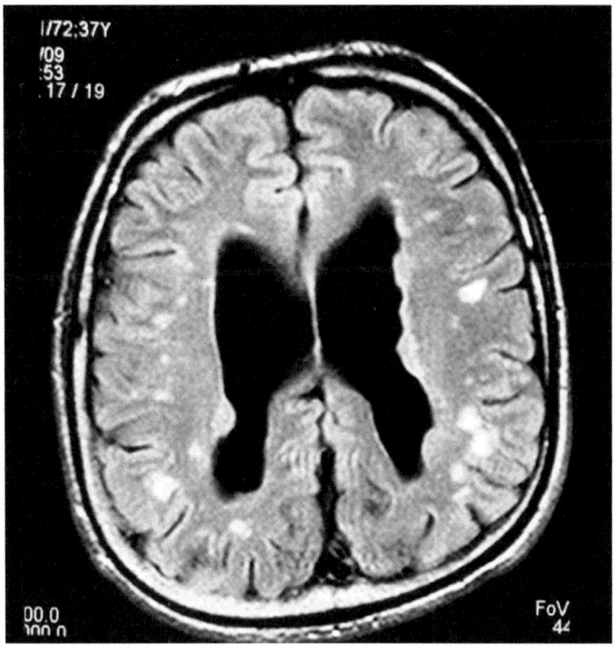

Fig. 6. MRI of the brain: Axial T1-weighted image shows multiple bilateral subependimal heterotopia of grey matter.

3. Discussion

In addition to clinical criteria set by Leonardi et al. (3) other authors present patients associated with other types of malformations. Kosak et al. describe two cases with hypotonia and hypospadias, one had intestinal malrotation with gastroesophageal reflux, and hypoplastic 5th finger of right hand with a cavernous hemangioma on dorsal side and other had scrotal cleft (2). Orstavik et al. describe two patients with anal malformations, in one case there was atresia of the anus with perianal fistula, while the other had anteriorly placed anus. In the third patient there was verified bilateral hydronephrosis (4). Zankl et al. describe a patient with secondary hypogammaglobulinemia due to loss through the gastrointestinal tract and with amelogenesis imperfecta (8). Wheeler et al. in his case describe a patient with deficiency of growth factors and consecutive growth failure at the age of 2, and also the unilateral hearing loss at the age of 6 (7). Several other authors describe presence of malformations of the skeletal muscle system in terms of syndactyly, brachydactyly, hypoplasic ribs, short neck, hemivertebrae and nail hypoplasia (1, 2, 3, 7). DeScipio et al., following a molecular and cytogenetic analysis in three families, verified subtelomeric deletion of chromosome 6p, and in one family also a duplication of chromosome 16q23, and as the three major genes that could be responsible for the disease stated FOXF1 and FOXQ1 and FOXC1 gene (1). Expression of these genes could result in different clinically presentation including malformations of the musculoskeletal system such as hemivertebrae, but no cases of scoliosis in patient with „3C" Syndrome has yet been reported.

Our patients was clinically presented with the following findings:

a. from the cranial malformations: down-slanting palpeberal fissurae, depressed nasal bridge, prominent forehead, operated cleft palate;
b. from the hearth malformations: operated ventricular septal defect with a small residual shunt at membranous part of interventicular septum;
c. from the cerebellar malformations: verified Dandy-Walker malformation with bilateral subependimal heterotopia of grey matter;
d. from other less frequent associated malformations we mention a complete syndactyly of 1st and 2nd finger on his right foot, congenital block of C6-C7 (body and articular processes), sinistro-convex scoliosis of thoracic spine segment, hypoplasia of 1st rib, liver hemangioma ando also, what is often described, a mental retardation.

The patient is under regular control of cardiologists and neurologists of the Referal Centre for epilepsy with continuous cardiac and antiepileptic therapy on which is his clinical condition fully satisfactory. Comparing the findings of our patients with the cases described in the literature we believe that all findings necessary for the diagnosis of Ritscher-Schinzel Syndrome (3C) manifested, noting that our patient had additional clinical features, presence subependimal heterotopia of grey matter, complex partial and generalized tonic-clonic epileptic seizures and scoliosis, all clinical presentations that have so far not been described accompanying Ritscher-Schinzel Syndrome.

4. Conclusion

Based on clinical examination, radiological and neuroradiological diagnostic procedures we belive that our patient meets all necessary criteria for the diagnosis of Ritscher-Schinzel syndrome. He is also the first patient who has, apart from criteria, gray matter heterotopia on MRI and epilepsy, and is also the first case described in Croatia, and so far the oldest patient described in the literature.

5. References

[1] DeScipio C., Schneider L., Young T.L. et al. Subtelomeric deletions of Chromosome 6p: Molecular and Catogenetic Characterization of Three New Cases With Ohenotypic Overlap With Ritscher-Schinzel (3C) Syndrome. Am J Med Genet 2005; 134A:3-11.
[2] Kosaki K, Curry C, Roeder E, Jones K. Ritscher-Schinzel (3C) syndrome: documentation of the phenotype. Am J Med Genet 1997;68:421-427.
[3] Leonardi M, Pai G, Wilkes B, Lebel R. Ritscher-Schinzel cranio-cerebello-cardiac (3C) syndrome: report of four new cases and review. Am J Med Genet 2001;102:237-242.
[4] Orstavik K, Bechensteen A, Fugelseth D, Orderud W. Sibs with Ritscher-Schinzel (3C) syndrome and anal malformations. Am J Med Genet 1998;75:300-303.
[5] Ritscher D, Schinzel A, Boltshauser E et al. Dandy-Walker (like) malformation, atrio-ventrikular septal defect and a similar pattern of minor anomalies in2 sisters: a new syndrome? Am J Med Genet 1987;26:481-491.
[6] Rusnak AJ, Hadfield MI, Chudley AE et al. Increased nuchal translucency thickness: a potential indicator for Ritscher-Schinzel syndrome. Fetal Diagn Ther 2008;24:395-399.

[7] Wheeler PG, Sadeghi-Nejad A, Elias ER. The 3C syndrome: evolution of the phenotype and growth hormone deficiency. Am J Med Genet 1999;87:61-64.

[8] Zankl A, Gungor T, Schinzel A. Cranio-cerebello-cardiac (3C) syndrome: Follow-up study of the original patient. Am J Med Genet 2003;118:55-59

4

Sensorimotor Integration in Adolescent Idiopathic Scoliosis Patients

Jean-Philippe Pialasse, Martin Descarreaux, Pierre Mercier, Jean Blouin and Martin Simoneau
Faculté de Médecine, Division de Kinésiologie, Université Laval - Vieillissement, Centre de Recherche FRSQ du Centre Hospitalier Affilié Universitaire de Québec
Canada

1. Introduction

Adolescent idiopathic scoliosis (AIS) is a multifactorial disorder with more questions than answers. In past years, research has mainly focused on 5 areas: genetic factors, neurological mechanism dysfunction, hormone/metabolic dysfunction, skeletal growth abnormalities, and biomechanical factors. As adolescents with any known functional or structural disorder in the somatosensory pathway are more susceptible to scoliosis during growth than healthy adolescents, it is possible that subclinical somatosensory impairment may be associated with AIS.

The aim of this chapter is to provide evidence that idiopathic scoliosis (IS) is likely related to neurological mechanism dysfunction. We recognize that no consistent neurological abnormalities have been identified in IS patients, but we nonetheless believe that curvature progression could result from specific neurological impairments. Consequently, we reviewed studies that assessed whether IS patients experience abnormal somatosensory processing. For instance, deficits in the structure and functioning of peripheral systems are of various natures in AIS. Lesions of the posterior column pathway have been implicated as a possible cause of scoliosis. In animal studies, scoliosis has been induced by damaging the posterior column pathway at the dorsal root and in the thoracic cord (Liszka, 1961; Pincott et al., 1984; Pincott & Taffs, 1982). These observations led some researchers to investigate whether IS patients would respond differently than healthy control participants to a mechanical stimulus (Barrack et al., 1988; Byl et al., 1997; Olafsson et al., 2002; Wyatt et al., 1986). No consensus has, however, been reached.

In recent years, several studies have reported sensorimotor impairments in IS patients. We believe that dysfunction of sensorimotor transformation mechanisms during growth results in IS or accelerates curvature progression as motor output could be inefficient, causing asymmetric axial muscle activation. This chapter reviews studies that investigated the potential implication of neurological mechanism dysfunction in IS patients.

1.1 Neurological abnormalities

Magnetic resonance imaging (MRI) and somatosensory evoked potentials (SEPs), 2 among various techniques, have been employed to verify whether scoliosis patients incur neurological abnormalities.

1.1.1 Cranio-cervical MRI

MRI discerns pathological and anatomical variations. These variations sometimes do not imply any visible clinical changes during standard patient examination besides the scoliosis. MRI of the spine and cranio-cervical region can detect aberrations, such as syringomyelia (Inoue et al., 2005; Inoue et al., 2003; Maiocco et al., 1997; Rajasekaran et al., 2010), cerebellar tonsil ectopia (<5 mm) (Cheng et al., 2003; Chu et al., 2007; Inoue et al., 2005; Inoue et al., 2003; Sun et al., 2007) and Arnold Chiari type I malformation (Krieger et al., 2011; Rajasekaran et al., 2010).

Considering that AIS patients are known to be taller than control subjects (Lam et al., 2011; Little et al., 2000) and curvature might be stretching the cord, tonsillar ectopia might be viewed as a consequence of scoliosis. Faster growth of the spine versus the spinal cord during childhood might also be a cause of tonsillar ectopia in some cases (Barson, 1970; Chu et al., 2006). Thus, it would be reasonable to question if ectopia is the result of scoliosis rather than its cause. In Arnold Chiari type I malformation, however, it is acknowledged that suboccipital craniectomy reduces spinal curvature, supporting the above statement (Colombo & Motta, 2011; Krieger et al., 2011).

A prospective study of 200 young Chinese adolescents (age: 10 to 20 years) by Cheng et al. (1999) involved 36 healthy participants, 135 AIS patients with Cobb's angle ranging from 10 to 45° and 29 AIS patients with Cobb's angle >45°. Tonsillar ectopia was detected in 7.3% of AIS patients. Remarkably, 27.6% of AIS patients with Cobb's angle >45° presented tonsillar ectopia. Furthermore, in this cohort, 3.7% of AIS patients had syringomyelia, and 17.2% had Cobb's angle >45°. None of the controls manifested syringomyelia. Tonsillar ectopia incidence in AIS patients was more frequent when syringomyelia was found (66.7% vs. 5.1%). Moreover, Cheng et al. (2003) demonstrated that 17.9% of AIS patients had tonsillar ectopia up to 5 mm below the basion-opisthion line, whereas control cerebellar tonsils were above it (mean=2.8 mm; range 0-10.5 mm).

In India, Rajasekaran et al. (2010) analyzed 177 young patients aged less than 21 years with scoliosis but not those with associated bone destruction, infectious causes, obvious spinal dysraphism or trauma. Patients were divided into 3 groups: congenital scoliosis patients (A), presumed infantile scoliosis, juvenile scoliosis or AIS (B), and other types of scoliosis, including neuromuscular scoliosis (C). MRI revealed intra-spinal abnormalities in group B. In this group, anomalies were observed in 14% of AIS, 27% of juvenile scoliosis, and 25% of infantile scoliosis patients. In group B, all patients with subtle sensorimotor impairments or aberrant abdominal reflexes had intra-spinal anomalies. The most common anomalies were syringomyelia associated with Arnold Chiari malformation and isolated syringomyelia. In addition, scoliosis occurred earlier (mean age=11.4 years) in patients with intra-spinal abnormalities compared to others (mean age=3.2 years). The incidence of abnormalities was also higher when Cobb's angle was greater. The best indicators of intra-spinal irregularities on MRI were: abnormal neurological findings, apical thoracic kyphosis, double curvature and early onset curvature. After excluding those with subtle neurological findings or atypical AIS curvature patterns (apical kyphosis), 4.2% of 71 AIS patients manifested abnormal MRI.

In Japan, Inoue et al. (2003) reported neurological anomalies detected by MRI in 13% of 71 AIS patients with a family history. Similarly, in preoperative MRI screening of 250 individuals, Inoue et al. (2005) found that 18% had neurological abnormalities, and scoliosis started earlier in these individuals. Neurological aberrations were noted in 18% of these 250 individuals after standard neurological examination. Among patients with abnormal neurological signs after standard neurological examination, 57% also had abnormal neurological MRI. These authors reported that the most predictable factors of neural axis malformation were sustained clonus (100% had malformation), asymmetrical superficial abdominal reflexes (71%), hyperreflexia (43%) and diminished sensation (13%).

In Europe, Hausmann et al. (2003) scanned 100 AIS patients before surgical correction. These patients did not feel pain or numbness, and their lower limb strength was normal. In addition, no abnormal neurological sign was observed after standard neurological examination. MRI revealed neurological anomalies in 3% of these patients.

In Turkey, however, Benli et al. (2002) found that preoperative MRI demonstrated neurological abnormalities in 7.1% of 84 AIS patients with absolute flexible thoracic curvatures (i.e., King-Moe type III).

In USA, Shen et al. (1996) reported 4% of abnormal MRI on preoperative screening among 72 AIS patients without any abnormal neurological results. Similarly, preoperative MRI screening of 140 neurologically normal AIS patients disclosed that 2.9% had neurological abnormalities (Winter et al., 1997). Furthermore, Do et al. (2001) reported abnormal findings in 2.1% in AIS patients after preoperative MRI.

Overall, the frequency of abnormal neurological results based on MRI scans varied slightly between studies: from 3% to 18% of AIS patients tested. This range may have been due to the study population. It could also have been related to the absence or presence of subtle neurological deficits and whether the authors classified such cases as AIS. Clinicians might have failed to detect subtle neurological deficits and classified patients as AIS when it was in fact neurological scoliosis.

Also, the definition of neurological abnormalities on MRI is important. When the pathology starts with Arnold Chiari type I malformation, with tonsils 5 mm or more below the basion-opisthion line, some will consider tonsillar ectopia <5 mm as normal and will not report it, whereas others will.

Globally, MRI findings from around the world give good external validity to these observations.

1.1.2 MRI and spinal cord length

Spinal cord length is not significantly different between AIS patients and controls (Chu et al., 2006). However, segmental spinal column lengthening at the thoracic level in AIS patients with severe curvatures gives a significantly reduced cord to vertebral length ratio. There is also no correlation between this ratio and tonsillar ectopia.

1.1.3 MRI of the brain

Other variations might be observed on more precise scrutiny at the brain level. MRI voxel-based morphometry has revealed less attenuation of white matter in the genu of the corpus callosum and left internal capsule in left thoracic AIS girls than in their controls (Shi et al.,

2009). These 2 structures are respectively responsible for interhemispheric communication and corticothalamic projectional fibers. Nevertheless, no difference has been discerned between right-sided thoracic AIS patients and control subjects. Geissele et al. (1991) reported asymmetry of the ventral pons in the area of the cortico-spinal tracts and an enlarged cisterna magna in AIS patients. Moreover, cortical thickness declined significantly with age in almost all cortical lobes except in the temporal lobe of normal subjects (Wang et al., 2012). In contrast, cortical thickness in right thoracic AIS patients did not decrease with age. Furthermore, some significant differences were found between the controls and AIS patients regarding the thickness of areas related to motor and vestibular function.

1.1.4 MRI of the vestibular apparatus

Significant effort has been made recently to develop tools to investigate the 3-D shape of the vestibular apparatus in AIS patients and healthy controls. 3-D measurement of vestibular system morphology in 20 right thoracic AIS patients and 20 healthy girls demonstrated that AIS patients had a smaller distance between centers of the lateral and superior canals and the angle with vertex at the center of the posterior canal in the left side of the vestibular system but not in the right side (Shi et al., 2011).

In addition, structural abnormality with communication between the lymphatic posterior and lateral semicircular canals with a frequency of 55% in 95 AIS patients was described, whereas it was only 15% in 445 participants who underwent MRI and computed tomography (Rousie et al., 1999). This abnormality is associated with the following signs: the absence of rotatory vertigo but frequent instability, transport sickness on head tilt to the side of the anomaly, spatial disorientation in new environments, and nystagmus.

1.1.5 SEPs and AIS

SEPs are frequently measured during corrective surgery. Moreover, SEPs are quantified in patients to determine whether IS is related to central nervous system (CNS) dysfunction. Abnormal SEPs can result from dysfunction at the level of the peripheral nerve, plexus, spinal root, spinal cord, brainstem, thalamocortical projections, or primary somatosensory cortex. Although most studies detected abnormal SEPs in IS patients, some failed to do so. For example, Brinker et al. (1992) and Olafsson et al. (2002) did not find abnormal SEPs in their AIS patients. In contrast, Fernandez-Bermejo et al. (1993) observed asymmetrical latency at the lumbar level in 20 out of 52 AIS patients. Moreover, Machida et al. (1994) noted abnormal SEP latency in chickens with experimentally-induced scoliosis and AIS patients. In this study, AIS patients with a single curvature had longer N37 latency when the tibial nerve was stimulated ipsilateral to the concave rather than the convex side. Moreover, N37 latency was delayed on both sides in AIS patients with double curvature. It is noteworthy that these authors observed abnormal SEP latency in 97% of their AIS patients (Machida et al., 1994).

A preoperative study revealed that only 3 out of 72 AIS patients (i.e., 4.2%) had abnormal SEPs on normal standard neurological examination (Shen et al., 1996). Two of these patients had asymmetrical P37 latency despite normal MRI. Other AIS patients presented subcortical responses after left tibial nerve stimulation but no cortical responses, indicating dysfunction of the ascending sensory pathways at the thalamocortical or cortical level. However, MRI pointed to Arnold Chiari type I malformation in these patients.

Hausmann et al. (2003) reported that 68% of 100 AIS patients with Cobb's angle ranging from 43° to 96° had abnormal SEPs before surgery, with 56% having body height corrected prolonged latency increased and 12% with pathological right and left differences.

Another study examined 147 AIS patients and 31 controls to determine whether the former have abnormal SEPs compared to the latter (Cheng et al., 1998). None of the AIS patients and controls had clinically-detectable neurological deficits. In this study, the authors analyzed P37 and N45 latencies and inter-side latency differences. The results revealed that inter-side latency differences in AIS patients were 1.1 (±1.6) ms and 1.2 (±1.6) ms for P37 and N45, respectively. In contrast, in the controls, inter-side latency was only 0.2 (±0.3) ms for P37 and N45. Overall, these findings demonstrated that inter-side latency differences were significantly larger in scoliosis patients, indicating asymmetric conduction velocity of electrical signals in somatosensory pathways compared to the controls. Absolute latencies and inter-side differences in latencies were abnormal in 11.6% of AIS patients. Consequently, this observation suggests that AIS could be divided into 2 subgroups, one with disorders of the somatosensory pathways, and the other with normal somatosensory pathways. In a subsequent prospective study, Cheng et al. (1999) attempted to correlate clinical scoliosis severity with structural abnormalities on MRI and SEP-detected functional disorders in the hind brain and spinal cord. In this investigation, 135 AIS patients and 36 healthy subjects consented to MRI and SEP examination. Abnormal SEPs were observed in 24 (14.6%) AIS patients. Approximately 12% and 28% of AIS patients with moderate and severe spine curvature had abnormal SEPs. The higher prevalence of abnormal somatosensory function in patients with severe curvature was significant. The authors calculated a significant correlation between tonsillar ectopia and abnormal SEPs (r=0.672); most of the patients (i.e., 66.7%) with tonsillar ectopia had abnormal SEPs. In contrast, in 160 patients without tonsillar ectopia, only 10% had abnormal SEPs. None of the controls had tonsillar ectopia or abnormal SEPs. In a subsequent study, the same research group calculated the spinal cord length to vertebral column length ratio, evaluated the position of the cerebellar tonsils, and correlated these data with SEPs (Chu et al., 2006). The results revealed that 43% of AIS patients (i.e., 6 of 14 patients) with Cobb's angle >40° and 14% of AIS patients (i.e., 2 of 14 patients) with Cobb's angle <40° had abnormal SEPs. Remarkably, there was no significant difference between cord to vertebral ratio and tonsillar level between patients with normal and abnormal SEPs. Finally, all controls had normal SEPs. In a parallel study, the same research group observed that 14.3% of 105 AIS patients with Cobb's angle ranging from 10° to 35° had abnormal SEPs (Guo et al., 2006). The novelty of this research was that it investigated if previously-reported balance control impairment in AIS patients was associated with scoliosis or abnormal somatosensory function. A significant difference in standing balance control was found between AIS patients with abnormal SEPs and the controls when relying on somatosensory input. Two years later, the same research group conducted another study in which SEPs were examined in 35 AIS patients with Cobb's angle <40°, 26 AIS patients with Cobb's angle >40°, and 36 controls. Overall, 23.0% of all AIS patients had abnormal SEPs; 9% and 42% had moderate and severe curvatures, respectively. Again, all controls had normal SEPs (Chu et al., 2008). It seems evident that some AIS patients have abnormal SEPs.

This review found that approximately 14 to 68% of AIS patients had afferent conduction abnormalities, whereas Machida et al. (1994) noted that 97% of AIS patients had aberrant SEPs.

1.2 Motor and balance control impairment

Herman et al. (1985) reported that AIS patients exhibited perceptual impairments, sensorimotor adaptation deficits and motor learning and balance control shortfalls. According to them, these deficits are the signature of disorders at higher integrative levels of the CNS. Furthermore, ocular and balance stability impairments in AIS patients designate the brainstem as a common target as it mediates sensory information for both the postural and oculomotor systems.

Transcranial magnetic stimulation explores motor responses as well as cortical inhibition and facilitation. A recent study showed no difference in motor responses to a single stimulation between AIS patients, congenital scoliosis patients and control individuals. It suggests that the motor circuit itself is not different. However, significant right/left asymmetry in cortical excitability was characterized by short-latency cortico-cortical inhibition and intra-cortical facilitation after paired pulse stimulation of the motor cortex (Domenech et al., 2010), reflecting a relative decrease in intra-cortical inhibition circuits of the motor cortex. Such dysregulation with hemispheric asymmetry in motor activity modulation of spinal posture at the intra-cortical level could cause or enhance the scoliotic deformity. Furthermore, the fact that congenital scoliosis patients have the same response as the controls tends to reinforce the view that the response is not a consequence of the deformation.

Spinal reflexes have been investigated during surgery (Maguire et al., 1993). Long-latency reflex activity has been observed in all AIS patients but not in non-AIS patients. The reflex, the result of polysynaptic spinal cord processing, might represent segmental disinhibition. It is unclear if this is the consequence of a segmental or supra-segmental abnormality, but the reflex is absent in normal subjects. Moreover, its absence in non-AIS patients confirms that it is not the result of the deformity itself.

AIS patients manifest greater balance instability than controls when sensory information is manipulated, and they have abnormal postural perception (Byl & Gray, 1993; Herman et al., 1985; Sahlstrand et al., 1978). However, without sensory manipulation, some studies did not observe greater body sway in AIS patients compared to their controls (Byl & Gray, 1993; Herman et al., 1985). Moreover, the assessment of balance control either with eyes open or closed showed larger Center of Pressure (CP) area and larger medio-lateral (ML) body sway in AIS patients with larger Cobb's angle (15°-25°) compared to AIS patients with smaller Cobb's angle (5°-14°) (Haumont et al., 2011).

Other studies have observed larger body sway area and CP displacement in AIS patients compared to their controls (Beaulieu et al., 2009; Byl et al., 1997). In the study by Beaulieu et al., AIS patients were divided into a pre-brace group (brace prescribed but not yet worn) and an observation group. This classification was adopted because more clinical criteria than Cobb's angle alone were considered (i.e., age, Risser sign, Cobb's angle, gibbosity and history of scoliosis in the immediate family). It turned out that pre-brace AIS patients had larger Cobb's angle than the observation group. The results revealed that pre-brace AIS patients had a smaller mean peak and larger mean distance than the controls (Beaulieu et al., 2009). Larger body sway area and CP displacement were noted in the observation group compared to the controls. The results suggest that the observation group could represent an intermediate sensorimotor condition between the control and the pre-brace AIS groups. The severity of scoliosis in pre-brace girls might be related to an increase in sensorimotor integration disorder.

Recently, Lao et al. (2008) reported dynamic balance control impairment during gait. These authors recorded significant differences between the right and left limbs for peak vertical force and antero-posterior (AP) maximal propulsive ground reaction force in AIS patients with abnormal SEPs. Besides, the data were more significant for the right limb compared to the left limb. Right and left limb asymmetries were also found in AIS patients with abnormal SEPs for minimum hip joint moment and maximum knee and ankle joint moments. The novelty of these results was the finding of greater gait impairments in AIS patients with abnormal SEPs. Similarly, they demonstrated that AIS patients with abnormal SEPs have poorer static balance control when they have to rely on somatosensory inputs (Guo et al., 2006).

2. Is AIS related to sensorimotor integration impairment?

Lesions of the posterior column pathway have been suggested to be a possible contributing factor in scoliosis. In animal studies, scoliosis has been induced by damaging the posterior column pathway at the dorsal root and in the thoracic cord (Liszka, 1961; Pincott & Taffs, 1982). This indicates that sensory problems could cause IS and it led some researchers to investigate whether IS patients would respond differently than age-matched controls to vibratory stimuli (Barrack et al., 1988; Byl et al., 1997; Olafsson et al., 2002; Wyatt et al., 1986). These studies were not, however, in agreement. For example, Wyatt et al. (1986) and Barrack et al. (1988) found that AIS had a lower proprioceptive threshold (more sensitive) whereas McInnes et al. (1991) reported that AIS patients had a significantly higher vibratory threshold (less sensitive) than control subjects. It is noteworthy that the proprioceptive system threshold can be evaluated via responses to vibration stimulation; they do not determine the capability of the brain to transform sensory perception into appropriate motor responses.

3. Integration and responses in sensory deprivation of visual and proprioceptive information

One way to assess the ability of the brain to transform available sensory inputs into appropriate motor commands is to manipulate sensory information and quantify its effect on balance control. Indeed, sensory deprivation in AIS patients exacerbates body sway oscillations (Sahlstrand et al., 1978; Simoneau et al., 2006a; Simoneau et al., 2006b). These studies clearly demonstrate sensorimotor integration impairments in AIS.

3.1 Sensory deprivation and balance control in AIS patients

More than 3 decades ago, Sahlstrand et al. (1978) explored the effect of removed vision and/or attenuated plantar sole mechanoreceptor information (i.e., participants stood on a compliant support base) on balance control in AIS patients. Their study revealed that attenuating sensory information originating from mechanoreceptors of the soles and/or occluding visual information increased the sway area of AIS patients to a greater extent than that of the controls. One limitation of this study is that standing on a compliant surface may affect balance stability itself (unstable support base). Therefore, standing on an unstable surface may exacerbate AIS patients' balance control problem.

To assess balance control, researchers usually quantify the kinematics of the CP as it depicts overall CP behaviour (e.g., total sway area, CP range, CP root mean square (RMS) velocity, etc.). This type of analysis, however, does not evaluate balance control commands. Consequently, Baratto et al. (2002) proposed a new approach to analyze the causes of overall CP behaviour. For instance, sway density curve analysis permits to determine whether body sway kinematics result from greater or more variable balance control commands.

A study in our laboratory (Simoneau et al., 2006b) expanded on the work of Sahlstrand et al. (1978) by deploying a different technique to manipulate lower limb proprioception: we applied tendon vibration to mask ankle proprioception. Furthermore, we assessed the underlying cause of greater body sway oscillations in AIS by quantifying the sway density curve. Eight scoliosis patients (7 females and 1 male; mean age: 16.4 years, Cobb's angle: 45.6°±7.5°) and 10 healthy young girls (average age 16.5 years) were tested. In this experiment, the study subjects stood barefoot on the force platform with their feet 10 cm apart and arms alongside their body. They maintained an upright standing posture while fixating on a small target in their central vision. They were subjected to 4 different experimental conditions. Three sensory deprivation conditions were created by manipulating sensory information: 1. no vision, 2. perturbed proprioception/vision and 3. perturbed proprioception/no vision. No sensory manipulation was the control condition.

By controlling the availability of sensory information and quantifying the outcome, i.e., CP range and CP RMS velocity, we could objectively ascertain the role of visual information and/or ankle proprioception on balance control. Overall, the results revealed that the CP range and CP RMS velocity of AIS patients were larger than those of the controls when ankle proprioception was attenuated. This was seen whether vision was available or not. An important observation, it suggests that despite the availability of vision, AIS patients rely much more on ankle proprioception to scale the amplitude of their balance control commands than control participants. It could be hypothesized that CP kinematics (greater CP range and CP RMS velocity) and greater balance control commands in AIS patients, compared to control participants, result from difficulty in reweighting gains of the vestibular system and the remaining sensory inputs after ankle proprioception alteration whether vision is available or not. Furthermore, sway density curve analysis demonstrated that these observations could be explained by amplitude rather than balance control command variation.

Overall, our interpretation of the results is that IS interferes with the neural mechanism that weighs the remaining sensory inputs. Such a mechanism is necessary to map these inputs into appropriate balance control commands. The remaining sensory information should come from the soles of the feet, the joints above the ankles, and the vestibular apparatus. Finally, we concluded that, compared to the controls, AIS patients rely much more on ankle proprioception to control the amplitude of balance control commands.

3.2 Sensory reweighting and balance control in AIS patients

A key finding of human balance control is that the integration of sensory information appears to be dynamically regulated to adapt to changing environmental conditions and the availability of sensory information; this process is called sensory reweighting. In another study conducted in our laboratory, we assessed the ability of AIS patients to perform sensory reweighting (Simoneau et al., 2006a). The framework to determine the ability of the brain to reweigh sensory information consists of monitoring balance stability during transient sensory perturbation, for example, when vision is removed and then becomes available again. In this circumstance, a decrease in balance stability (e.g., a sudden increase in body sway) could result from difficulties in dynamically reweighting sensory information when it is made available after a period of deprivation.

In this experiment, 8 scoliosis patients (7 females and 1 male; mean age: 16.3±2.3 years, Cobb's angle: 45.6°±7.5°) and 9 healthy adolescent girls (average age 16.5 ±1.7 years) were tested.

Participants stood barefoot on a force platform with their feet 10 cm apart and their arms alongside their body. They maintained an upright posture while fixating on a small target in central vision. All subjects performed 6 trials in each experimental condition. Each trial lasted 30 s and was divided into 2 epochs of 15 s. During the first interval, sensory information (vision and/or proprioception) was occluded (vision) or masked (ankle proprioception, tendon vibration applied at the ankles). In the second epoch, sensory information (vision and/or ankle proprioception) was returned; participants opened their eyes and/or tendon vibrations were stopped. This procedure aimed to assess the immediate effect of change in the availability of sensory inputs on balance control. The different sensory transition conditions were: 1. reintegration of vision under normal proprioception (RV-P), i.e., no vision/proprioception to vision/proprioception, 2. reintegration of proprioception under vision (RP-V), i.e., perturbed proprioception/vision (PP-V) to RP-V, and 3. reintegration of proprioception without vision (RP-NV), i.e., perturbed proprioception/no vision (PP-NV) to RP-NV. The ability of participants to control their balance was also evaluated in trials without any sensory manipulation for 30 s (control condition). The experimental conditions were randomized within the experimental session and across participants.

ML and AP velocities of the CP were calculated according to the finite difference technique. To characterize balance control, we computed CP RMS velocity along the ML and AP axes. This parameter measures the variability of CP velocity. To study the mechanisms causing more variable CP velocity during sensory transition, we analyzed the sway density curve (Baratto et al., (2002). Peaks of the sway density curve correspond to time instants in which the CP and presumably associated balance motor commands are relatively stable. Mean peak represents the time spent by CP inside the 3-mm radius circle centered at the time of peak on the sway density curve. Consequently, peak amplitude estimates the variability of balance control commands.

In the control condition, for both axes, compared to the controls, AIS patients showed greater CP RMS velocity and it was larger for the AP than for the ML axis. Sway density curve analysis revealed that in the absence of sensory manipulation, AIS patients' balance control commands were greater and more variable than those of the controls for mean distance and mean peak.

Balance stability analysis after the reintegration of vision showed that AIS patients had greater CP RMS velocity than the controls along both axes (Fig. 1, upper panel). Analysis of the sway density curve and time spent within the zones of stability (Fig. 1, lower panel) revealed that the balance control commands of AIS patients were much more variable than those of the controls as they spent less time within the 3-mm radius circle (lower mean peaks).

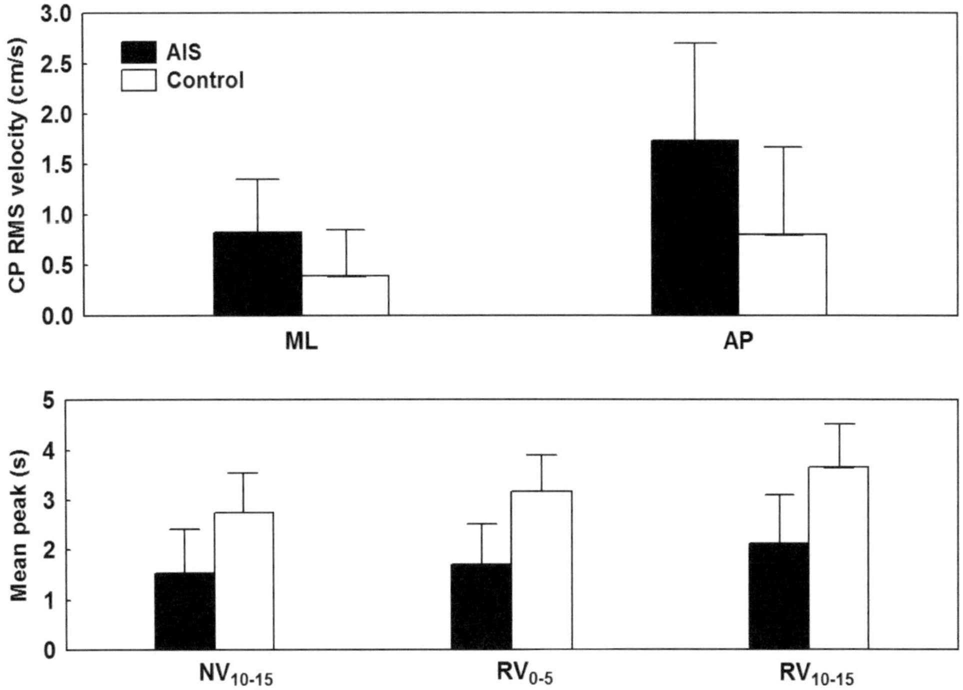

Fig. 1. Balance control performance during reintegration of vision. Upper panel - Group means of CP RMS velocity along the ML and AP axes for the proprioception/no vision to proprioception/reintegration vision condition. The lower panel illustrates Group by Epoch interaction for time spent within the zones of stability (mean peak) for the last 5-s epoch of the proprioception/no vision interval (NV_{10-15}) and the first 5-s epoch (RV_{0-5}) and last 5-s epoch (RV_{10-15}) of the proprioception/vision reintegration intervals. In both panels, the error bars indicate 95% confidence intervals. Cited from Simoneau et al. 2006a BMC Neuroscience under Creative Commons licence.

Balance stability analysis after reintegration of proprioception when vision was available revealed that CP RMS velocity increased in AIS patients but not in the controls (Fig. 2, upper panel: PP-V_{10-15} to RP-V_{0-5}). Across time (RP-V_{0-5} versus RP-V_{10-15}), however, AIS patients improved their balance as CP RMS velocity decreased. Sway density curve analysis indicated that balance motor commands in AIS patients were much more variable than in the controls: their mean peak increased slightly across time; therefore, the CP of AIS patients did not spend much time within the stability area compared to the controls (Fig. 2, lower panel).

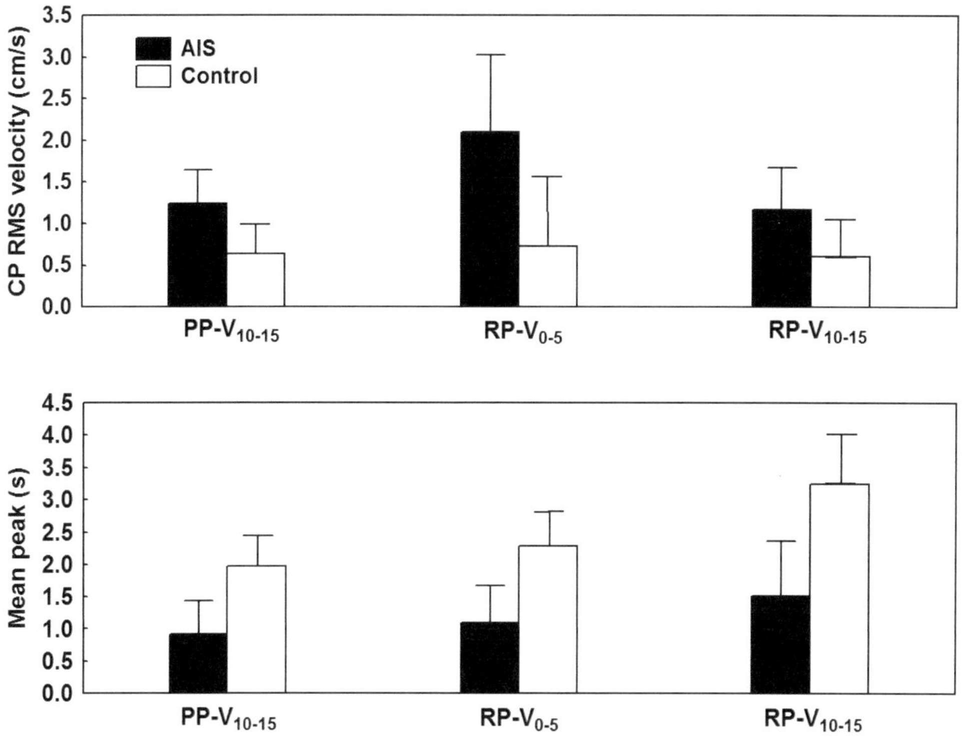

Fig. 2. Balance control performance during reintegration of ankle proprioception when vision is available. The upper panel illustrates Group by Epoch interaction for CP RMS velocity for the last 5-s epoch of the sensory deprivation interval ($PP\text{-}V_{10-15}$ perturbed proprioception/vision) and for the first and last 5-s epoch of the sensory reintegration interval ($RP\text{-}V_{0-5}$ and $RP\text{-}V_{10-15}$ reintegration proprioception/vision). The lower panel shows Group by Epoch interaction for time spent within the zone of stability for the same 5-s epochs as in the upper panels. In all panels, the error bars correspond to 95% confidence intervals. Cited from Simoneau et al. 2006a BMC Neuroscience under Creative Commons licence.

A significant group difference was also demonstrated when participants had to reintegrate ankle proprioception in the absence of vision. For instance, balance stability analysis after the reintegration of proprioception without vision indicated that AIS patients' CP RMS velocity was larger than that of the controls and differed across time (Fig. 3, upper panel). Moreover, the sway density curve (Fig. 3, lower panel) disclosed that balance control commands in AIS patients were more variable than in the controls during the first 5 s of the sensory reintegration interval ($RP\text{-}NV_{0-5}$) as their mean peak did not increase from $PP\text{-}NV_{10-15}$ to $RP\text{-}NV_{0-5}$ ($p>0.05$). In contrast, control participants reduced the variability of their balance control commands as their mean peak increased from $PP\text{-}NV_{10-15}$ to $RP\text{-}NV_{0-5}$ ($p<0.01$).

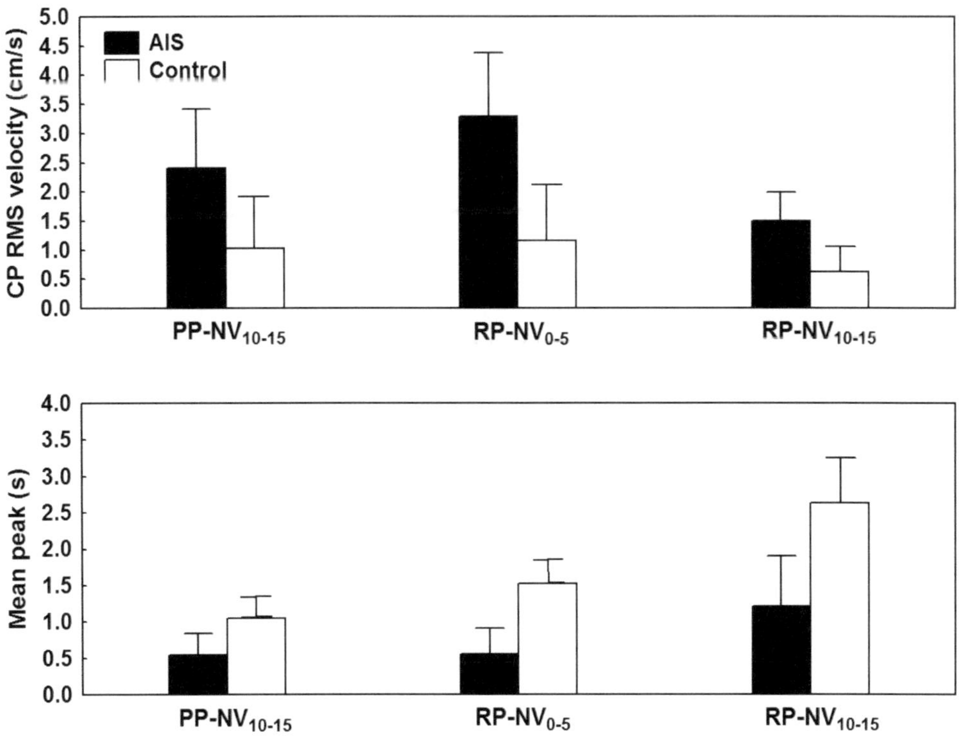

Fig. 3. Balance control performance during reintegration of ankle proprioception in the absence of vision. The upper panel presents Group by Epoch interaction for CP RMS velocity for the last 5-s epoch of the sensory deprivation interval ($PP\text{-}NV_{10\text{-}15}$ perturbed proprioception/no-vision) and for the first and last 5-s epoch of the sensory reintegration interval ($RP\text{-}NV_{0\text{-}5}$ and $RP\text{-}NV_{10\text{-}15}$ reintegration proprioception/no-vision condition). The lower panel illustrates Group by Epoch interaction for time spent within the zone of stability for the same 5-s epochs as in the upper panels. In all panels, the error bars indicate 95% confidence intervals. Cited from Simoneau et al. 2006a BMC Neuroscience under Creative Commons licence.

The originality of our results is that AIS patients showed greater CP RMS velocity after the reintegration of proprioception information from muscles acting at the ankle joint. This was observed whether or not vision was available. In contrast, the controls were able to maintain or rapidly reduce their CP RMS velocity when proprioceptive information from the lower leg muscles returned to normal. Furthermore, in the absence of vision, AIS patients exhibited increased CP RMS velocity after the reintegration of ankle proprioception. The increase in CP RMS velocity observed in the context of sensory transition (i.e., sensory information returned to normal; no tendon vibration and/or eyes open) indicates that the central sensory reweighing mechanisms are less effective in AIS patients. Moreover, the greater CP RMS velocity noted during sensory reintegration suggests that AIS patients' balance control commands were inappropriate. Analysis of their sway density plots confirmed that AIS patients had greater mean peak (balance control command variability) and mean distance (balance control command amplitude). This could result from improper transformation of sensory orientation cues into corrective balance control commands.

4. The vestibular system

Although the etiopathology of scoliosis is not well understood (Jensen & Wilson, 1979; Manzoni & Miele, 2002), we believe that impaired responses of the vestibulo-spinal tracts could contribute to spine curvature and its progression. This hypothesis derives from clinical and animal studies which demonstrated that stimulation of vestibular nuclei (vestibulo-spinal tract) activated the back muscles (Ali et al., 2003; Ardic et al., 2000; Britton et al., 1993; Schwartz-Giblin et al., 1984a; Schwartz-Giblin et al., 1984b; Siegel & Tomaszewski, 1983). In addition, oculo-motor and postural vestibular deficits have been reported to range from 50 to 85% in AIS, whereas these deficits represent 12 and 17% in the controls (Manzoni & Miele, 2002). It has been shown that some AIS patients have a lower gain of vestibulo-ocular reflexes (VOR) and a larger phase lead compared to age-matched controls. Moreover, AIS patients have a reduced duration of post-rotatory vestibular and optokinetic nystagmus as well as self-motion perception, with a significant relationship between the time constant of vestibular-elicited nystagmus and magnitude of the curvature; the shorter the time constant, the larger the curvature (Manzoni & Miele, 2002). Moreover, these authors have reported that AIS patients with abnormal VOR showed a more progressive curve during growth. Finally, weaker predominance of the right vestibular apparatus is sometimes reported in AIS patients (Manzoni & Miele, 2002).

Various procedures - calorimetric test, vestibular-evoked myogenic potential (VEMP), vestibular chair and galvanic vestibular stimulation (GVS) - can evaluate vestibular system integrity (Schubert & Minor, 2004). The calorimetric test is a gold standard for the identification of peripheral unilateral vestibular hypofunction by simply introducing warm or cold water in the external auditory canal. Unfortunately, this technique only stimulates the lateral semicircular canal and to a lesser extent than a physiological stimulus (Schubert & Minor, 2004). In contrast, VEMP stimulates only the otoliths and detects unilateral hypofunction with clicking sounds and by recording associated sternocleidomastoid muscle myogenic potentials (Schubert & Minor, 2004). The vestibular chair provides a physiological stimulus by rotating the seated patient around a vertical axis through the vertex. It explores both sides of the semicircular canals, VOR and vestibular integration (Blouin et al., 1997; Schubert & Minor, 2004). On the other hand, GVS is a procedure that can explore the semicircular canals and otoliths (Cathers et al., 2005). GVS generates ML body sway responses (Day et al., 1997; Fitzpatrick & Day, 2004) and AP body sway responses (Scinicariello et al., 2002; Severac Cauquil et al., 1998). It can create eye movements when high stimulation is delivered (Aw et al., 2006; Kim et al., 2006). GVS is an attractive tool because it probes vestibular function and reveals balance control system operation in response to pure vestibular perturbation, at least immediately after GVS onset. The direction of body sway responses after GVS varies with head orientation (Fitzpatrick & Day, 2004). Moreover, electrode positioning also influences the direction of the postural response. Different GVS configurations exist. For example, during bilateral bipolar stimulation, the most common configuration, an anodal electrode is located on the mastoid process behind one ear with the cathodal electrode behind the other ear. On the other hand, during bilateral monopolar GVS, both electrodes have the same polarity, and a reference electrode is located on the forehead, for example. Because GVS produces a signal of head movement, the direction of the postural response depends upon head orientation, During monopolar GVS, body sway will be along the AP axis whereas it will be along the ML axis during bilateral bipolar stimulation (Fitzpatrick & Day, 2004).

4.1 Cognitive exploration and the vestibular chair

Although various studies have proven that some AIS patients have abnormal VOR (Manzoni & Miele, 2002), little attention has been devoted to assessing the capacity of AIS patients to integrate vestibular information for cognitive processing of space perception. Consequently, we investigated the ability of AIS patients to process vestibular information for space updating (Simoneau et al., 2009). In this experiment, seated AIS patients and controls experienced torso rotations of different directions and amplitudes in the dark and produced saccades that would reproduce their perceived spatial characteristic of the rotations (vestibular condition). Furthermore, we controlled for possible alteration of the oculomotor and vestibular systems by measuring subject accuracy in performing saccades toward memorized peripheral targets in the absence of body rotation and gain of their vestibulo-ocular reflex. Ten IS patients (9 females, mean age: 17.4 years, Cobb's angle: 28-51) and 13 age-matched healthy individuals (11 females, mean age: 16.4 years) were tested. The participants sat on a chair in a completely dark room and were able to rotate around its central vertical axis, located in the center of a black cylinder with a radius of 1.5 m. The pseudo-randomly selected magnitudes of whole-body rotation were 10°, 20° or 30°. Whole-body rotation was clockwise for half of the trials and counter-clockwise for the other half. Horizontal eye movements were recorded by electro-oculography.

The experimental session consisted of a main experimental condition that tested the ability of participants to process vestibular inputs (i.e., cognitive vestibular condition) and 2 control conditions, one that examined the subjects' capacity to produce accurate saccadic eye movements (i.e., visual condition) and the other that controlled for possible alteration of the vestibular system (i.e., vestibulo-ocular reflex condition). The participants were passively rotated in the cognitive vestibular condition. Eye movements were attenuated during body rotations by asking them to look at a chair-fixed diode positioned straight ahead. After rotation, they produced a saccade to shift their gaze to their initial position (Fig. 4: "vestibular memory-contingent saccade" paradigm (Bloomberg et al., 1988)). Saccade amplitude (i.e., perceived body rotation amplitude) was measured at the end of the first saccade (defined as the first instant that eye velocity dropped below 5°/s after saccade onset). Therefore, participants had to process and memorize the vestibular signals generated during whole-body rotation to produce a saccade of equal magnitude but in the opposite direction of the rotations.

Cognitive vestibular gain analysis (Fig. 5) showed that both groups underestimated whole-body rotation, as demonstrated by their average ratios which were inferior to 1. Nonetheless, AIS patients underestimated the magnitude of whole-body rotation to a greater extent than control participants (mean of 0.65 and 0.82 for the AIS and control groups, respectively; main Group effect: $F_{1,20}=5.57$, $p<0.05$). For both groups, the directions of chair rotation and their amplitude had no effect on cognitive vestibular gains.

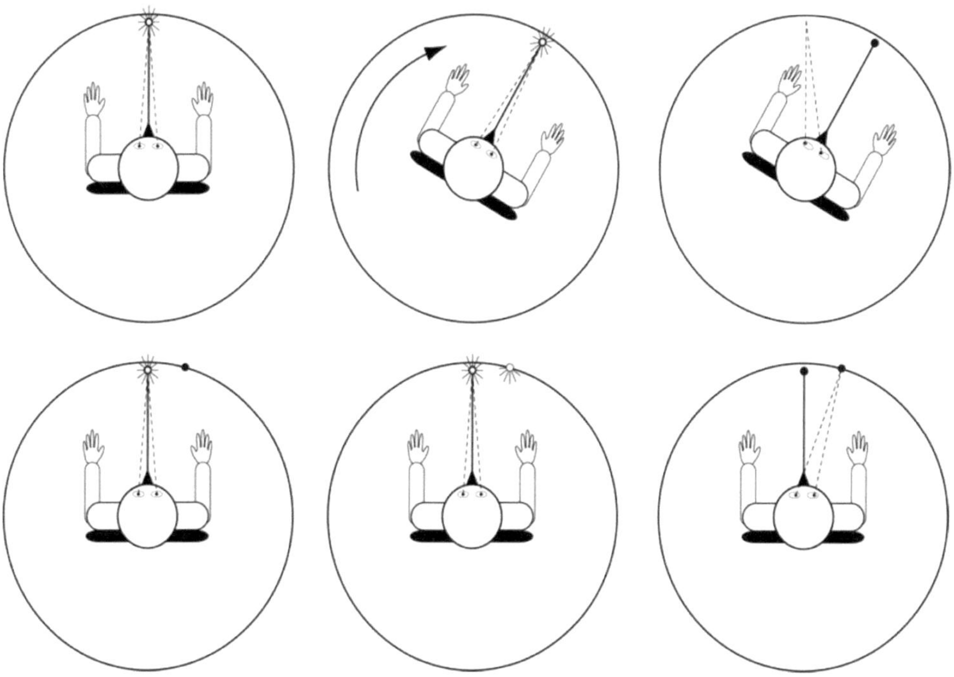

Fig. 4. Schema of the experimental set-up: the upper panels depict the vestibular condition, and the lower panels, the visual condition. Participants looked at a chair-fixed light (CFL) before being submitted to whole-body rotation (upper left panel). Then, whole-body rotation mainly stimulated the horizontal semicircular canals (upper middle panel). After rotation, the CFL was turned off and the participants performed a saccade to the starting position (upper right panel). In the visual condition, participants looked at the CFL (lower left panel). Then, the peripheral target lit up for 0.2 s (lower middle panel). Finally, after 1 s, the CFL was turned off and the participants performed a saccade to the peripheral target (lower right panel). Cited from Simoneau et al. 2009 BMC Neuroscience under Creative Commons licence.

Saccades in the absence of whole-body rotation were accurate, with no significant difference in amplitude between groups ($t=1.88$, $df=20$, $p>0.05$). Furthermore, analysis revealed that the VOR gain of AIS patients did not differ from that of control participants, regardless of rotation direction (no main Group or Direction effect and no Group by Direction interaction: $p>0.05$). The performance of accurate saccades by AIS patients to memorize the targets excluded any saccadic motor deficit. This observation substantiates previous results suggesting that the network assisting the control of vestibular memory-guided saccades is different from the one governing visual memory-guided saccades (Israel et al., 1995; Pierrot-Deseilligny et al., 1991). Moreover, the fact that AIS patients had normal VOR gains confirms that the vestibular system in these patients is normal. Overall, this study revealed that, compared to the controls, AIS patients underestimated the amplitude of rotations, indicating impairment of their ability to memorize and process vestibular signals. It is possible that severe spinal deformity was partly due to impaired vestibular information travelling from the cerebellum to the vestibular cortical network or alteration in the cortical mechanisms processing vestibular signals. However, these results do not allow us to make claims as to whether deficits in the cognitive processing of vestibular signals should be considered as a potential factor leading to curvature progression in scoliosis patients. Further studies may determine if this deficit and melatonin signalling dysfunction in AIS can predict curve progression in patients with small spinal deformity.

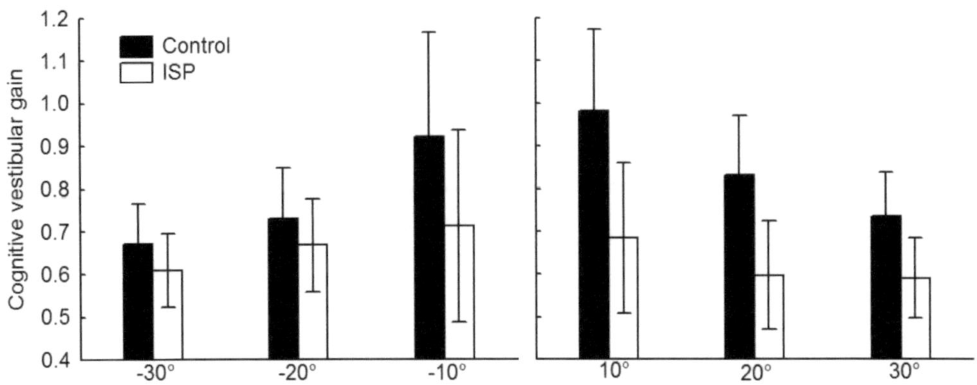

Fig. 5. Vestibular cognitive gain with chair rotations of 10, 20 and 30° in both directions (error bars represent ±95% confidence intervals). Cited from Simoneau et al. 2009 BMC Neuroscience under Creative Commons licence.

4.2 Integration and motor responses

Vestibular information is also used to maintain posture and balance. To this end, vestibulo-motor responses during head movements are sent to the postural muscles through the vestibulo-spinal and reticulo-spinal tracts.

4.2.1 GVS

GVS serves to manipulate vestibular sensory information (i.e., semicircular canals and otoliths) and to evoke vestibulo-motor responses. Binaural bipolar GVS stimulation is known to provoke body sway towards the anode side (Ardic et al., 2000; Marsden et al., 2003; Marsden et al., 2002).

4.2.2 Do AIS patients have abnormal vestibulo-motor responses?

After the literature review presented above concerning the possible implication of sensorimotor impairments in IS, we hypothesized that AIS patients will show vestibulo-motor responses along the frontal plane that differ from control values. If this hypothesis is confirmed, during and after GVS, the amplitude of postural responses of AIS patients should be different from that of the controls.

We, therefore, conducted a pilot study to verify the hypothesis. Eight AIS patients [mean Cobb's angle: 40.5° (±5.9°), mean age: 15.5 (±1.4) years, mean height: 165.5 (±9.0) cm, mean weight: 59.3 (±14.5) kg] and 8 control participants [mean age: 12.4 (±2.0) years, mean height: 158.3 (±7.1) cm, mean weight: 49.7 (±7.7) kg] were tested. Both groups underwent 15 trials that lasted 8 s. Participants had their eyes closed at all times. GVS was a step response that lasted 2 s and had an amplitude of 1 mA. GVS direction was randomized: left GVS (L-GVS) anode left and cathode right, and right GVS (R-GVS) anode right and cathode left.

To quantify lateral displacement of the body along the frontal plane, 3 electromagnetic sensors (Polhemus Liberty Model, sampling frequency 120 Hz) were located on the participants' forehead, 7th cervical vertebra and 1st lumbar vertebra. So far, qualitative analysis revealed that the kinematic responses of healthy controls are similar to those of adult individuals (Day et al., 1997; Marsden et al., 2003; Marsden et al., 2002; Marsden et al., 2005). For instance, the maximum displacement of each body part (i.e., head, upper and lower trunk) along the frontal plane is less than 1 cm and is reached during GVS (Fig. 6). It is noteworthy that control participants returned to their initial position approximately 1 s after the end of GVS.

In AIS patients, maximal lateral displacement along the frontal plane was approximately 2 times greater than in the controls (Fig. 7). Furthermore, after GVS, AIS patients required much more time to return to their initial position and some oscillations were even observed (Fig. 7).

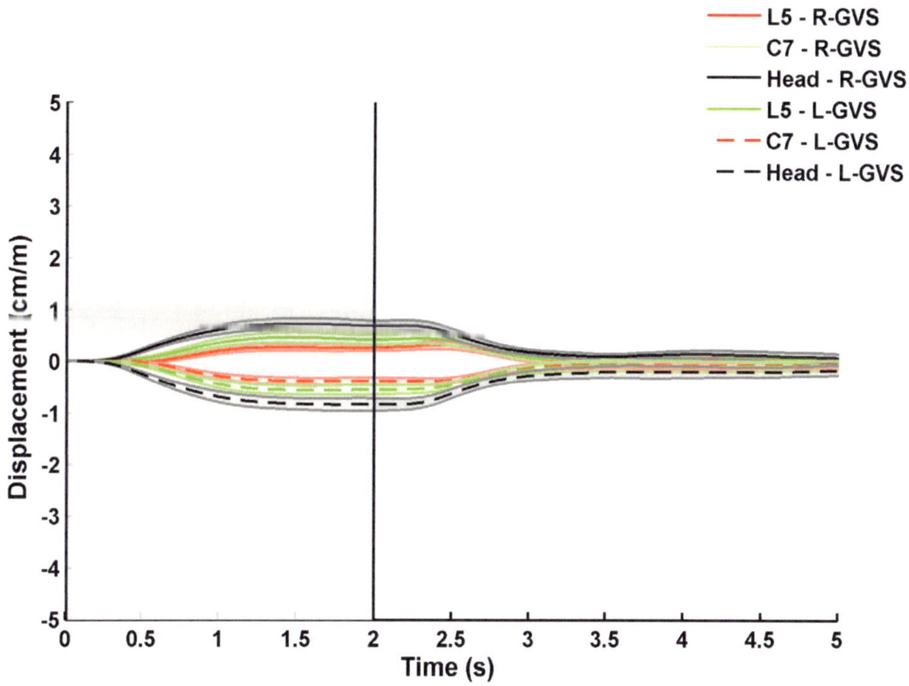

Fig. 6. Mean lateral displacement along the frontal plane for the control group (0 s corresponds to GVS onset, and the vertical line indicates when GVS stops). The solid lines are for right to left GVS (R-GVS), and the dashed lines are for left to right GVS (L-GVS). The shaded areas represent standard errors.

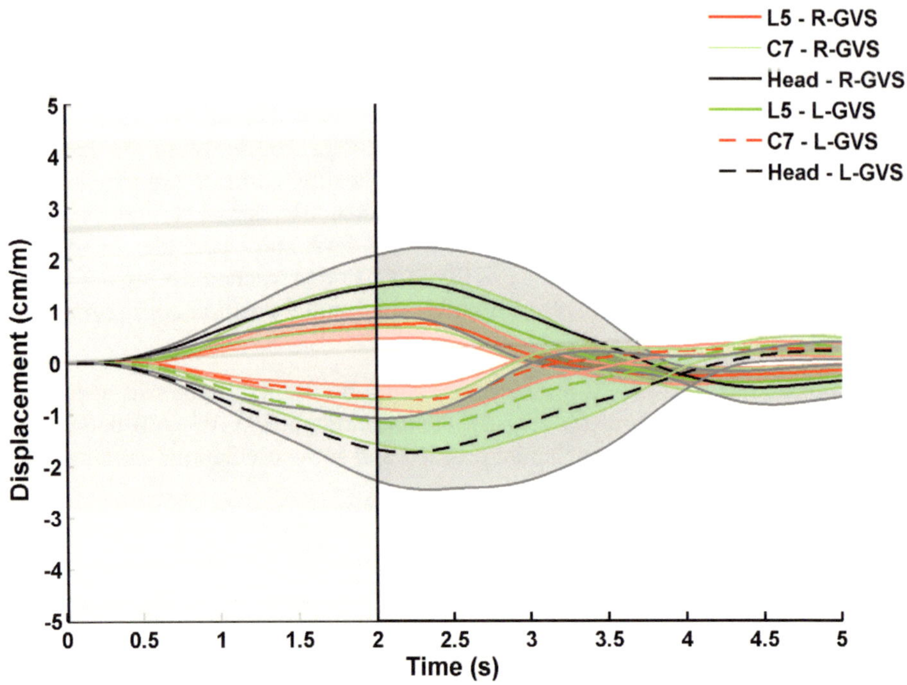

Fig. 7. Mean lateral displacement along the frontal plane for the AIS group (0 s corresponds to GVS onset, and the vertical line indicates when GVS stops). The solid lines are for right to left GVS (R-GVS), and the dashed lines are for left to right GVS (L-GVS). The shaded areas represent standard errors.

These results clearly show that stimulation of the vestibular apparatus in AIS patients evokes a larger kinematics response than in the controls. In addition, because AIS patients required more time than the controls to return to equilibrium after GVS cessation, this observation suggests that AIS patients have more difficulties in reweighting sensory information.

The results of this pilot study support our previous results. Using a different sensory channel (vestibular rather than vision and proprioception), we showed that the cortical mechanisms reweighting sensory information are altered in AIS patients (Simoneau et al., 2006a; Simoneau et al., 2006b).

5. Conclusion

Although the aetiology of IS remains unknown, a growing body of evidence indicates that spinal deformity could be the expression of a subclinical nervous system disorder. Consequently, impairment of sensorimotor transformation may lead to abnormal postural tone and may create spinal curvature during growth.

Future research should assess whether sensory integration and motor response impairments correlate with neuroanatomical changes in the CNS.

6. Acknowledgments

We would like to express our gratitude to all study subjects and their parents for their participation and patience. In addition, we thank *La Fondation Yves Cotrel – Institut de France, Fonds de la recherche en santé du Québec, Fondation de recherche en chiropratique du Québec* and *the Natural Sciences and Engineering Research Council of Canada* for financial support.

7. References

Ali, A.S.; Rowen, K.A. & Iles, J.F. (2003). Vestibular actions on back and lower limb muscles during postural tasks in man. *The Journal of Physiology*, Vol. 546, No. Pt 2, (January 2003), pp. 615-624, ISSN 0022-3751.

Ardic, F.N.; Latt, L.D. & Redfern, M.S. (2000). Paraspinal muscle response to electrical vestibular stimulation. *Acta Oto-Laryngologica*, Vol. 120, No. 1, (January 2000), pp. 39-46, ISSN 0001-6489.

Aw, S.T.; Todd, M.J. & Halmagyi, G.M. (2006). Latency and initiation of the human vestibuloocular reflex to pulsed galvanic stimulation. *Journal of Neurophysiology*, Vol. 96, No. 2, (August 2006), pp. 925-930, ISSN 0022-3077.

Baratto, L.; Morasso, P.G.; Re, C. & Spada, G. (2002). A new look at posturographic analysis in the clinical context: sway-density versus other parameterization techniques. *Motor Control*, Vol. 6, No. 3, (July 2002), pp. 246-270, ISSN 1087-1640.

Barrack, R.L.; Wyatt, M.P.; Whitecloud, T.S., 3rd; Burke, S.W.; Roberts, J.M. & Brinker, M.R. (1988). Vibratory hypersensitivity in idiopathic scoliosis. *Journal of Pediatric Orthopedics*, Vol. 8, No. 4, (July-August 1988), pp. 389-395, ISSN 0271-6798.

Barson, A.J. (1970). The vertebral level of termination of the spinal cord during normal and abnormal development. *Journal of Anatomy*, Vol. 106, No. Pt 3, (May 1970), pp. 489-497, ISSN 0021-8782.

Beaulieu, M.; Toulotte, C.; Gatto, L.; Rivard, C.H.; Teasdale, N.; Simoneau, M. & Allard, P. (2009). Postural imbalance in non-treated adolescent idiopathic scoliosis at different periods of progression. *European Spine Journal*, Vol. 18, No. 1, (January 2009), pp. 38-44, ISSN 0940-6719.

Benli, I.T.; Un, A.; Karaaslan, S.; Cinemre, O.; Gurses, L. & Hekimoglu, B. (2002). [Neural axis abnormalities detected by preoperative magnetic resonance imaging in patients with type III idiopathic scoliosis]. *Acta Orthop Traumatol Turc*, Vol. 36, No. 4, (January 2002), pp. 354-361, ISSN 1017-995X.

Bloomberg, J.; Jones, G.M.; Segal, B.; McFarlane, S. & Soul, J. (1988). Vestibular-contingent voluntary saccades based on cognitive estimates of remembered vestibular information. *Advances in Oto-Rhino-Laryngology*, Vol. 41, (January 1988 1988), pp. 71-75, ISSN 0065-3071.

Blouin, J.; Gauthier, G.M. & Vercher, J.L. (1997). Visual object localization through vestibular and neck inputs. 2: Updating off-mid-sagittal-plane target positions. *Journal of Vestibular Research*, Vol. 7, No. 2-3, (March-June 1997), pp. 137-143, ISSN 0957-4271.

Brinker, M.R.; Willis, J.K.; Cook, S.D.; Whitecloud, T.S., 3rd; Bennett, J.T.; Barrack, R.L. & Ellman, M.G. (1992). Neurologic testing with somatosensory evoked potentials in idiopathic scoliosis. *Spine*, Vol. 17, No. 3, (March 1992), pp. 277-279, ISSN 0362-2436.

Britton, T.C.; Day, B.L.; Brown, P.; Rothwell, J.C.; Thompson, P.D. & Marsden, C.D. (1993). Postural electromyographic responses in the arm and leg following galvanic vestibular stimulation in man. *Experimental Brain Research*, Vol. 94, No. 1, (January 1993), pp. 143-151, ISSN 0014-4819.

Byl, N.N. & Gray, J.M. (1993). Complex balance reactions in different sensory conditions: adolescents with and without idiopathic scoliosis. *Journal of Orthopaedic Research*, Vol. 11, No. 2, (March 1993), pp. 215-227, ISSN 0736-0266.

Byl, N.N.; Holland, S.; Jurek, A. & Hu, S.S. (1997). Postural imbalance and vibratory sensitivity in patients with idiopathic scoliosis: implications for treatment. *Journal of Orthopaedic and Sports Physical Therapy*, Vol. 26, No. 2, (August 1997), pp. 60-68, ISSN 0190-6011.

Cathers, I.; Day, B.L. & Fitzpatrick, R.C. (2005). Otolith and canal reflexes in human standing. *The Journal of Physiology*, Vol. 563, No. Pt 1, (February 2005), pp. 229-234, ISSN 0022-3751.

Cheng, J.C.; Chau, W.W.; Guo, X. & Chan, Y.L. (2003). Redefining the magnetic resonance imaging reference level for the cerebellar tonsil: a study of 170 adolescents with normal versus idiopathic scoliosis. *Spine*, Vol. 28, No. 8, (April 2003), pp. 815-818, ISSN 0362-2436.

Cheng, J.C.; Guo, X. & Sher, A.H. (1998). Posterior tibial nerve somatosensory cortical evoked potentials in adolescent idiopathic scoliosis. *Spine*, Vol. 23, No. 3, (February 1998), pp. 332-337, ISSN 0362-2436.

Cheng, J.C.; Guo, X.; Sher, A.H.; Chan, Y.L. & Metreweli, C. (1999). Correlation between curve severity, somatosensory evoked potentials, and magnetic resonance imaging in adolescent idiopathic scoliosis. *Spine*, Vol. 24, No. 16, (August 1999), pp. 1679-1684, ISSN 0362-2436.

Chu, W.C.; Lam, W.W.; Chan, Y.L.; Ng, B.K.; Lam, T.P.; Lee, K.M.; Guo, X. & Cheng, J.C. (2006). Relative shortening and functional tethering of spinal cord in adolescent idiopathic scoliosis?: study with multiplanar reformat magnetic resonance imaging and somatosensory evoked potential. *Spine*, Vol. 31, No. 1, (January 2006), pp. E19-E25, ISSN 0362-2436.

Chu, W.C.; Man, G.C.; Lam, W.W.; Yeung, B.H.; Chau, W.W.; Ng, B.K.; Lam, T.P.; Lee, K.M. & Cheng, J.C. (2007). A detailed morphologic and functional magnetic resonance imaging study of the craniocervical junction in adolescent idiopathic scoliosis. *Spine*, Vol. 32, No. 15, (July 2007), pp. 1667-1674, ISSN 0362-2436.

Chu, W.C.; Man, G.C.; Lam, W.W.; Yeung, B.H.; Chau, W.W.; Ng, B.K.; Lam, T.P.; Lee, K.M. & Cheng, J.C. (2008). Morphological and functional electrophysiological evidence of relative spinal cord tethering in adolescent idiopathic scoliosis. *Spine*, Vol. 33, No. 6, (March 2008), pp. 673-680, ISSN 0362-2436.

Colombo, L.F. & Motta, F. (2011). Consensus conference on Chiari: a malformation or an anomaly? Scoliosis and others orthopaedic deformities related to Chiari 1 malformation. *Neurological Sciences*, Vol. 32, No. Suppl. 3 (September 2011), ISSN 1590-1874.

Day, B.L.; Severac Cauquil, A.; Bartolomei, L.; Pastor, M.A. & Lyon, I.N. (1997). Human body-segment tilts induced by galvanic stimulation: a vestibularly driven balance protection mechanism. *The Journal of Physiology*, Vol. 500, No. Pt 3, (May 1997), pp. 661-672, ISSN 0022-3751.

Do, T.; Fras, C.; Burke, S.; Widmann, R.F.; Rawlins, B. & Boachie-Adjei, O. (2001). Clinical value of routine preoperative magnetic resonance imaging in adolescent idiopathic scoliosis. A prospective study of three hundred and twenty-seven patients. *Journal of Bone and Joint Surgery*, Vol. 83-A, No. 4, (April 2001), pp. 577-579, ISSN 0021-9355.

Domenech, J.; Tormos, J.M.; Barrios, C. & Pascual-Leone, A. (2010). Motor cortical hyperexcitability in idiopathic scoliosis: could focal dystonia be a subclinical etiological factor? *European Spine Journal*, Vol. 19, No. 2, (February 2010), pp. 223-230, ISSN 0940-6719.

Fernandez-Bermejo, E.; Garcia-Jimenez, M.A.; Fernandez-Palomeque, C. & Munuera, L. (1993). Adolescent idiopathic scoliosis and joint laxity. A study with somatosensory evoked potentials. *Spine*, Vol. 18, No. 7, (June 1993), pp. 918-922, ISSN 0362-2436.

Fitzpatrick, R.C. & Day, B.L. (2004). Probing the human vestibular system with galvanic stimulation. *Journal of Applied Physiology*, Vol. 96, No. 6, (June 2004), pp. 2301-2316, ISSN 0161-7567.

Geissele, A.E.; Kransdorf, M.J.; Geyer, C.A.; Jelinek, J.S. & Van Dam, B.E. (1991). Magnetic resonance imaging of the brain stem in adolescent idiopathic scoliosis. *Spine*, Vol. 16, No. 7, (July 1991), pp. 761-763, ISSN 0362-2436.

Guo, X.; Chau, W.W.; Hui-Chan, C.W.; Cheung, C.S.; Tsang, W.W. & Cheng, J.C. (2006). Balance control in adolescents with idiopathic scoliosis and disturbed somatosensory function. *Spine*, Vol. 31, No. 14, (June 2006), pp. E437-E440, ISSN 0362-2436.

Haumont, T.; Gauchard, G.C.; Lascombes, P. & Perrin, P.P. (2011). Postural instability in early-stage idiopathic scoliosis in adolescent girls. *Spine*, Vol. 36, No. 13, (February 2011), ISSN 0362-2436.

Hausmann, O.N.; Boni, T.; Pfirrmann, C.W.; Curt, A. & Min, K. (2003). Preoperative radiological and electrophysiological evaluation in 100 adolescent idiopathic scoliosis patients. *European Spine Journal*, Vol. 12, No. 5, (October 2003), pp. 501-506, ISSN 0940-6719.

Herman, R.; Mixon, J.; Fisher, A.; Maulucci, R. & Stuyck, J. (1985). Idiopathic scoliosis and the central nervous system: a motor control problem. The Harrington lecture, 1983. Scoliosis Research Society. *Spine*, Vol. 10, No. 1, (January-February 1985), pp. 1-14, ISSN 0362-2436.

Inoue, M.; Minami, S.; Nakata, Y.; Otsuka, Y.; Takaso, M.; Kitahara, H.; Tokunaga, M.; Isobe, K. & Moriya, H. (2005). Preoperative MRI analysis of patients with idiopathic scoliosis: a prospective study. *Spine*, Vol. 30, No. 1, (January 2005), pp. 108-114, ISSN 0362-2436.

Inoue, M.; Nakata, Y.; Minami, S.; Kitahara, H.; Otsuka, Y.; Isobe, K.; Takaso, M.; Tokunaga, M.; Itabashi, T.; Nishikawa, S. & Moriya, H. (2003). Idiopathic scoliosis as a presenting sign of familial neurologic abnormalities. *Spine*, Vol. 28, No. 1, (January 2003), pp. 40-45, ISSN 0362-2436.

Israel, I.; Rivaud, S.; Gaymard, B.; Berthoz, A. & Pierrot-Deseilligny, C. (1995). Cortical control of vestibular-guided saccades in man. *Brain*, Vol. 118, No. Pt 5, (October 1995), pp. 1169-1183, ISSN 0006-8950.

Jensen, G.M. & Wilson, K.B. (1979). Horizontal postrotatory nystagmus response in female subjects with adolescent idiopathic scoliosis. *Physical Therapy*, Vol. 59, No. 10, (October 1979), pp. 1226-1233, ISSN 0031-9023.

Kim, H.J.; Choi, J.Y.; Son, E.J. & Lee, W.S. (2006). Response to galvanic vestibular stimulation in patients with unilateral vestibular loss. *Laryngoscope*, Vol. 116, No. 1, (January 2006), pp. 62-66, ISSN 0023-852X.

Krieger, M.D.; Falkinstein, Y.; Bowen, I.E.; Tolo, V.T. & McComb, J.G. (2011). Scoliosis and Chiari malformation Type I in children. *Journal of Neurosurgery: Pediatrics*, Vol. 7, No. 1, (January 2011), pp. 25-29, ISSN 1933-0707.

Lam, T.P.; Hung, V.W.; Yeung, H.Y.; Tse, Y.K.; Chu, W.C.; Ng, B.K.; Lee, K.M.; Qin, L. & Cheng, J.C. (2011). Abnormal bone quality in adolescent idiopathic scoliosis: a case-control study on 635 subjects and 269 normal controls with bone densitometry and quantitative ultrasound. *Spine*, Vol. 36, No. 15, (July 2011), pp. 1211-1217, ISSN 0362-2436.

Lao, M.L.; Chow, D.H.; Guo, X.; Cheng, J.C. & Holmes, A.D. (2008). Impaired dynamic balance control in adolescents with idiopathic scoliosis and abnormal somatosensory evoked potentials. *Journal of Pediatric Orthopedics*, Vol. 28, No. 8, (December 2008), pp. 846-849, ISSN 1539-2570.

Liszka, O. (1961). Spinal cord mechanisms leading to scoliosis in animal experiments. *Acta Medica Polona*, Vol. 2, (January 1961), pp. 45-63, ISSN 0001-608X.

Little, D.G.; Song, K.M.; Katz, D. & Herring, J.A. (2000). Relationship of peak height velocity to other maturity indicators in idiopathic scoliosis in girls. *Journal of Bone and Joint Surgery*, Vol. 82, No. 5, (May 2000), pp. 685-693, ISSN 0021-9355.

Machida, M.; Dubousset, J.; Imamura, Y.; Iwaya, T.; Yamada, T.; Kimura, J. & Toriyama, S. (1994). Pathogenesis of idiopathic scoliosis: SEPs in chicken with experimentally induced scoliosis and in patients with idiopathic scoliosis. *Journal of Pediatric Orthopedics*, Vol. 14, No. 3, (May-June 1994), pp. 329-335, ISSN 0271-6798.

Maguire, J.; Madigan, R.; Wallace, S.; Leppanen, R. & Draper, V. (1993). Intraoperative long-latency reflex activity in idiopathic scoliosis demonstrates abnormal central processing. A possible cause of idiopathic scoliosis. *Spine*, Vol. 18, No. 12, (September 1993), pp. 1621-1626, ISSN 0362-2436.

Maiocco, B.; Deeney, V.F.; Coulon, R. & Parks, P.F., Jr. (1997). Adolescent idiopathic scoliosis and the presence of spinal cord abnormalities. Preoperative magnetic resonance imaging analysis. *Spine*, Vol. 22, No. 21, (November 1997), pp. 2537-2541, ISSN 0362-2436.

Manzoni, D. & Miele, F. (2002). Vestibular mechanisms involved in idiopathic scoliosis. *Archives Italiennes de Biologie*, Vol. 140, No. 1, (January 2002), pp. 67-80, ISSN 0003-9829.

Marsden, J.F.; Blakey, G. & Day, B.L. (2003). Modulation of human vestibular-evoked postural responses by alterations in load. *The Journal of Physiology*, Vol. 548, No. Pt 3, (May 2003), pp. 949-953, ISSN 0022-3751.

Marsden, J.F.; Castellote, J. & Day, B.L. (2002). Bipedal distribution of human vestibular-evoked postural responses during asymmetrical standing. *The Journal of Physiology*, Vol. 542, No. Pt 1, (July 2002), pp. 323-331, ISSN 0022-3751.

Marsden, J.F.; Playford, D.E. & Day, B.L. (2005). The vestibular control of balance after stroke. *Journal of Neurology, Neurosurgery and Psychiatry*, Vol. 76, No. 5, (May 2005), pp. 670-678, ISSN 0022-3050.

McInnes, E.; Hill, D.L.; Raso, V.J.; Chetner, B.; Greenhill, B.J. & Moreau, M.J. (1991). Vibratory response in adolescents who have idiopathic scoliosis. *Journal of Bone and Joint Surgery*, Vol. 73, No. 8, (September 1991), pp. 1208-1212, ISSN 0021-9355.

Olafsson, Y.; Odergren, T.; Persson, H.E. & Saraste, H. (2002). Somatosensory testing in idiopathic scoliosis. *Developmental Medicine and Child Neurology*, Vol. 44, No. 2, (February 2002), pp. 130-132, ISSN 0012-1622.

Pierrot-Deseilligny, C.; Rivaud, S.; Gaymard, B. & Agid, Y. (1991). Cortical control of memory-guided saccades in man. *Experimental Brain Research*, Vol. 83, No. 3, (1991), pp. 607-617, ISSN 0014-4819.

Pincott, J.R.; Davies, J.S. & Taffs, L.F. (1984). Scoliosis caused by section of dorsal spinal nerve roots. *Journal of Bone and Joint Surgery. British Volume*, Vol. 66, No. 1, (January 1984), pp. 27-29, ISSN 0301-620X.

Pincott, J.R. & Taffs, L.F. (1982). Experimental scoliosis in primates: a neurological cause. *Journal of Bone and Joint Surgery. British Volume*, Vol. 64, No. 4, (January 1982), pp. 503-507, ISSN 0301-620X.

Rajasekaran, S.; Kamath, V.; Kiran, R. & Shetty, A.P. (2010). Intraspinal anomalies in scoliosis: An MRI analysis of 177 consecutive scoliosis patients. *Indian Journal of Orthopaedics*, Vol. 44, No. 1, (January 2010), pp. 57-63, ISSN 0019-5413.

Rousie, D.; Hache, J.C.; Pellerin, P.; Deroubaix, J.P.; Van Tichelen, P. & Berthoz, A. (1999). Oculomotor, postural, and perceptual asymmetries associated with a common cause. Craniofacial asymmetries and asymmetries in vestibular organ anatomy. *Annals of the New York Academy of Sciences*, Vol. 871, (May 1999), pp. 439-446, ISSN 0077-8923.

Sahlstrand, T.; Ortengren, R. & Nachemson, A. (1978). Postural equilibrium in adolescent idiopathic scoliosis. *Acta Orthopaedica Scandinavica*, Vol. 49, No. 4, (August 1978), pp. 354-365, ISSN 0001-6470.

Schubert, M.C. & Minor, L.B. (2004). Vestibulo-ocular physiology underlying vestibular hypofunction. *Physical Therapy*, Vol. 84, No. 4, (April 2004), pp. 373-385, ISSN 0031-9023

Schwartz-Giblin, S.; Femano, P.A. & Pfaff, D.W. (1984a). Axial electromyogram and intervertebral length gauge responses during lordosis behavior in rats. *Experimental Neurology*, Vol. 85, No. 2, (August 1984a), pp. 297-315, ISSN 0014-4886.

Schwartz-Giblin, S.; Halpern, M. & Pfaff, D.W. (1984b). Segmental organization of rat lateral longissimus, a muscle involved in lordosis behavior: EMG and muscle nerve recordings. *Brain Research*, Vol. 299, No. 2, (May 1984b), pp. 247-257, ISSN 0006-8993.

Scinicariello, A.P.; Inglis, J.T. & Collins, J.J. (2002). The effects of stochastic monopolar galvanic vestibular stimulation on human postural sway. *Journal of Vestibular Research*, Vol. 12, No. 2-3, (July 2002), pp. 77-85, ISSN 0957-4271.

Severac Cauquil, A.; Gervet, M.F. & Ouaknine, M. (1998). Body response to binaural monopolar galvanic vestibular stimulation in humans. *Neuroscience Letters*, Vol. 245, No. 1, (March 1998), pp. 37-40, ISSN 0304-3940.

Shen, W.J.; McDowell, G.S.; Burke, S.W.; Levine, D.B. & Chutorian, A.M. (1996). Routine preoperative MRI and SEP studies in adolescent idiopathic scoliosis. *Journal of Pediatric Orthopedics*, Vol. 16, No. 3, (May-June 1996), pp. 350-353, ISSN 0271-6798.

Shi, L.; Wang, D.; Chu, W.C.; Burwell, G.R.; Wong, T.T.; Heng, P.A. & Cheng, J.C. (2011). Automatic MRI segmentation and morphoanatomy analysis of the vestibular system in adolescent idiopathic scoliosis. *Neuroimage*, Vol. 54, No. Suppl. 1 (January 2011), pp. S180-188, ISSN 1053-8119.

Shi, L.; Wang, D.; Chu, W.C.; Burwell, R.G.; Freeman, B.J.; Heng, P.A. & Cheng, J.C. (2009). Volume-based morphometry of brain MR images in adolescent idiopathic scoliosis and healthy control subjects. *AJNR. American Journal of Neuroradiology*, Vol. 30, No. 7, (August 2009), pp. 1302-1307, ISSN 0195-6108.

Siegel, J.M. & Tomaszewski, K.S. (1983). Behavioral organization of reticular formation: studies in the unrestrained cat. I. Cells related to axial, limb, eye, and other movements. *Journal of Neurophysiology*, Vol. 50, No. 3, (September 1983), pp. 696-716, ISSN 0022-3077.

Simoneau, M.; Lamothe, V.; Hutin, E.; Mercier, P.; Teasdale, N. & Blouin, J. (2009). Evidence for cognitive vestibular integration impairment in idiopathic scoliosis patients. *BMC Neuroscience*, Vol. 10, No. (August 2009), p. 102, ISSN 1471-2202.

Simoneau, M.; Mercier, P.; Blouin, J.; Allard, P. & Teasdale, N. (2006a). Altered sensory-weighting mechanisms is observed in adolescents with idiopathic scoliosis. *BMC Neuroscience*, Vol. 7, No. (October 2006), p. 68, ISSN 1471-2202.

Simoneau, M.; Richer, N.; Mercier, P.; Allard, P. & Teasdale, N. (2006b). Sensory deprivation and balance control in idiopathic scoliosis adolescent. *Experimental Brain Research*, Vol. 170, No. 4, (April 2006), pp. 576-582, ISSN 0014-4819.

Sun, X.; Qiu, Y.; Zhu, Z.; Zhu, F.; Wang, B.; Yu, Y. & Qian, B. (2007). Variations of the position of the cerebellar tonsil in idiopathic scoliotic adolescents with a cobb angle >40 degrees: a magnetic resonance imaging study. *Spine*, Vol. 32, No. 15, (July 2007), pp. 1680-1686, ISSN 0362-2436.

Wang, D.; Shi, L.; Chu, W.C.; Burwell, R.G.; Cheng, J.C. & Ahuja, A.T. (2012). Abnormal cerebral cortical thinning pattern in adolescent girls with idiopathic scoliosis. *Neuroimage*, Vol. 59, No. 2 (January 2012), ISSN 1053-8119.

Winter, R.B.; Lonstein, J.E.; Heithoff, K.B. & Kirkham, J.A. (1997). Magnetic resonance imaging evaluation of the adolescent patient with idiopathic scoliosis before spinal instrumentation and fusion. A prospective, double-blinded study of 140 patients. *Spine*, Vol. 22, No. 8, (April 1997), pp. 855-858, ISSN 0362-2436.

Wyatt, M.P.; Barrack, R.L.; Mubarak, S.J.; Whitecloud, T.S. & Burke, S.W. (1986). Vibratory response in idiopathic scoliosis. *Journal of Bone and Joint Surgery. British Volume*, Vol. 68, No. 5, (November 1986), pp. 714-718, ISSN 0301-620X.

Section 2

Assessment of Idiopathic Scoliosis

5

Virtual Anatomy of Spinal Disorders by 3-D MRI/CT Fusion Imaging

Junji Kamogawa and Osamu Kato
Shiraishi Hospital/Spine & Sports Center
Japan

1. Introduction

Both CT and MRI are widely known to be important tools in diagnosing spinal disorders. However, even when three-dimensional data are collected, images are often presented in two dimensions and in monochrome. Furthermore, CT and MRI represent different types of information, and it is very difficult for doctors to mentally fuse these images. We have been working to overcome these challenges, and reported the first 3-D MRI/CT fusion images of the cranio-vertebral junction (Kamogawa, 2009). We have since continued to develop the technique, and have used it to visualize the lumbar nerve root (Misaki, 2009; Yamanaka 2010).

However, there are two major problems related to ensuring image quality for accurate diagnosis. The first is the optimal operation of MRI machines in order to obtain the best MRI sequences for each patient. Although it is simple to obtain clear CT images of spinal bone, it is very difficult to obtain such images of neural anatomy (spinal cord, cauda equina and spinal nerve roots) by MRI. Second, we must precisely superimpose the two images (MRI and CT) using computer software to evaluate complex spinal disorders.

In this chapter, the methods adopted at our hospital for obtaining, evaluating and displaying 3-D MRI/CT fusion imaging are discussed, focusing on their application to the field of spinal surgery.

2. Aims

There are numerous conditions of the spine that cannot readily be diagnosed using regular 2-D MRI. One such condition is spinal deformity (including malformation and tumor) with a focus on bone architecture; another is the secondary changes in the structure or environment of the spinal canal, which is the space inside the spinal column that supplies the nerve tissue. These secondary changes are involved in numerous disorders, such as chondrogenesis, bulging disk, thickened ligament flavum and varix (Table 1).

The power of fusion imaging is particularly apparent in the visualization of conditions of the nerve root. Nerve roots are important from a clinical perspective because they are the source of particularly severe pain, and because tethering of a nerve root during procedures to correct the spinal column can cause paralysis. The nerve roots are normally distal to the lateral canal of the spinal column, but this area is difficult to assess by either myelography or CT myelography (Fig. 1). Fusion imaging offers a solution to the problem of this hidden imaging zone, in which assessment has not been possible using the techniques available to date.

A. Spinal deformity
  1. Congenital scoliosis
  2. Adult Deformity
    - Degenerative scoliosis
    - Spondylolisthesis and retrolisthesis
    - Rotatory subluxation
  3. Trauma

B. The secondary changes in structure or environment of the spinal canal
  1. Siatica due to
    - Single pathological nerve root on degenerative lumbar scoliosis
    - Lumbar lateral canal stenosis
    - Far-out syndrome, Double-crash lesion
    - Spondylolysis
    - Varix
  2. Adhesion due to
    - Epi-dural membrane formation on dural sac
    - Failed back surgery syndrome
    - Re-operation

C. Tumor

Table 1. Indication for Fusion Imaging.

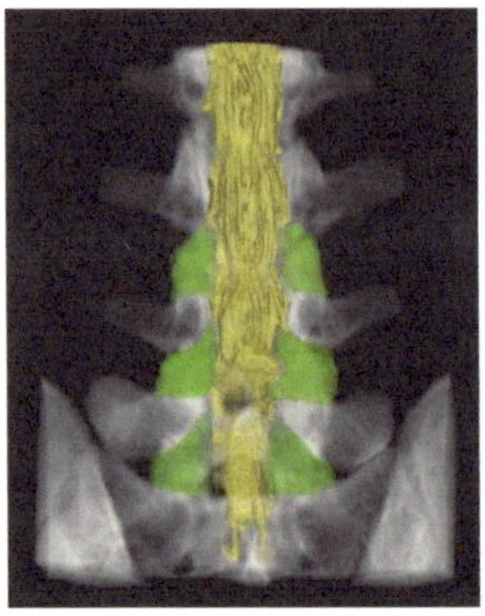

Fig. 1. Hidden imaging zone. Even with myelography or CT myelography (yellow area), the green areas do not show up in detail.

3. Machines

We used an Asteion 4® 4-row CT unit (TOSHIBA, Tochigi, Japan), an Echelon Vega® 1.5-T MRI unit (HITACHI, Tokyo, Japan), and Synapse Vincent® workstation software (FUJIFILM, Tokyo, Japan). Parameters for CT were as follows: tube voltage, 120 kV; tube current, 260 mA; slice thickness, 1 mm; rotational speed, 0.75 s/rotation; and slice thickness for reconstruction, 0.5 mm. The MRI sequences are shown in Table 2.

	BASG	RSSG
Mode	3D coronal	3D coronal
FOV	250 mm	384 mm
TR	10.4 ms	18.0 ms
TE	5.2 ms	9.2 ms
Flip angle	45°	10°
Slice thickness	1.3 mm	1.5 mm
Recon-pitch	0.65 mm	0.75 mm
Recon-slice	100	90
Scan time	6′40″	6′45″

BASG® (Balanced Sarge by HITACHI)
RSSG® (RS Sarge by HITACHI)

Table 2. Sequences of MRI

4. Steps for producing 3-D MRI/CT fusion images (procedure for obtaining the image in case 1)

4.1 Data reading

First, the workstation reads both CT and MRI DICOM data.

4.2 Registering

We use the "Superposition" application to automatically place the MRI data onto the CT data. When we use this tool, as it is not exclusively for spinal use, misalignment between the two modalities is possible. We must therefore correct the gap manually on the sagittal, coronal and axial planes (Fig. 2). An automatic superposition tool specifically for use with the spine has not yet been developed.

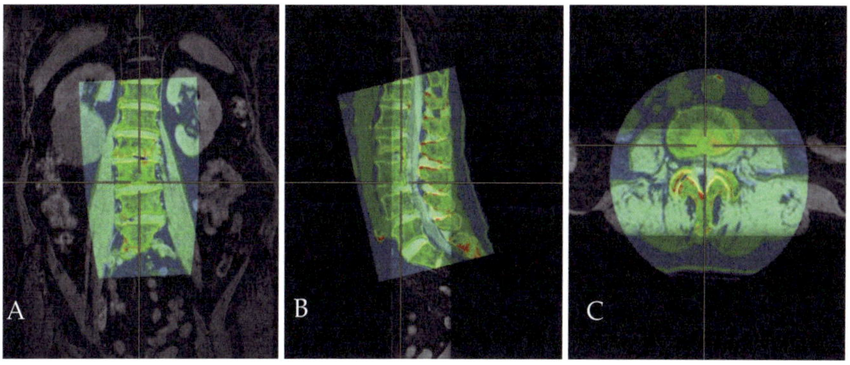

Fig. 2. Superposition of MRI and CT. The monochrome image is CT, and the green MRI image is superposed onto the CT image. Coronal (A), sagittal (B) and axial (C) planes.

4.3 Isolation of vertebral body for 3-D CT

First, we must remove unneeded information (e.g., calcification of aorta) (Fig. 3A, B). We must then separate each L1-5 vertebra in turn from the whole lumbar spine structure in order to use the "Mask editing" application (Fig. 4). For one vertebra, we use the "Slice out", "Closing and Painting", and "Surfacing" tools, and it takes about 10 minutes to manually finish one vertebra. The technique for individually isolating the vertebra is extremely useful, as the shape of the apophyseal joint (facet) is clarified at a glance (Fig. 3C, D, E). Colors are then added (Fig. 3F). Using this technique, the vertebrae can be made translucent at any density.

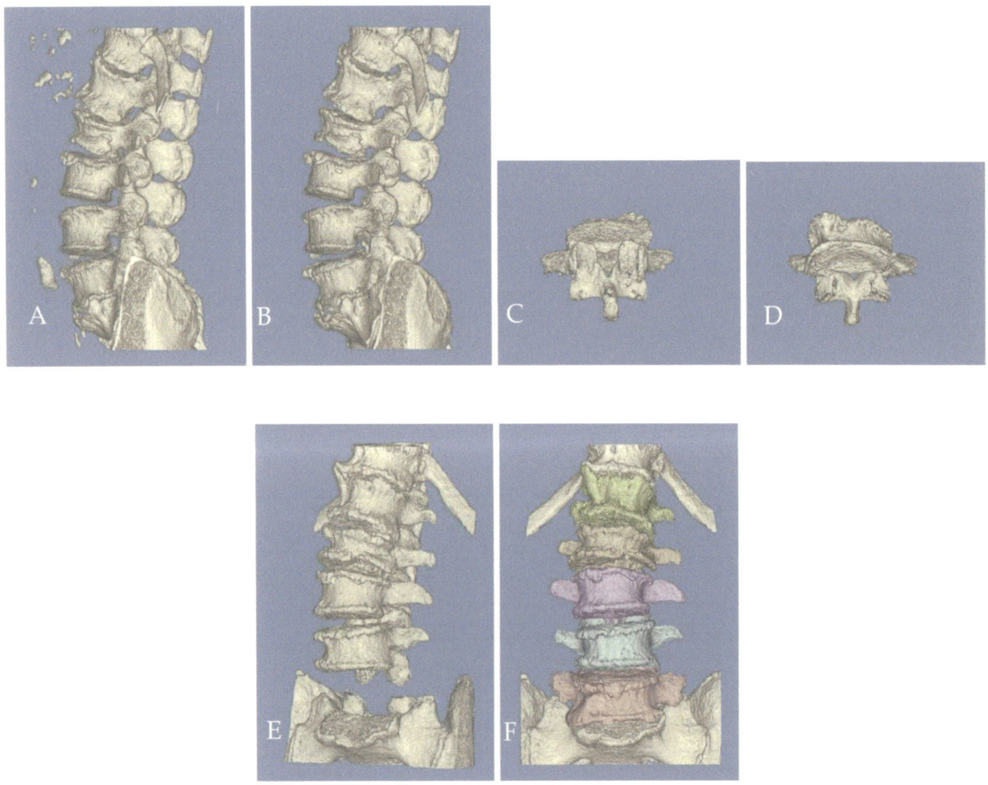

Fig. 3. 3-D CT reconstruction and vertebral isolation. Removal of unnecessary information: before (A) and after (B). Facet surface and neural arch can be evaluated (C, D). Whole lumbar spine without L5 vertebra (E). Finally, color was added (F).

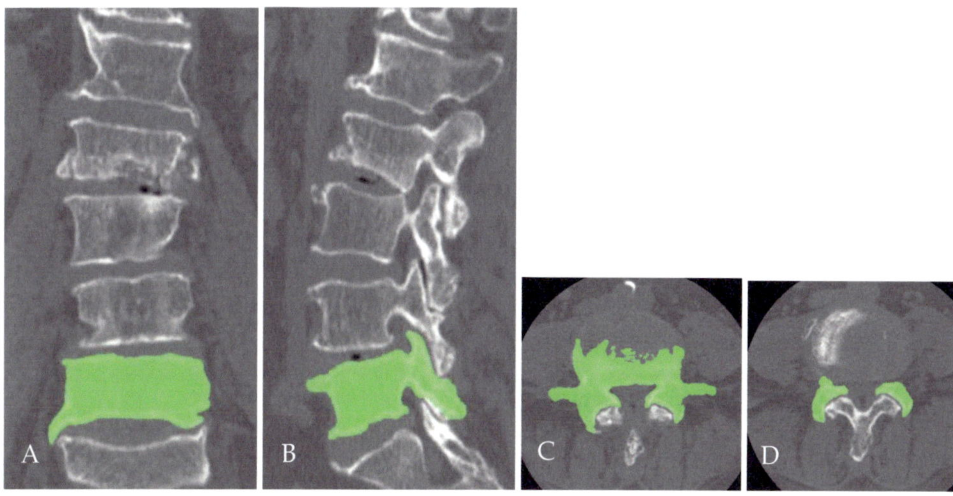

Fig. 4. Extraction of individual vertebrae. Details of the superior and inferior articular process (facet) are carefully colored. Coronal (A), sagittal (B) and axial (C, D) planes.

4.4 3-D representation of spinal cord

We produce a 3-D representation of both the dural sac and the spinal cord using an RSSG® sequence (HITACHI) with a single click on the Workstation (Fig. 5A).

4.5 Mapping spinal nerve roots from 3-D MRI

It is very difficult to obtain and map the spinal nerve roots. We use two MRI sequences: 3-D myelography of 1.3 mm slice thickness (Balanced SG® by HITACHI) and 3-D myelography of 1.5 mm slice thickness (RSSG® by HITACHI). There are many methods for obtaining clear images of spinal nerves on MRI. Careless operation of the MRI will result in failure to obtain nerve information. First, we place dots on the nerve roots in MPR (multiplanar reconstruction) using the "Center line editing" application. We then observe a straight nerve converted by the straight CPR (curved planar reformation) method. Next, we use "Contour editing" 7-10 times in order to repair the edge of the straight nerve. After obtaining the finished 3-D nerve root, it is necessary to cut the unnecessary image near the root edge. We place the finished 3-D nerve on the MPR screen like tracing paper (Fig. 6), filling in the dots manually. Finally, we obtain a finished 3-D nerve root (Fig. 5B, C, D). It takes about 20 minutes for a radiographer to produce an image of one nerve root, and we typically prepare images of six nerve roots for both sides of the lumbar spine (the main pathological root, and the top and bottom roots) for degenerative lumbar scoliosis.

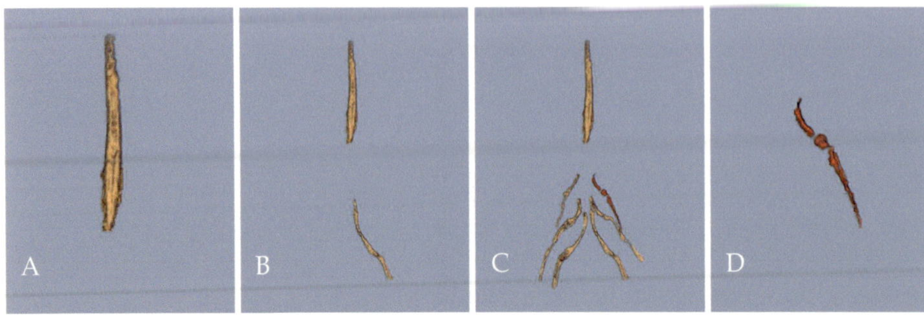

Fig. 5. Nerve tissue extraction. Dural sac and spinal cord (A). Each individual nerve root is extracted (B, C). The nerve root, which is the focus of disease (orange), is swollen and the pressure has led to constriction (C, D).

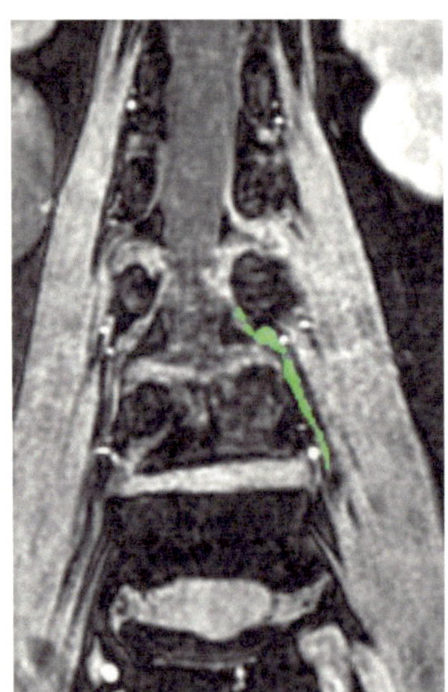

Fig. 6. Mapping of spinal nerve roots. The green area shows the nerve root being identified.

4.6 Final superposition

We place the 3-D MRI images onto 3-D CT images, and observe the entire lumbar spine in any direction (Fig. 7). A total of 5-8 h is required to produce 3-D fusion imaging.

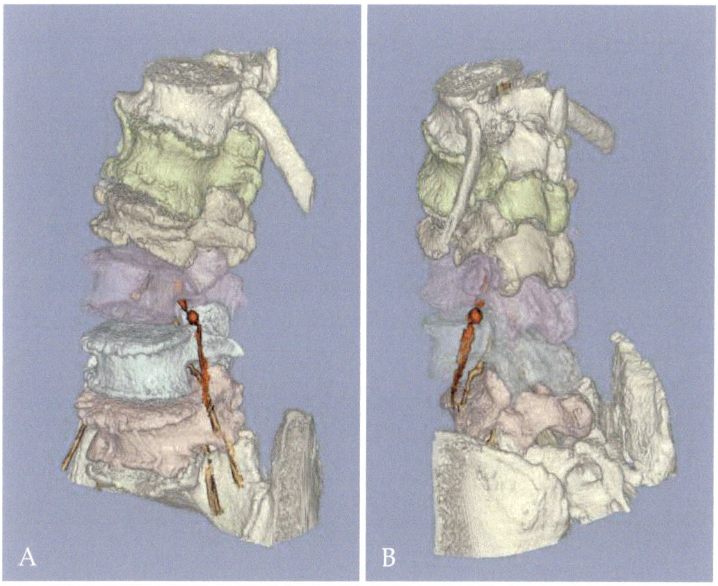

Fig. 7. Completed 3-D fusion imaging. The bones can be made semi-transparent and vertebrae can be removed at will, and assessment can be performed from any direction. The orange shows the main pathological nerve root. Left anterior oblique view (A) and left posterior oblique view (B).

5. Case presentation

5.1 Case 1

A 72-year-old female, degenerative lumbar scoliosis with L2 compression fracture

The main clinical findings were severe sciatica of the left thigh, a feeling of heaviness in the lower back, and gait disturbance for 5 meters. Marked radicular pain of the left L3 nerve root was confirmed, while selective left L3 root block caused reproducible pain, and reduced her distress for 2 days. No images depicted accurate information of her chief complaint, and plain roentgenography is shown in Fig. 8. 3-D MRI/CT Fusion Imaging revealed compression of the left L3 nerve root at the intraforaminal zone. We were able to evaluate the lesion from any direction at a glance, and were able to obtain clear evidence to suggest sciatica due to the L3 nerve root (Fig. 9).

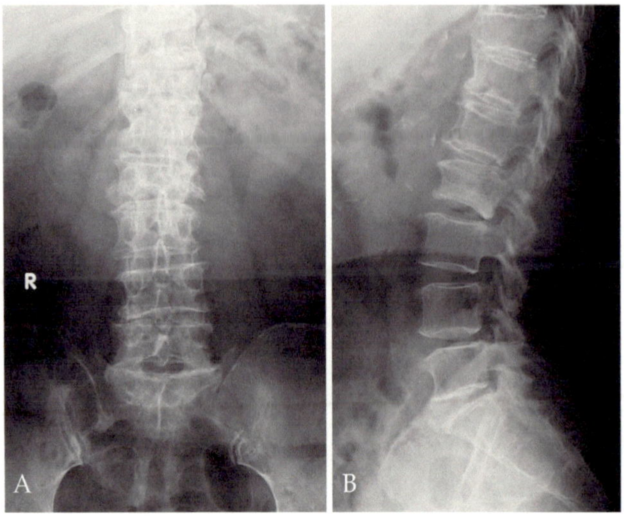

Fig. 8. Plain X-ray image. Previous compression fracture of L2 can be seen. AP view (A) and lateral view (B).

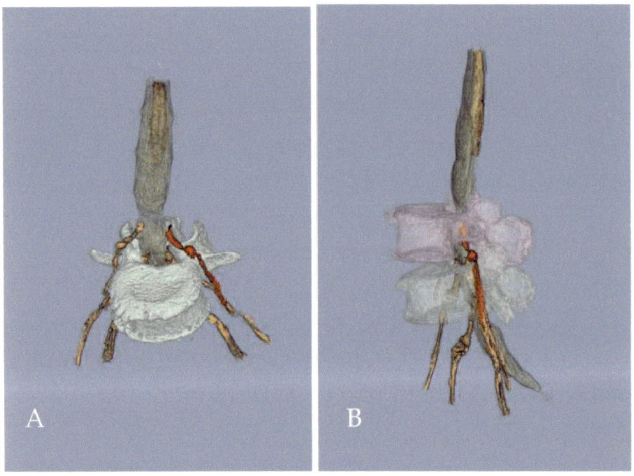

Fig. 9. Left L3 root and relationship with surrounding bony structure. The L3 root can be seen to be under pressure in the foraminal zone (orange). This image is greatly useful in selecting the operative procedure. Anterosuperior view (A) and lateral view (B).

5.2 Case 2

A 9-year-old male, congenital scoliosis

Morphology classification is difficult by plain X-ray alone (Fig. 10). However, using a workstation to isolate the vertebral anomaly and observe it from various angles allows the morphology of the anomaly to become evident (Fig. 11). Particular attention needs to be paid to isolation of the individual vertebrae. Furthermore, the presence of any abnormalities in the nerves can be appreciated through fusion imaging (Fig. 12). This is the optimal imaging for preoperative planning.

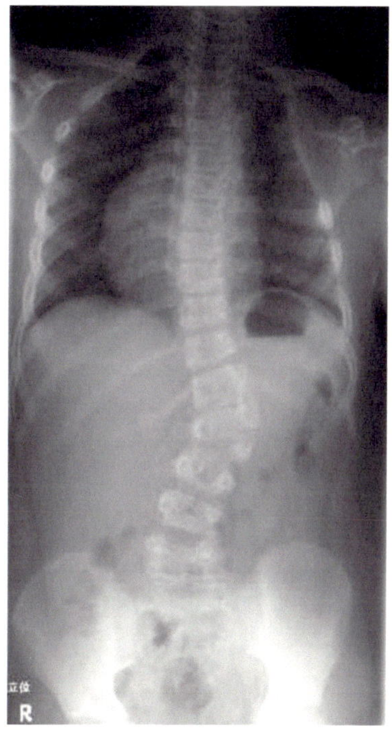

Fig. 10. Plain X-ray image. The details of vertebrae are unclear.

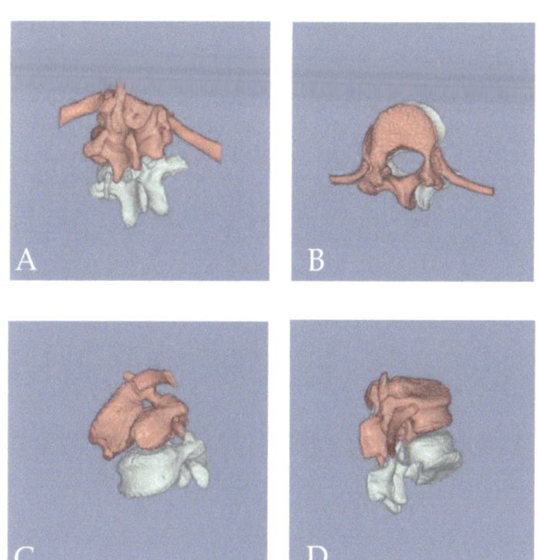

Fig. 11. Isolation of block vertebrae. This is extremely useful for gaining an understanding of the condition and planning osteotomy. Posterior view (A), superior view (B), left lateral view (C) and right lateral view (D).

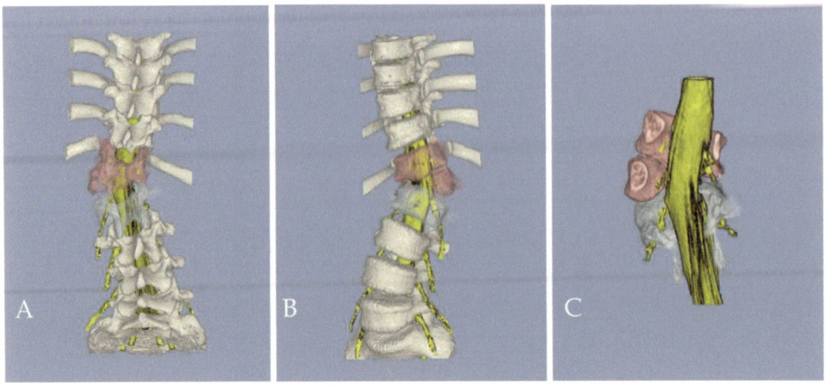

Fig. 12. Completed 3-D fusion imaging. If the bone is made semi-transparent, details of the nerve tissue at the surgical site can be seen. Posterior view (A) and anterior view (B). Magnified view (C). The bone are partly cut off to evaluate the nerve roots. The patient was examined for MRI without a sedative.

5.3 Case 3

A 27-year-old female, spondylolisthesis

Plain X-ray (Fig. 13) can confirm Meyerding grade III spondylolisthesis. However, none of the previously available scans can clearly depict the travel or condition of the bilateral L5 nerve root. Use of fusion imaging allows a detailed appreciation of the condition of the L5 nerve root. This is the useful imaging for preoperative evaluation (Fig. 14).

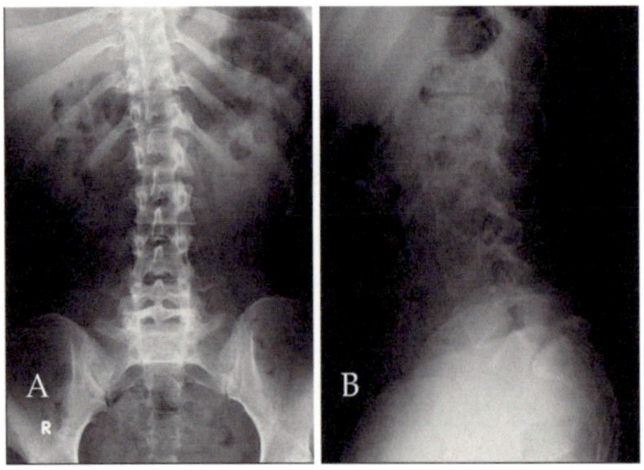

Fig. 13. Plain X-ray image. Spondylolysis of L5 can be seen. AP view (A) and lateral view (B).

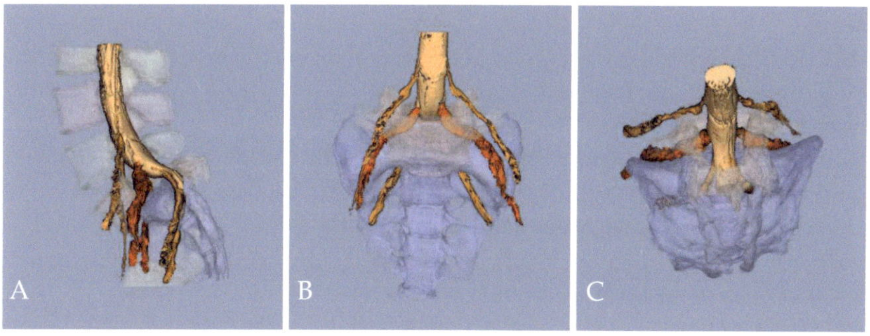

Fig. 14. Completed 3-D fusion imaging. The bone has been made semi-transparent. Bilateral L5 nerve roots are considerably swollen, and the travel of the nerve root is clear at a glance. The relationship between the L5 vertebra and the L5 root is clearly visible. Left lateral view (A), AP view (B) and posterosuperior view (C).

6. Conclusion

The ultimate purpose of our research is to produce images that can easily be interpreted by anyone at a glance without the use of contrast media. When we examine patients suffering from sciatica and back pain, or those who have no normal spinal canal structure due to deformities, it is very difficult to obtain useful images showing the neurological details. MRI is particularly poor for torsion, curved and rotational deformities of the spine.

In recent years, researchers have attempted to produce clear 3-D images of self-operating organs such as the heart, large and small intestines, and blood vessels using multi-row, top-of-the-line CT with the use of contrast media. On the other hand, the fields of spinal surgery that deal with non-self-operating, complex motions require only 4-16-row CT, but high-quality MRI units are vital. There are global standards of quality for CT among the disciplines of internal medicine, brain surgery and radiology; however, no such global standards yet exist for MRI in spinal surgery. The reason for this is that although taking CT images is straightforward and the image quality does not vary substantially with different imaging methods, the necessary conditions and methods for MRI are complex, and even a good MRI device can be difficult to operate. The nerve roots of cervical vertebrae can be visualized by utilizing particular conditions (data not shown).

Why is it so difficult to obtain clear MR images of the spine? It is vitally important to obtain MRI data to produce fusion images, and there are numerous reasons for the poor results of MRI to date (Table 3).

There may well be spinal pathology that are only detected after the start of spinal surgery. Nonetheless, if it were possible to demonstrate that the patient's detailed anatomy could not be seen satisfactorily in preoperative images, it may also be possible to better interpret preoperative images. This was the purpose of devising fusion imaging. After the spinal anatomy is clearly visualized, the pathology can be described, and effective surgical plans can be formulated. Although our technique is associated with problems such as reproducibility, convenience and applicability, we intend to continue with further development in the future.

1. Hardware
   - MRI devices have their own characteristics that vary between manufacturers, and each individual device has its own quirks.
2. Technical (device operation)
   - 2-1. It is difficult to determine the optimal MRI sequence for the spinal nerve root.
   - 2-2. Which direction is best for cutting the body to visualize the spinal nerve root?
   - 2-3. Affinity between the patient and MRI machine
3. Spinal deformity
   - No capability for scoliosis or rotatory subluxation
4. Physical object
   - Smaller objects give poorer images.
5. Scan time
   - We give the image quality priority over time.
6. Socio-economic
   - It is inexpensive for patients to undergo MRI examinations in Japan because of the universal health insurance system.
7. Cooperation with laboratory technicians
   - The spinal surgeon and radiologist must be consistent in the areas they want to observe.

Table 3. Why is it not possible to achieve clear MRI images?

7. References

Kamogawa, J., Katagi, R., Kodama, K. et al. (2009). The 3D-MRI/MRA/CT Fusion Imaging in spine and spinal cord disorders focusing on upper cervical spine: Report of two cases. *Spine & Spinal Cord*, Vol.22, No.8, pp.979-982 (In Japanese)

Kawakami, N., Tsuji, T., Imagama, S. et al.(2009). Classification of Congenital Scoliosis and Kyphosis: A New Approach to the Three-Dimensional Classification for Progressive Vertebral Anomalies Requiring Operative Treatment. *Spine* Vol.34, No.17, pp. 1756-1765

Kikuchi, S., Hasue, M. (1996) Radicular symptoms of lumbo-sacral spine -*Anatomic consideration*-, textbook, KANEHARA & Co., Ltd., Tokyo

Misaki, H., Kamogawa, J., Katagi,R. et al. (2009). Image assessment of the neural impairment at the adjacent level after lumbar decompression surgery. A case report with new trial using 3D-MRI/CT Fusion Imaging. *Spine & Spinal Cord*, Vol.22, No.10, pp. 1171-1175 (In Japanese)

Yamanaka, Y., Kamogawa, J., Katagi,R. et al.(2010), 3-D MRI/CT fusion imaging of the lumbar spine. *Skeletal Radiol* Vol.39, No.3, pp. 285-288.

6

Quantitative MRI for Scoliosis Follow-Up

Périé Delphine
Ecole Polytechnique de Montréal, Montréal,
Research center, CHU Sainte-Justine, Montréal,
Canada

1. Introduction

Scoliosis deformities progress more during skeletal growth (Bjerkreim et Hassan, 1982; Weinstein et Ponseti, 1983). This progression is believed to be governed by the "Hueter-Volkmann Law" (Hueter, 1862; Volkmann, 1882), which states that growth depends on the amount of compression on the growth plate, is retarded by increased compression and accelerated by reduced compression (Arkin et Katz, 1956; Roaf, 1960; Hert et Liskova, 1964; Gooding et Neuhauser, 1965; McCall et al., 1981; Scoles et al., 1991). Thus, scoliosis would produce asymmetric loading, which would cause asymmetric vertebral growth resulting in a "vicious cycle" (Mente et al., 1997; Mente et al., 1999; Roaf, 1960; Roaf, 1963; Stokes et al., 1996). Because of the interdependence between the mechanical properties of intervertebral discs and adjacent vertebral bone (Keller et al., 1993), this process may also occur in the discs (Stokes et al., 1996). Moreover, muscles undergo these asymmetric loading and might be also implicated in this vicious cycle. But the remaining question is why does scoliosis progress in some people but either does not progress or spontaneously corrects itself in others? Biomarkers of early scoliosis progression are needed for better therapeutic guidance.

Over other medical imaging techniques, magnetic resonance imaging (MRI) has the advantage of not utilizing ionising radiation and of exploring several physical phenomenons such as relaxation times, magnetization transfer, or diffusion. The first paragraph of this chapter introduces these MRI parameters and presents how they are acquired in vivo. The second paragraph presents the studies on the MRI parameters of bone in order to show how these parameters are good candidates for the investigation of the bone health with scoliosis. The third chapter describes the studies on the relationships between MRI parameters and biochemical or mechanical properties of the intervertebral disc in order to demonstrate that MRI offers great potential as a sensitive and non-invasive technique for describing the alterations in biochemical and material properties within scoliotic intervertebral discs. The fourth paragraph focuses on the relationships between MRI parameters and muscle properties, and the possible applications to scoliosis. The last paragraph focuses on the potential of quantitative MRI to become a very important diagnostic and treatment assessment tool in scoliosis.

2. Quantitative MRI

2.1 NMR phenomenon

The NMR phenomenon appears when a system of nuclei in a static magnetic field experiences a perturbation. As long as the transverse magnetization exists, an electrical voltage is induced in a dedicated antenna, the coil. The signal intensity, that is the magnitude of the induced voltage, allows the image to be coded. The density and the relaxation of water protons primarily dominate the high soft-tissue contrast of MRI. The proton density represents the hydrogen concentration within the tissue and reflects the water content. The relaxation process of the tissue is described by T1 that represents the recovery of the longitudinal magnetization and T2 that represents the decay of the transverse magnetization. The spin-lattice relaxation in the rotating frame, $T1\rho$, detects low-frequency physicochemical interactions between water and extracellular matrix molecules, as well as changes in macromolecular content, without problems of spin dephasing due to inhomogeneous magnetic fields inherent of T2 contrast. The magnetization transfer MT measures the cross-relaxation and chemical exchange processes between free and macromolecule-bound water protons in tissues. Diffusion tensor imaging takes advantage of the thermally induced random Brownian motion that causes microscopic diffusion of water molecules.

2.2 Acquisition protocol

Using a MRI 3T whole-body system (Philips Achieva X-Serie), a protocol for quantitative MRI was optimized for the spine (Périé et al., 2006; Recuerda et al., 2012; Manac'h et al., 2012). Images for the quantification of T1 (Figure 1-a) and T2 (Figure 1-b) are acquired using a multiple inversion recovery turbo spin-echo (TSE) sequence for T1 and a multi-echo turbo spin-echo (TSE) sequence for T2. $T1\rho$ is quantified using a RF-spoiled turbo gradient-echo sequence with six different spin-lock durations varying between 1ms and 50ms. The MTR is obtained using two gradient echo sequences, one with the off-resonance pulse applied at 1100Hz down to the free water proton resonance frequency (Ms, Figure 1-c) and the other one without it (Mo, Figure 1-d) (Wang et al., 2010). A spin-echo EPI diffusion-weighted sequence (TR/TE=2000/40 ms, Figure 1-e) with 15 non-collinear diffusion and a b value of 1000s/mm^2 is used to quantify the apparent diffusion coefficient ADC, the fractional anisotropy FA and the eigenvectors of the diffusion tensor.

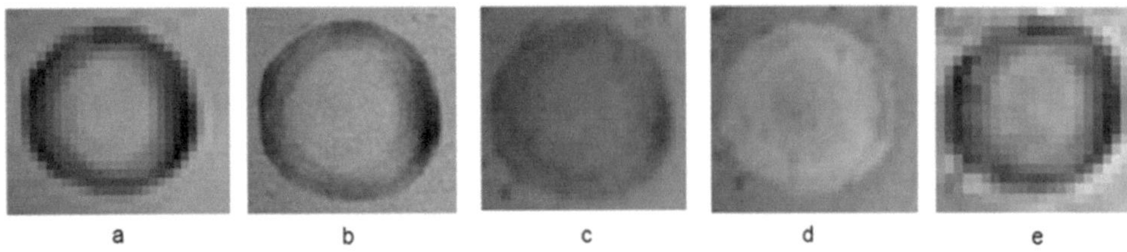

Fig. 1. T1 weighted image (a), T2 weighted image (b), MT image with the off-resonance pulse (c), MT image without the off-resonance pulse (d) and Diffusion weighted image (e) for an isolated intervertebral disc (Manac'h et al., 2012).

2.3 Parameter computation

The relaxation times T1 and T2 are extracted from the signal intensity by curve fitting using Equation 1 and Equation 2 respectively (Wright et al., 2008). T1ρ values are calculated on a pixel-by-pixel basis by a linear regression of intensity data to an exponential decay function using Equation 3 (Johannessen et al., 2006). MT ratio is calculated from Equation 4 (Henkelman et al., 2001). Diffusion parameters (Tensor D, apparent diffusion coefficient ADC and fraction of anisotropy FA) are calculated using Equations 5-7 (Le Bihan et al., 1986; Kingsley et al., 2006). Fibres directions are obtained, in a pixel-by-pixel computation, from the corresponding eigenvalues and eigenvectors of the diffusion tensor (Figure 2).

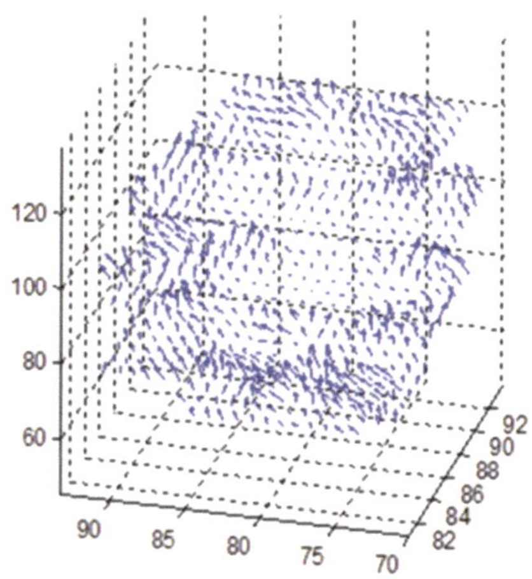

Figure 2: 3D mapping of Diffusion eigenvectors within the intervertebral disc.

$$SI_{TI} = S_0 . \left\{1 - (1 - \cos(\alpha))E_{TI}\left(1 - E_{TW} f^N \left(1 - \frac{E_{TE/2}}{2}\right)\right)\right\} \quad (1)$$

with $f(x) = 1 - E_{TE}.x$, $E_{TI} = e^{-\frac{TI}{T1}}$, $E_{TW} = e^{-\frac{TW}{T1}}$, $E_{TE} = e^{-\frac{TE}{T1}}$ and N=8

$$SI_{TE} = SI_{(TE=0)} . e^{-TE/T2} \quad (2)$$

Where SI is the signal intensity, TW is the time in ms between the last refocusing pulse and the next inversion pulse, and N is the number of refocusing pulses.

$$S(TSL) = S_0 e^{-TSL/T1\rho} \quad (3)$$

$$MTR = \frac{M_0 - M_s}{M_0} \quad (4)$$

$$\begin{bmatrix} \ln\left(\frac{SI_b}{SI_{b=0}}\right)^1 \\ \vdots \\ \ln\left(\frac{SI_b}{SI_{b=0}}\right)^6 \end{bmatrix} = - \begin{bmatrix} b_{xx}{}^1 & 2b_{xy}{}^1 & 2b_{xz}{}^1 & b_{yy}{}^1 & 2b_{yz}{}^1 & b_{zz}{}^1 \\ \vdots & \vdots & \vdots & \vdots & \vdots & \vdots \\ b_{xx}{}^6 & 2b_{xy}{}^6 & 2b_{xz}{}^6 & b_{yy}{}^6 & 2b_{yz}{}^6 & b_{zz}{}^6 \end{bmatrix} \mathbf{x} \begin{bmatrix} D_{xx} \\ D_{xy} \\ D_{xz} \\ D_{yy} \\ D_{yz} \\ D_{zz} \end{bmatrix} \quad (5)$$

$$ADC = \frac{\lambda_1+\lambda_2+\lambda_3}{3} \tag{6}$$

$$F_A = \sqrt{\frac{3[(\lambda_1-ADC)^2+(\lambda_2-ADC)^2+(\lambda_3-ADC)^2]}{[\lambda_1^2+\lambda_2^2+\lambda_3^2]}} \tag{7}$$

Where SI represents the signal intensity at the corresponding b-value $\boldsymbol{b}$ and b_{ij} represent the projected b-value obtained from the diffusion-encoding directions, λi are the eigenvalues of the diffusion tensor D.

3. MRI parameters of bone

It has been shown that for early scoliosis, the mechanical properties of the apical vertebral body are modified (Périé et al., 2001). Computed tomography (CT) examination was performed on eleven girls presenting idiopathic scoliosis. A finite element mesh of the vertebral body, the mapping of the CT number on each CT slice and predictive relationships between the CT number and the Young's modulus of bone (Hobatho et al., 1996) allowed the 3D analysis of the bone mechanical property distribution within the vertebral body. Geometrical and mechanical centres were calculated. Compared to the geometrical centre, the mechanical centre was shifted forward to the concavity in the coronal plane and to the back in the sagittal plane. This modification of the mechanical properties seemed to appear in the scoliotic vertebral body before any geometrical deformation such as wedging. Moreover, the comparison between the centre shift forward and the one year curvature evolution wearing the Cheneau-Toulouse-Munster brace showed that if the shift forward was important then the curvatures were stabilised or aggravated, and if the shift forward was low then the curvatures were reduced. This parameter has the potential of being a biomarker of the progression of scoliosis. However, its measurement requires invasive CT acquisitions that cannot be used for longitudinal studies of adolescents with idiopathic scoliosis. Thus the question is can we determine this biomarker from a non invasive medical image technique such as MRI (Figure 3)?

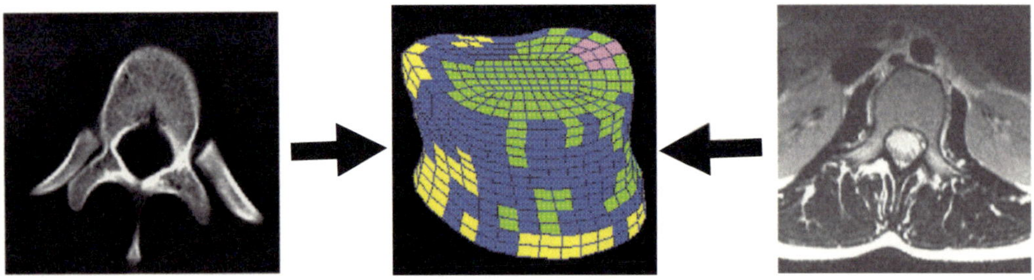

Fig. 3. 3D mapping of the mechanical properties of vertebral bone from CT images (left). Is it possible to determine these properties from MR images (right)?

MRI has the potential to give information pertaining to both trabecular bone mineral density (BMD) and bone structure. The effective transverse relaxation time T2* of bone marrow, measured from the signal intensity (Equation 8), is shortened in the presence of trabecular bone. The variations in magnetic susceptibility at the interface of solid and soft tissues causes local magnetic field inhomogeneities which induce a dephasing of the transverse magnetization, and thus a change in the effective transverse relaxation time T2*. Strong correlations were found between BMD, as measured from CT, and 1/T2*, as measured from MRI, on cadaveric human vertebral bodies (Majumdar et al., 1991). Correlations were also found between the Young's modulus E and 1/T2 on cancellous bone (Chung et al., 1993), and between T2* and 1/E (Equation 9, Jergas et al., 1995). A combination of 1/T2* and MRI-derived bone volume fraction further improved the prediction of yield stress and ultimate strength (Lammentausta et al., 2006).

$$SI = I_0 e^{-TE/T2^*} \tag{8}$$

$$\frac{1}{E} = a\,T_2^* + \frac{b}{T_2^*} + n \tag{9}$$

T2* is not a simple derivate of bone density, it is influenced by the number, thickness, geometric shape and spatial arrangement of trabecular elements in a defined volume. Structural parameters (fractional area, trabecular width, trabecular number, fractal dimension, trabecular spacing) depend on the pulse sequence (gradient echo or spin-echo) and echo time used to obtain the MR images, and also on the choice of the threshold used to segment the images (Majumdar et al., 1995; Link et al., 1998). Cortical bone mineral content, trabecular bone mineral density and volume fraction, trabecular thickness and number, and fractal dimension all decreased with age (Wehrli et al., 1995; Majumdar et al., 1997).

However, this use of MRI for the assessment of mechanical properties of bone tissues was applied only to the effect of osteoporosis. As CT measurements showed changes in the mechanical properties of bone with early scoliosis (Périé et al., 2001), and as CT measurements were found correlated to MRI measurements (Majumdar, 1991), MRI and T2* mapping should be an effective tool to assess the changes in bone with idiopathic scoliosis. The longitudinal relaxation time T1 has been measured recently from ultrashort TE MR imaging on bovine femur and this parameter was found to be sensitive to the water content within the bone tissue (Kokabi et al., 2011). However, ultrashort TE MRI reduces the signal to noise ratio and might be difficult to apply in vivo on scoliotic patients.

4. MRI parameters of intervertebral discs

Spinal deformities affect both the structural and the biochemical composition of the intervertebral disc (Bushell et al., 1979; Jongeleenen et al., 2006) and lead to its degeneration. Adolescent Idiopathic Scoliosis is marked by a wedging of the intervertebral disc linked with a displacement of the nucleus pulposus (Figure 4, Périé et al., 2001) and changes in the glycosaminoglycan and water content repartition (Urban et al., 2001; Schenzka et al., 1991; Kouwenhoven et Castelein, 2008).

The measure of the concentrations of specific molecules reflecting matrix synthesis and degradation in normal and scoliotic intervertebral discs showed higher collagen Type II synthetic levels and increased total protein content with no matrix turnover (Antoniou et al., 1998). These results suggest that scoliotic changes are due to an altered and ineffective synthetic response to a pathologic mechanical environment. These biochemical changes within the intervertebral disc are known to be related to the MR parameters T1, T2, MT and ADC.

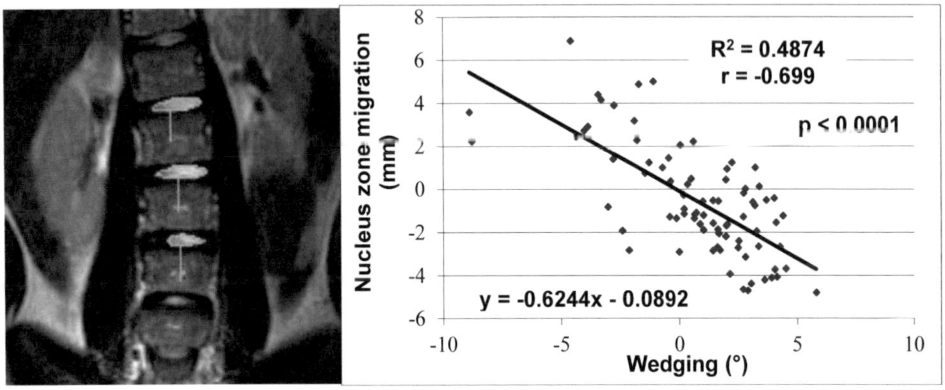

Fig. 4. Segmentation of the nucleus pulposus zone from T2-weighted images (left) and correlation between nucleus zone migration and intervertebral wedging in adolescent idiopathic scoliosis (Périé et al., 2001).

In the intervertebral disc in vitro, T1, T2 and MT were found to be correlated to the water content and GAG content, but not to the collagen content or percentage of denatured type II collagen (Tertti et al., 1991; Antoniou et al., 1998), whereas the apparent diffusion coefficient was directly related to proteoglycans content and inversely related to collagen denaturation (Antoniou et al., 2004). However, a moderate negative correlation was found between 1/T2 and water content whereas there was no significant correlation between 1/T2 and proteoglycan content (Weidenbaum et al., 1992). In normal nucleus pulposus, T1 and T2 decrease with age, with no significant correlation between proton density and age (Jenkins et al., 1989), but with a significant correlation between signal intensity and age (Sether et al., 1990). Changes in water content due to degeneration have a greater influence on T1 in the nucleus pulposus than in the annulus fibrosus (Chatani et al., 1993; Antoniou et al., 1998). In vitro collagenase treatment significantly increased the proportion of denatured collagen, and decreased T1, T2 and ADC, with no significant effect on MT (Antoniou et al., 2004). The diffusion parameters were found to be more sensitive to the trypsin digestion of isolated discs than the relaxation times T1 and T2. However, these parameters were sensitive to the hydration process (Manac'h et al., 2012). Significant differences were found on the MR parameters by region (higher T1, T2 and ADC in the nucleus than in the annulus), loading state (higher T1 and ADC in the loaded disc than in the unloaded), Thompson grade (T2, ADC), and direction of diffusion (Chiu et al., 2001). After compression, the water diffusion either increases in creep (load steps) experiments (Chiu et al., 2001), or decreases in stress-relaxation (displacement steps) experiments (Burstein et al., 1993). The orientations of diffusion anisotropy in the annulus fibrosus exhibited a layered morphology that agreed with light micrographs of the corresponding samples, and the behaviour of the orientation angles was consistent with the known collagen fibber architecture (Hsu and Setton, 1999). All these studies showed that the MRI parameters are sensitive to both the biochemical content and the structure of the intervertebral disc.

Some authors have shown that MRI offers great potential as a sensitive and non-invasive technique for describing the alterations in the mechanical properties of intervertebral discs or cartilage. Correlations were found in cartilage between the longitudinal relaxation time T1gd as measured by Gadolinium-Enhanced MRI and the local stiffness as measured by mechanical indentation (Samosky et al., 2005), or unconfined compression (Chen et al., 2003; Kurkijarvi et al., 2004; Nieminen et al., 2004; Lammentausta et al., 2006). The spin-lock longitudinal relaxation time T1ρ was strongly correlated to the compressive modulus and the hydraulic permeability in cartilage (Wheaton et al., 2005) and to the swelling pressure in human nucleus pulposus (Nguyen et al., 2008). On bovine nucleus pulposus, significant correlations were found between the hydraulic permeability and the relaxation times or the diffusion trace (Périé et al., 2006). Moreover, the compressive modulus of nucleus pulposus was found to be correlated to the longitudinal relaxation times T1 and T1ρ, while the hydraulic permeability of annulus fibrosus was found to be inversely correlated to T1ρ (Mwale et al., 2008). Multi linear regressions showed that 50 to 80% of the compressive modulus and the permeability of isolated intervertebral discs can be explained by MRI parameters (T1, T2, MT, ADC, FA) within both the annulus fibrosus and the nucleus pulposus. However, multicollinearity was present among the independent variables, suggesting that T1 and T2 were likely candidates for elimination in the equation. Thus the compressive modulus and the permeability of isolated intervertebral discs can be assessed mostly by MT and diffusion sequences (Recuerda et al., 2012).

However, before the use of this technique to quantify the mechanical properties of intervertebral discs in vivo on patients suffering from various spine diseases, the relationships have to be defined for each degeneration type of the tissue that mimics the pathology (Recuerda et al., 2012). Another issue is that the intervertebral disc is submitted to complex loading stimuli in vivo. Does the mechanical loading of the disc influence the MRI acquisition of the relaxation times, magnetization transfer and diffusion parameters? An apparatus allowing the compression of isolated intervertebral discs was designed and manufactured in ABS. Intervertebral discs were dissected from fresh young bovine tail, measured for their thickness and submitted to static compression (5, 10, 20 and 40% deformation) just before the MRI acquisition. The short term static compression of the intervertebral disc did not lead to any significant change of the MRI parameters, except for the diffusion that decreased in the direction of the compressive stress (Manac'h et al., 2012).

Quantitative MRI of the intervertebral disc was also performed in vivo. Diurnal variations, significantly less pronounced in degenerative than in normal intervertebral disc, were characterized by lower T1 and higher T2 measured in the evening than in the morning (Karakida et al., 2003; Boos et al., 1993), whereas lower T2 were found after bed rest (LeBlanc et al., 1994). T2 and ADC turned out to be sensitive parameters in investigating changes in the MR characteristics of the intervertebral disc matrix between morning and evening (Ludescher et al., 2008). A significant and strong correlation was found between in vivo T1ρ values and discography opening pressure measurements suggesting that T1ρ is a quantitative measure of degeneration (Borthakur et al., 2011). A relationship was also found between in vivo MRS spectroscopy (water content, proteoglycan content), imaging parameters (T1ρ, Pfirrmann Grade), and discography results suggesting that MRS-quantified water, proteoglycans and MR T1ρ relaxation time may potentially serve as biomarkers of symptomatic intervertebral disc degeneration (Zuo et al., 2011). An abnormal loading representing an increase of the intradiscal pressure from 0.5MPa to 1-2MPa was created in vivo by walking for 1h30 with a back pack of 20kg. Quantitative MRI was done on the lumbar spine before and after the loading that entailed a significant decreased in T1 while T2 increased significantly (Table 1, preliminary work from the author, unpublished data). Mean ADC and MT values were constant. Qualitatively, there were differences in the distribution of each parameter, even for ADC, confirmed by the smaller slope of the cumulative histogram after loading (Figure 5).

	Before loading	After loading
T1	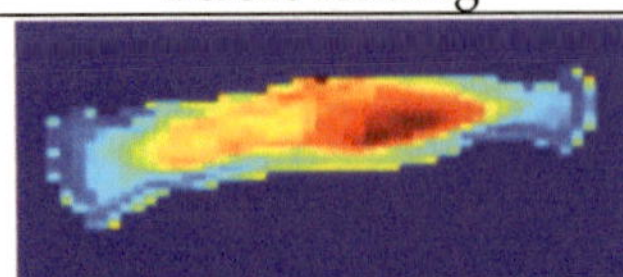	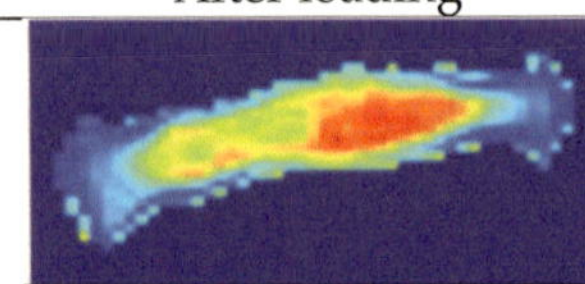
T2	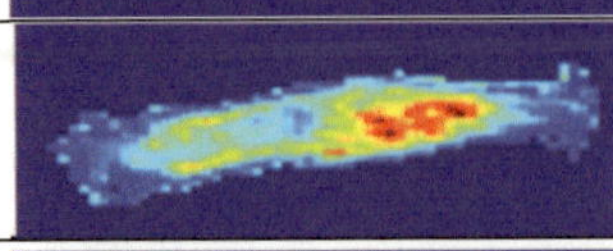	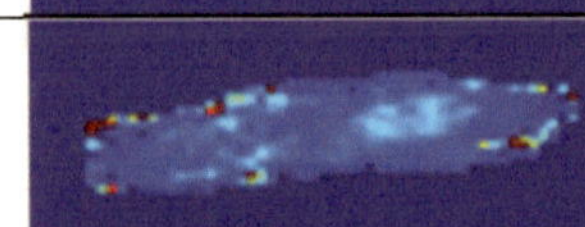
ADC	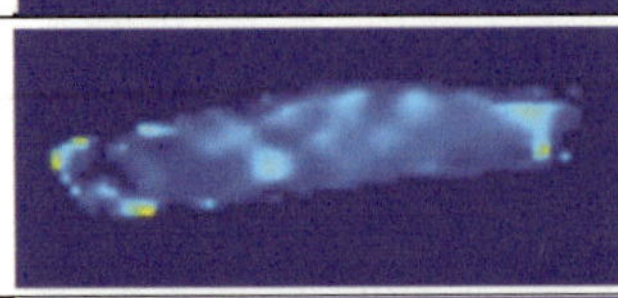	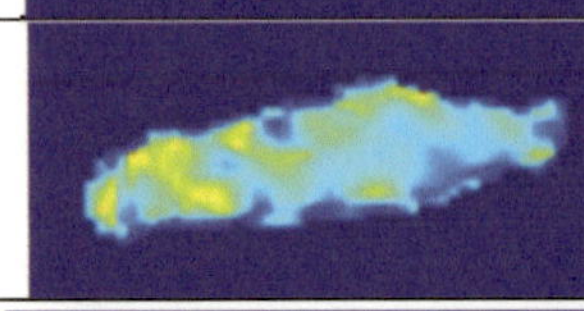
MT	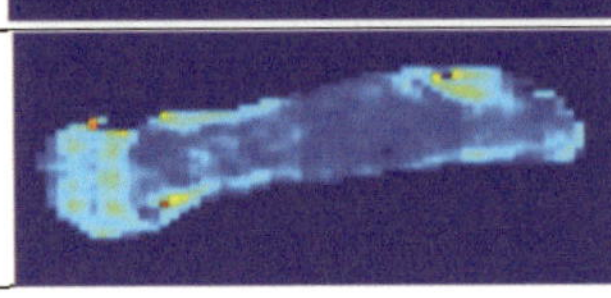	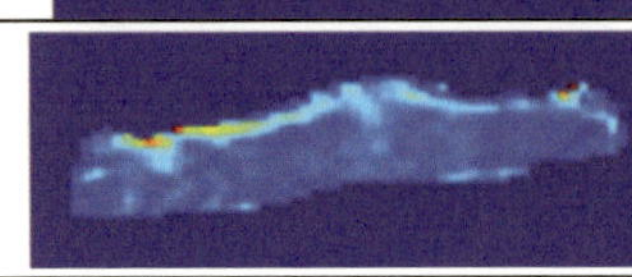

Table 1: Mapping of the L4-L5 intervertebral disc of a healthy subject, before and after the loading that consisted in walking with a 20kg back pack for one hour.

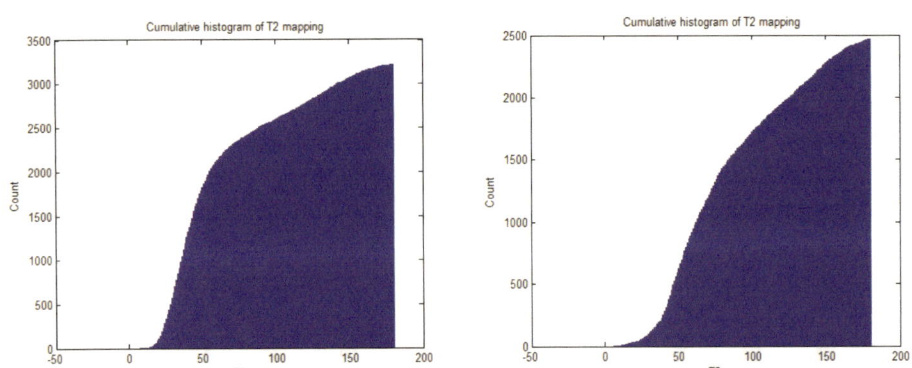

Fig. 5. Cumulative histogram of T2 in L5/S1 intervertebral disc before (left) and after (right) loading.

5. MRI parameters of muscles

Idiopathic scoliosis disrupts the symmetry of the paraspinal muscle activities, decreases the total mechanical work, increases the oxygen consumption and energy cost and decreases muscles efficiency (Tsai et al.; Mahaudens et al.; Khosla et al., 1980). Biopsy studies shows abnormalities regarding the architecture of the paraspinal muscles of scoliotic subjects (Kennelly et Stokes, 1993), their protein synthesis (Gibson et al., 1988) and their muscle fiber type composition (Meier et al., 1997; Mannion et al., 1998; Sirca et al., 1985). In scoliotic subjects, the proportion of type I muscle fibers is smaller on the concave side than on the convex side whereas in normal subjects, a symmetric distribution is observed. Moreover, the cross sectional area of type II muscle fibers is larger on the concave side than on the convex side (Mannion et al., 1998; Bylund et al., 1987; Zetterberg et al., 1983). A larger electromyographic (EMG) signal has often been observed in idiopathic scoliosis on the convex side of the curves (Odermatt et al., 2003; Cheung et al., 2006). However, during isometric efforts in extension, EMG parameters could not discriminate between the back muscles of scoliotic subjects and those of control subject regarding fiber type composition, neuromuscular efficiency and muscle fatigue at the level of the apex, maybe due to compensatory strategies at lower level of the spine (Goudreault et al., 2005).

Several specific magnetic resonance imaging (MRI) techniques were developed for muscle applications, such as MR spectroscopy to quantify adenosine-5 triphosphate, lactates or creatine (Jeneson et Bruggeman, 2004) and MR elastography (Bensamoun et al., 2007, 2008) to visualize and measure the deformation waves within the tissue submitted to mechanical excitations and to assess their mechanical properties. However, MR spectroscopy is limited by a low resolution, the acquisition of a single voxel and results difficult to interpret. A special apparatus is needed for MR elastography to create the vibrations, which means extra cost and time to prepare the patient.

Studies on the human skeletal muscles demonstrated that ADC may be used to analyze the spatial architecture (Heemskerk et al., 2005) and to indicate the change in micro-structure associated with passive extension and contraction (Hatakenaka et al., 2008). Also, T2 increases with the muscle activation as a result of the shift of the osmotically driven intracellular fluid, and could be used to demonstrate aberrant muscle activation (Kinusaga et al., 2006; Patten et al., 2003). It is well established that MR parameters are linked to the mechanical and biochemical properties of cartilage tissues. Does a relationship exist between the mechanical properties and the MR parameters of muscles?

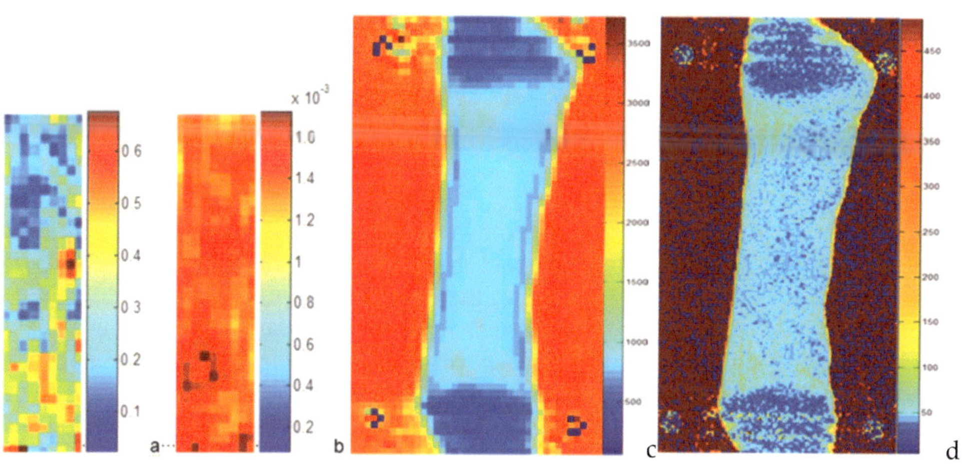

Fig. 6. FA map (a), ADC map (b), T1 map (c) and T2 map (d) of the rabbit semi-membranous muscle (rigor mortis).

Leg and arm muscles of adult rabbits were dissected, and tested 12 hours post mortem, in a state of rigor mortis, or 72 hours post mortem, in a state of post-rigor mortis (Grenier et al., 2012). The tests consisted of a quantitative MRI acquisition (T1, T2, MTR, ADC, FA, Figure

6) and a uniaxial tensile test until failure (Young's modulus E). The results showed that multiple linear regressions exist between E, MTR and ADC (Equation 10) and that MRI would be a sensitive and non-invasive tool for the characterisation of muscle properties in the back muscles.

$$E\,[Pa] = (36{,}6\,[Pa] - 37{,}5\,[Pa] \times MTR\,[\%]) \times 10^{4} - 128{,}1 \times 10^{12}\,[Kg/s{*}m^{3}] \times ADC[m^{2}/s] \quad (10)$$

6. qMRI in idiopathic scoliosis

MRI can be a powerful tool for the diagnosis of spine pathologies and can potentially help to monitor their progression in vivo (Majumdar, 2006; Endean et al., 2010, Mwale et al., 2008). For instance, MRI gives reliable non-invasive 3D images of the intervertebral disc (Pfirmann et al., 2001) allowing longitudinal follow-up studies and T2-weighted images are used to assess the intervertebral disc degeneration (Majumdar et al., 2006; Pfirmann et al., 2001; Antoniou et al., 1998), but is limited to the detection of late stages of the spine pathologies (Pfirmann et al., 2001).

The distribution of the MRI signal intensity was not exploited so far to analyze the local changes in the intervertebral disc structure and biochemistry with degeneration. Only the mean signal intensity or disc height or disc volume were analysed from clinical images. A prospective study was realized on the MR T2-weighted images of 32 volunteers with scoliosis and 15 control volunteers (Figure 9).

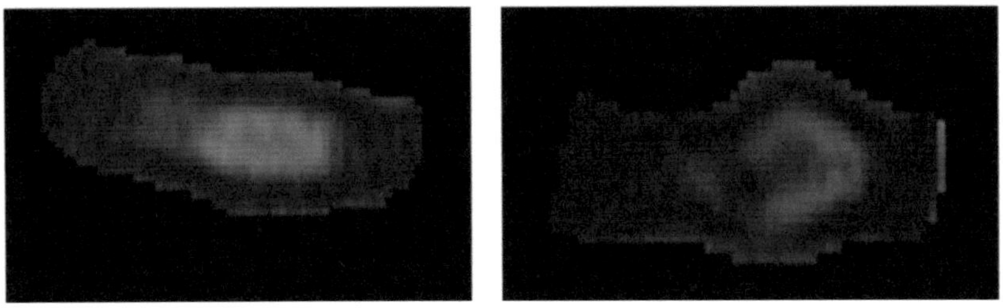

Fig. 9. Segmented intervertebral discs for control (left) and scoliosis (right) volunteer on sagittal T2-weighted images.

The pathologic subjects were separated into two severity groups. The Gaussian distribution of the MRI signal intensity was analyzed by normalized histograms. The following descriptive statistics were computed within the intervertebral disc, nucleus pulposus and annulus fibrosus of each subject in order to analyze the Gaussian distribution of their MR signal intensity. The standard error of the mean depicts how sample mean approximates the true population mean. The confidence interval of the mean describes the range in which the true population mean will fall for a percentage of all possible samples drawn from the population. The sum of square defines the sum of squared deviations from the mean. The Skewness gives an index on the symmetry of the Gaussian distribution of the histogram. The Kolmogorov-Smirnov distance is the maximum cumulative distance between the histogram distribution and the Gaussian distribution of intensity data. Their 75th percentile was also computed. The center weighted by the MRI intensity within the intervertebral disc and the volume ratio of the nucleus pulposus within the total intervertebral disc were computed. There were significant variations of indices between scoliosis and control groups and between low and high severity groups. These newly developed MRI parameters allowed the quantitative analysis of spinal deformities involved in scoliosis of different severities (Gervais et al., 2012).

This promising technique was limited by the low resolution of the clinical T2-weighted images, which induces considerable segmentation errors or a poor and limited visual interpretation. Acquiring high resolution matrices is time consuming and induces high cost. A new mathematical technique based on multidimensional Dual-Kriging was developed (Aissiou et al., 2012). T1, T2, MTR and Diffusion sequences were used to acquire two different matrices with different sizes (128x128 and 256x256). The Kriging system parameters and the polynomial degree were optimized, and low resolution images (128x128) were interpolated to high resolution (256x256) in 2D (Figure 10-12) and 3D (Figure 13). Kriging system provided relatively high performances and low error within the regions of interest. Components contours tend to be corrected and better defined, following the Kriging interpolation. Progressive Dual-Kriging is a flexible technique that can be optimized to interpolate 2D and 3D qMRI data based on the signal distribution. The computation is extremely fast and the interpolation is better fitted to the signal distribution as opposed to the Zero-Padding technique.

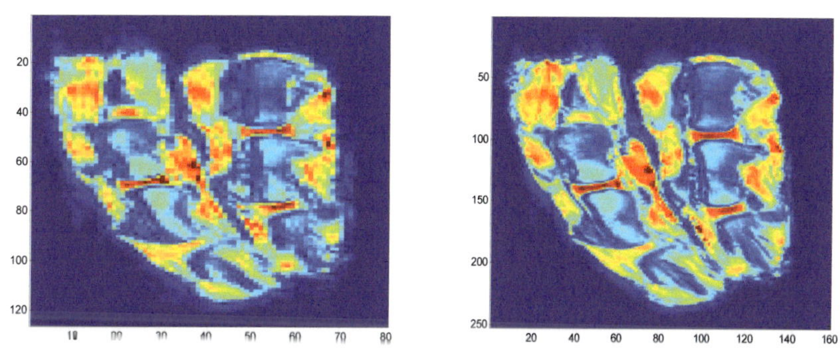

Fig. 10. T1 before kriging (left) and after kriging (right) of two bovine tail segments.

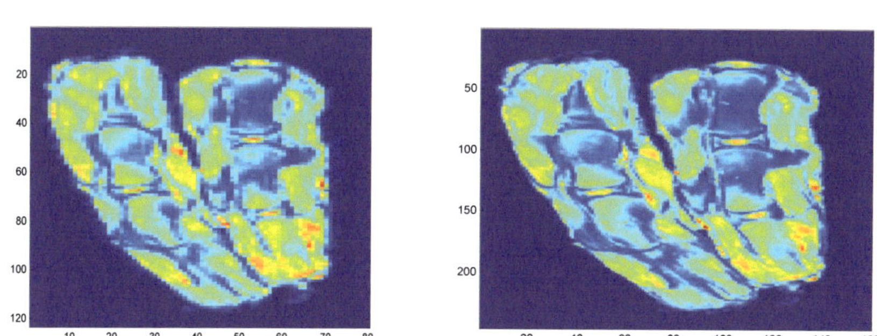

Fig. 11. T2 before kriging (left) and after kriging (right) of two bovine tail segments.

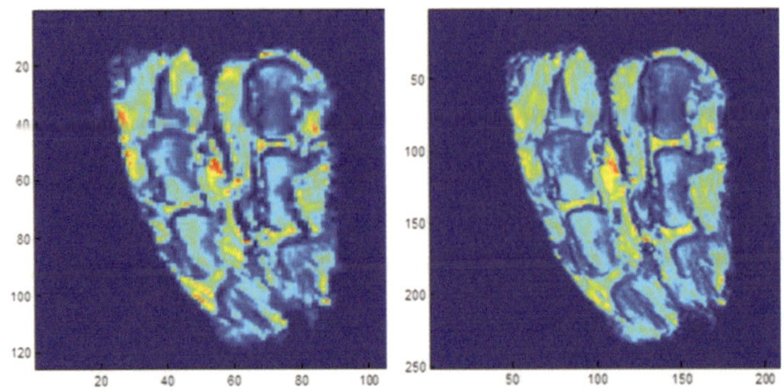

Fig. 12. MTR before kriging (left) and after kriging (right) of two bovine tail segments.

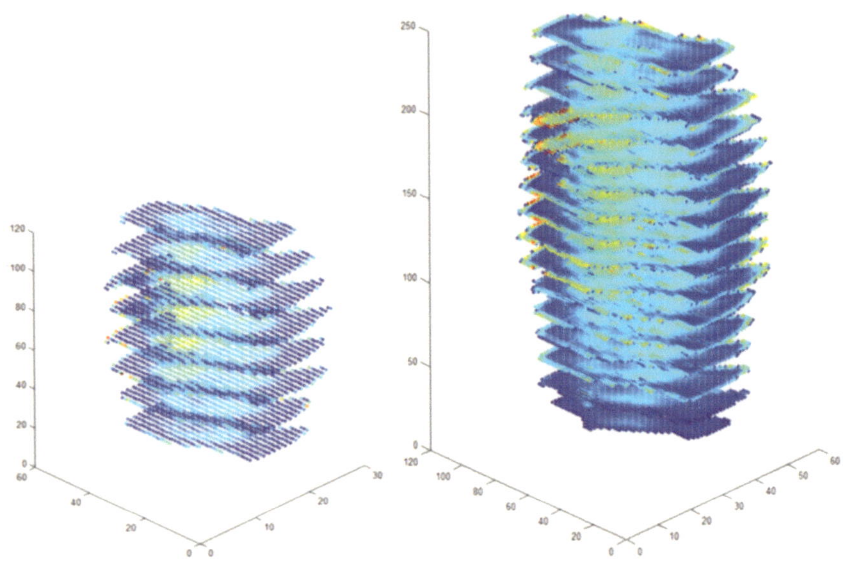

Figure 13: Non-parametric volume Kriging (with signal inversion and substraction) of a human intervertebral disc from an in vivo quantitative MRI acquisition (T2 map).

The two techniques presented in this paragraph, analysis of the MR signal distribution within the tissue of interest using descriptive statistics of histograms and kriging of the images to increase their resolution, can be applied to quantitative MR images of scoliotic spines. A quantitative MRI protocol takes about 40 minutes in vivo, including T1 or T1rho, T2, MT and diffusion sequences, 8 sagittal slices 3mm thick, resolution of 1mmx1mm. This resolution can be improved automatically during the post-treatment of the images. Automatic segmentation of the discs components can be done on the color maps of the relaxation times and MT ratio, not yet on the diffusion maps, not yet on the muscles. The parameters are automatically calculated, and the follow-up of these parameters on scoliotic patients would confirm or reject that they are biomarkers of the progression of the pathology.

7. Conclusion

Quantitative MRI associated with kriging techniques to improve the image resolution, automatic segmentation techniques and tools for the analysis of the distribution of each parameter in a region of interest has the potential to become a very important diagnostic and treatment assessment tool in scoliosis. This region of interest can be located within the intervertebral disc, annulus fibrosus or nucleus pulposus, within the vertebral bone, or within the muscle, for a same MRI acquisition in the sagittal plane. It could replace discography before fusion surgery, help identify the degenerated tissues, help compare different types of surgery with respect to future adjacent degeneration, or be used to monitor the changes after any treatment proposed. Moreover, these MRI parameters could be identified as biomarkers of scoliosis progression.

8. Acknowledgment

The author would like to thank Maximilien Recuerda, Julien Gervais, Yann-Guirec Manac'h, Mohamed Aissiou, for their contribution to the works presented in this chapter, Guillaume Gilbert and Gilles Beaudoin for their support for all MRI data acquisitions and analysis. The work from the author presented in this chapter was supported in part by the NSERC (Discovery grant), the Scoliosis Research Society (Young Investigator Research grant), the CHU Sainte-Justine (Start-up grant) and the Ecole Polytechnique de Montreal (Start-up grant).

9. References

Aissiou M., Gilbert G., Gervais J., Beaudoin G., Trocchu F., Périé D., *Progressive Dual Kriging for 2D and 3D qMRI data interpolation.* Medical Physics, submitted.

Antoniou J, Pike GB, Steffen T, et al. *Quantitative magnetic resonance imaging in the assessment of degenerative disc disease.* Magn Reson Med. 1998;40(6):900-7.

Arkin AM, Katz JF. (1956), *The effects of pressure on epiphyseal growth. The mechanism of plasticity of growing bone.* J Bone Joint Surg [Am] 38:1056-76.

Bensamoun, S. F., Ringleb, S. I., Chen, Q., Ehman, R. L., An, K. N., and Brennan, M., 2007, "*Thigh Muscle Stiffness Assessed with Magnetic Resonance Elastography in Hyperthyroid Patients before and after Medical Treatment,*" J Magn Reson Imaging, 26(3), pp. 708-13.

Bensamoun, S. F., Glaser, K. J., Ringleb, S. I., Chen, Q., Ehman, R. L., and An, K. N., 2008, "*Rapid Magnetic Resonance Elastography of Muscle Using One-Dimensional Projection,*" J Magn Reson Imaging, 27(5), pp. 1083-8.

Bjerkreim I, Hassan I. (1982), *Progression in untreated idiopathic scoliosis after end of growth.* Acta Orthop Scand 53:897-900.

Borthakur A, Maurer PM, Fenty M, Wang C, Berger R, Yoder J, Balderston RA, Elliott DM. T1ρ magnetic resonance imaging and discography pressure as novel biomarkers for disc degeneration and low back pain. Spine 2011;36(25):2190-6.

Bushell GR, Ghosh P, Taylor TK, Sutherland JM. *The collagen of the intervertebral disc in adolescent idiopathic scoliosis.* J Bone Joint Surg Br. 1979;61-B(4):501-8.

Bylund P, Jansson E, Dahlberg E, Eriksson E: *Muscle fiber types in thoracic erector spinae muscles. Fiber types in idiopathic and other forms of scoliosis.* Clin Orthop 1987:222-228.

Chen CT, Fishbein KW, Torzilli PA, Hilger A, Spencer RG, Horton WE. *Matrix fixed-charge density as determined by magnetic resonance microscopy of bioreactor-derived hyaline cartilage correlates with biochemical and biomechanical properties.* Arthritis Rheum 2003, 48(4):1047-56.

Cheung J, Veldhuizen AG, Halberts JP, Sluiter WJ, Van Horn JR. *Geometric and electromyographic assessments in the evaluation of curve progression in idiopathic scoliosis.* Spine 2006;31:322–9.

Chung H, Wehrli FW, Williams JL, Kugelmass SD. *Relationship between NMR transverse relaxation, trabecular bone architecture, and strength.* Proc Natl Acad Sci USA 1993, 90(21):10250-4.

Endean A, Palmer KT, Coggon D. *Potential of Magnetic Resonance Imaging Findings to Refine Case Definition for Mechanical Low Back Pain in Epidemiological Studies: A Systematic Review.* Spine (Phila Pa 1976). 2010.

Gaudreault N, Arsenault AB, Larivière C, DeSerres SJ, Rivard CH. *Assessment of the paraspinal muscles of subjects presenting an idiopathic scoliosis: an EMG pilot study.* BMC Musculoskelet Disord. 2005 Mar 10;6:14.

Gervais J., Périé D., Aubin C.E., Parent S., Labelle H., *MRI signal distribution within the intervertebral disk as a descriptive factor of spine deformities.* Spine, submitted.

Gibson JNA, McMaster MJ, Scrimgeour CM, Stoward PJ, Rennie MJ: *Rates of protein synthesis in paraspinal muscles: Lateral disparity in children with idiopathic scoliosis.* Clinical Science 1988, 75:79-83.

Gooding CA, Neuhauser EBD. (1965), *Growth and development of the vertebral body in the presence and absence of normal stress.* AJR Am J Roentgenol 93:388-94.

Grenier R., Gilbert G., Beaudoin G., Curnier D., Périé D., *Assessment of mechanical properties of muscles using Quantitative MRI.* Journal of Biomechanical Engineering, submitted.

Hatakenaka, M., Yabuuchi, H., Matsuo, Y., Okafuji, T., Kamitani, T., Setoguchi, T., Nishikawa, K., and Honda, H., 2008, "*Effect of Passive Muscle Length Change on Apparent Diffusion Coefficient: Detection with Clinical Mr Imaging,*" Magn Reson Med Sci, 7(2), pp. 59-63.

Heemskerk, A. M., Strijkers, G. J., Vilanova, A., Drost, M. R., and Nicolay, K., 2005, "*Determination of Mouse Skeletal Muscle Architecture Using Three-Dimensional Diffusion Tensor Imaging,*" Magn Reson Med, 53(6), pp. 1333-40.

Henkelman, R.M., Stanisz, G.J., and Graham, S.J. 2001. *Magnetization transfer in MRI: a review.* NMR in Biomedicine 14:57-64.

Hert J, Liskova M. (1964), *Regulation of the longitudinal growth of the long bone by mechanical influence.* Acta Univ Carol Med 20(Suppl):32-4.

Hueter C. (1862), *Anatomische Studien an den Extremitaetengelenken Neugeborener und Erwachsener.* Virkows Archiv Path Anat Physiol 25:572-99.

Jeneson, J. A., and Bruggeman, F. J., 2004, "*Robust Homeostatic Control of Quadriceps Ph During Natural Locomotor Activity in Man,*" Faseb J, 18(9), pp. 1010-2.

Jergas MD, Majumdar S, Keyak JH, Lee IY, Newitt DC, Grampp S, Skinner HB, Genant HK. *Relationships between young modulus of elasticity, ash density, and MRI derived effective transverse relaxation T2* in tibial specimens.* J Comput Assist Tomogr 1995, 19(3):472-9.

Johannessen W, Auerbach JD, Wheaton AJ, et al. *Assessment of human disc degeneration and proteoglycan content using T1rho weighted magnetic resonance imaging.* Spine 2006:31:1253–1257.

Jongeleenen CMJ. *Biomechanics in the intervertebral disc : A literature review.* BMTE 0618. 2006:24.

Keller T.S., Ziv I., Moeljanto E., Spengler D.M. (1993), *Interdependence of lumbar disc and subdiscal bone properties: a report of the normal and degenerated spine.* J Spinal Disord. 6(2):106-13.

Kennelly KP, Stokes MJ: *Pattern of asymmetry of paraspinal muscle size in adolescent idiopathic scoliosis examined by real-time ultrasound imaging. A preliminary study.* Spine 1993, 18(7):913-917.

Khosla, S., Tredwell, S. J., Day, B., Shinn, S. L., and Ovalle, W. K., Jr., 1980, "*An Ultrastructural Study of Multifidus Muscle in Progressive Idiopathic Scoliosis. Changes Resulting from a Sarcolemmal Defect at the Myotendinous Junction,*" J Neurol Sci, 46(1), pp. 13-31.

Kingsley, P.B. 2006. *Introduction to diffusion tensor imaging mathematics: Part I. Tensors, rotations, and eigenvectors.* Concepts in Magnetic Resonance Part A 28A:101-122.

Kingsley, P.B. 2006. *Introduction to diffusion tensor imaging mathematics: Part II. Anisotropy, diffusion-weighting factors, and gradient encoding schemes.* Concepts in Magnetic Resonance Part A 28A:123-154.

Kinugasa, R., Kawakami, Y., and Fukunaga, T., 2006, "*Mapping Activation Levels of Skeletal Muscle in Healthy Volunteers: An Mri Study,*" J Magn Reson Imaging, 24(6), pp. 1420-5.

Kokabi N, Bae W, Diaz E, Chung CB, Bydder GM, Du J. of bovine cortical bone: the effect of water loss on the T1 and T2* relaxation times. Magn Reson Med. 2011 Aug;66(2):476-82.Kouwenhoven JWM, Castelein RM. *The Pathogenesis of Adolescent Idiopathic Scoliosis Review of the Literature.* Spine. 2008;33(26):2898-908.

Kurkijarvi JE, Nissi MJ, Kiviranta I, Jurvelin JS, Nieminen MT. *Delayed gadolinium-enhanced MRI of cartilage (dGEMRIC) and T2 characteristics of human knee articular cartilage: topographical variation and relationships to mechanical properties.* Magn Reson Med 2004, 52(1):41-6.

Lammentausta E, Hakulinen MA, Jurvelin JS, Nieminen MT. *Prediction of mechanical properties of trabecular bone using quantitative MRI.* Phys Med Biol. 2006; 51(23):6187-98.

Lammentausta E, Kiviranta P, Nissi MJ, Laasanen MS, Kiviranta I, Nieminen MT, Jurvelin JS. *T2 relaxation time and delayed gadolinium-enhanced MRI of cartilage (dGEMRIC) of human patellar cartilage at 1.5 T and 9.4 T: Relationships with tissue mechanical properties.* J Orthop Res 2006, 24(3):366-74.

Le Bihan, D., Breton, E., Lallemand, D., Grenier, P., Cabanis, E., and Laval-Jeantet, M. 1986. *MR imaging of intravoxel incoherent motions: application to diffusion and perfusion in neurologic disorders.* Radiology 161:401-407.

Link TM, Majumdar S, Lin JC, Newitt D, Augat P, Ouyang X, Mathur A, Genant HK. *A comparative study of trabecular bone properties in the spine and femur using high resolution MRI and CT.* J Bone Miner Res 1998, 13(1):122-32.

Ludescher B, Effelsberg J, Martirosian P, Steidle G, Markert B, Claussen C, Schick F. T2- and diffusion-maps reveal diurnal changes of intervertebral disc composition: an in vivo MRI study at 1.5 Tesla. J Magn Reson Imaging. 2008 Jul;28(1):252-7.

Mahaudens, P., and Mousny, M., "*Gait in Adolescent Idiopathic Scoliosis Kinematics, Electromyographic and Energy Cost Analysis,*" Stud Health Technol Inform, 158(pp. 101-6.

Majumdar S, Thomasson D, Shimakawa A, Genant HK. *Quantitation of the susceptibility difference between trabecular bone and bone marrow: experimental studies.* Magn Reson Med 1991, 22(1): 111-27.

Majumdar S, Newitt D, Jergas M, Gies A, Chiu E, Osman D, Keltner J, Keyak J, Genant H. *Evaluation of technical factors affecting the quantification of trabecular bone structure using magnetic resonance imaging.* Bone 1995, 17(4):417-30.

Majumdar S, Genant HK, Grampp S, Newitt DC, Truong VH, Lin JC, Mathur A. *Correlation of trabecular bone structure with age, bone mineral density, and osteoporotic status: in vivo studies in the distal radius using high resolution magnetic resonance imaging.* J Bone Miner Res 1997, 12(1):111-8.

Majumdar S. *Magnetic resonance imaging and spectroscopy of the intervertebral disc.* NMR Biomed. 2006;19:894-904.

Manac'h YG., Gilbert G, Beaudoin G., Périé D, *Sensitivity of quantitative MRI to mechanical compression of isolated intervertebral discs.* Magnetic Resonance Imaging, submitted.

Mannion AF, Meier M, Grob D, Muntener M: *Paraspinal muscle fibre type alterations associated with scoliosis: An old problem revisited with new evidence.* Eur Spine J 1998, 7(4):289-293.

McCall IW, Galvin E, O'Brien JP, Park WM. (1981), *Alterations in vertebral growth following prolonged plaster immobilization.* Acta Orthop Scand 52:327-30.

Meier MP, Klein MP, Krebs D, Grob D, Muntener M: *Fiber transformations in multifidus muscle of young patients with idiopathic scoliosis.* Spine 1997, 22(20):2357-2364.

Mente P.L., Stokes I.A., Spence H., Aronsson D.D. (1997), *Progression of vertebral wedging in an asymmetrically loded rat tail model.* Spine. 1997 22(12):1292-6.

Mente P.L., Aronsson D.D., Stokes I.A., Iatridis J.C. (1999), *Mechanical modulation of growth for the correction of vertebral wedge deformities.* J Orthop Res. 17(4):518-24.

Mwale F., Demers C.N., Michalek A.J., Beaudoin G., Goswami T., Beckman L. Iatridis J.C., Antoniou J. *Evaluation of Quantitative Magnetic Resonance Imaging, Biochemical and Mechanical Properties of Trypsin-Treated Intervertebral Discs Under Physiological Compression Loading.* J. Magn. Reson. Imag. 2008, 27:563–73.

Mwale F, Iatridis JC, Antoniou J. *Quantitative MRI as a diagnostic tool of intervertebral disc matrix composition and integrity.* Eur Spine J. 2008;17 Suppl 4:432-40.

Nguyen AM, Johannessen W, Yoder JH, Wheaton AJ, Vresilovic EJ, Borthakur A, Elliott DM. *Noninvasive quantification of human nucleus pulposus pressure with use of T1rho-weighted magnetic resonance imaging.* J Bone Joint Surg Am. 2008, 90(4):796-802.

Nieminen MT, Toyras J, Laasanen MS, Silvennoinen J, Helminen HJ, Jurvelin JS. *Prediction of biomechanical properties of articular cartilage with quantitative magnetic resonance imaging.* J Biomech 2004, 37(3):321-8.

Odermatt D, Mathieu PA, Beausejour M, Labelle H, Aubin CE. *Electromyography of scoliotic patients treated with a brace.* J Orthop Res 2003;21:931–6.

Patten, C., Meyer, R. A., and Fleckenstein, J. L., 2003, "*T2 Mapping of Muscle*," Semin Musculoskelet Radiol, 7(4), pp. 297-305.

Périé D, Sales de Gauzy J, Curnier D, Hobatho MC. *Intervertebral disc modeling using a MRI method: migration of the nucleus zone within scoliotic intervertebral discs.* Magn Reson Imaging. 2001;19(9):1245-8.

Périé D., Iatridis J.C., Beaudoin G., Goswami T., Mwale F., Antoniou J. *Assessment of compressive modulus and hydraulic permeability of intervertebral nucleus pulposus using quantitative MRI.* Journal of Biomechanics 2006, 39(8):1392-400.

Pfirrmann CW, Metzdorf A, Zanetti M, Hodler J, Boos N. *Magnetic resonance classification of lumbar intervertebral disc degeneration.* Spine (Phila Pa 1976). 2001;26(17):1873-8.

Recuerda M., Gilbert G., Beaudoin G., Périé D., *Quantitative MRI for the assessment of mechanical properties of intervertebral discs.* BMC Musculoskeletal Disorders, submitted.

Roaf R. (1960), *Vertebral growth and its mechanical control.* J Bone Joint Surg [Br] 42:40–59.

Roaf R. (1963), *The treatment of progressive scoliosis by unilateral growth-arrest.* J Bone Joint Surg [Br] 45:637-51.

Samosky JT, Burstein D, Eric Grimson W, Howe R, Martin S, Gray ML. *Spatially-localized correlation of dGEMRIC-measured GAG distribution and mechanical stiffness in the human tibial plateau.* J Orthop Res. 2005, 23(1):93-101.

Schlenzka D, Poussa M, Seitsalo S, Osterman K. *Intervertebral disc changes in adolescents with isthmic spondylolisthesis.* J Spinal Disord. 1991;4(3):344-52.

Scoles PV, Latimer BM, DiGiovanni BF, Vargo E, Bauza S, Jellema LM. (1991), Vertebral alterations in Scheuermann's kyphosis. Spine 16:509-15.

Sirca A, Kostevc V: *The fibre type composition of thoracic and lumbar paravertebral muscles in man.* J Anat 1985, 141:131-137.

Stokes IA, Spence H, Aronsson DD, Kilmer N. (1996), *Mechanical modulation of vertebral body growth. Implications for scoliosis progression.* Spine 21(10):1162-7.

Urban MR, Fairbank JCT, Bibby SRS, Urban JPG. *Intervertebral disc composition in neuromuscular scoliosis - Changes in cell density and glycosaminoglycan concentration at the curve apex.* Spine. 2001;26(6):610-7.

Tsai, Y. T., Leong, C. P., Huang, Y. C., Kuo, S. H., Wang, H. C., Yeh, H. C., and Lau, Y. C., "*The Electromyographic Responses of Paraspinal Muscles During Isokinetic Exercise in Adolescents with Idiopathic Scoliosis with a Cobb's Angle Less Than Fifty Degrees,*" Chang Gung Med J, 33(5), pp. 540-50.

Volkmann R. (1882) *Verletzungen und Krankenheiten der Bewegungsorgane. In: von Pitha und Billroth: Handbuch der allgemeinen und speciellen* Chirurgie Bd II Teil II. Stuttgart: Ferdinand Enke.

Wang, C., Witschey, W., Goldberg, A., Elliott, M., Borthakur, A., and Reddy, R. 2010. *Magnetization transfer ratio mapping of intervertebral disc degeneration.*

Weinstein SL, Ponseti IV. (1983), *Curve progression in idiopathic scoliosis.* J Bone Joint Surg [Am] 65:447-55.

Wehrli FW, Ford JC, Haddad JG. *Osteoporosis: clinical assessment with quantitative MR imaging in diagnosis.* Radiology 1995, 196(3):631-41.

Wheaton AJ, Dodge GR, Elliott DM, Nicoll SB, Reddy R. *Quantification of cartilage biomechanical and biochemical properties via T1rho magnetic resonance imaging.* Magn Reson Med. 2005, 54(5):1087-93.

Wright, P., Mougin, O., Totman, J., Peters, A., Brookes, M., Coxon, R., Morris, P., Clemence, M., Francis, S., Bowtell, R., et al. 2008. *Water proton measurements in brain tissue at 7, 3, and 1.5T using IR-EPI, IR-TSE, and MPRAGE: results and optimization.* Magnetic Resonance Materials in Physics, Biology and Medicine 21:121-130.

Zetterberg C, Aniansson A, Grimby G: *Morphology of the paravertebral muscles in adolescent idiopathic scoliosis.* Spine 1983, 8(5):457-462.

Zuo J, Joseph GB, Li X, Link TM, Hu SS, Berven SH, Kurhanewitz J, Majumdar S. In-vivo Intervertebral Disc Characterization using Magnetic Resonance Spectroscopy and T1ρ Imaging: Association with Discography and Oswestry Disability Index and SF-36. Spine 2011 [Epub ahead of print].

7

Moiré Topography: From Takasaki Till Present Day

Flávia Porto[1,2,3], Jonas L. Gurgel[3,4],
Thaís Russomano[5] and Paulo T.V. Farinatti[2]
[1]*Post-Graduate Stricto Sensu in Exercise and Sports Sciences, Gama Filho University (UGF)*
[2]*Physical Activity and Health Promotion Laboratory, Institute of Physical Education and Sports, Rio de Janeiro State University (UERJ)*
[3]*Biomechanics Research Group of Fluminense Federal University (UFF)*
[4]*Academic Master of Science in Health Care (UFF)*
[5]*Microgravity Centre of Pontifical Catholic University (PUCRS)*
Brazil

1. Introduction

The introduction of the Moiré phenomenon in scientific studies occurred in 1874, when Raylegh compared the overlapping of two equal gratings (Ikeda & Terada, 1981).

Since Takasaki (Takasaki, 1970) proposed Moiré topography (MT) for the analysis of the surface of the human body, other authors have published studies with the objective to explain, improve and apply the method in individuals with different characteristics, as well as using other possible techniques that involve MT (Adler et al., 1984, Breque et al., 2004, Castro, 2007, Drerup, 1981, Hertz, 2005, Kim & al., 2004, Kim et al., 2001, Lino & Fabbro, 2004, Porto et al., 2007, Rössler et al., 2006, Yeras et al., 2003). Takasaki himself also seemed to be concerned with the evolution of the technique and its several clinical applications (Takasaki, 1973, 1982, 1976), after his first publication in 1970.

To this day however, few devices are commercially available on the market for the evaluation of the topography of the human body - although the advantages of MT are well recognized as a diagnostic and prophylactic tool, especially for postural deviations of the vertebral column. Perhaps, this limited use of MT is due to a lack of knowledge about the physical phenomenon of Moiré and, consequently, its potential clinical applications.

This Chapter therefore aims to present a literature review regarding the main characteristics of the Moiré phenomenon, and its use as a topographical method for clinical diagnosis of postural deviations.

2. Materials and methods

This research survey was divided in two phases in order to form the body of analysis for this study. In the first phase, a search of studies related to MT was performed from the sources PubMed, Science Direct and Academic Google. Also, the tool of Multiple Search was used from the website of the Library Irmão José Ótão of the Pontifical Catholic University of Rio Grande do Sul, Brazil (PUCRS, Brazil). This tool allows multiple searches to be carried out with only one command from several available sources of information in the Library of PUCRS. It can retrieve at once complete scientific articles from electronic databases, such as Proquest, Ebsco, Biological Abstracts and Scielo. In addition to this, some works were acquired by means of direct contact with authors via e-mail. The second phase consisted of a literature survey based on the list of references of each paper found in phase one.

The search and selection criterion of the articles for this study was performed through the use of key words in Portuguese and English, including: Moiré, Moiré topography, Shadow Moiré and Moiré Technique. Physics text books and article review were also consulted to clarify the concepts in Optics.

All scientific papers obtained through the literature search were submitted to the technique of Scanning (GOODMAN, 1976 apud (Kleiman, 1989)), consisting of a superficial reading of articles with the intention of better selecting useful works for the study. Some articles published prior to 1980, although not up to date in terms of scientific discoveries, were still considered because of their importance for the characterization of the state-of-the-art of MT. These were obtained through the Commutation Service, available from the homepage of the Library Irmão José Ótão of PUCRS.

A content analysis, adapted from the proposal of Bardin (Bardin, 2000) and having been used in other studies (Porto, 2003), was applied to the selected material. The characteristics of the analysis adopted were: 1) the description of the Moiré phenomenon and the origin of the technique name; 2) the evaluation techniques based on this physical phenomenon, including instruments used, calibration of these equipment, analysis of the image and the care required in the performance of MT application; 3) areas of clinical use.

This study approached the subject according to the following topics: physical principle of Moiré; techniques based on the Moiré phenomenon; calibration of the equipment for MT; analysis of the topograms (Moiré pictures); application of the method; and the care needed in applying MT.

3. Results and discussion

3.1 The physical principle

According to Oster (Oster, 1988), the Moiré phenomenon - also called, standard or fringes of Moiré - occurs when one set of curves is overlapped over another set of curves, forming a completely new set. This overlapping of the gratings (or curves) must be less than an angle of 45° in order to generate interference. This interference formed by the intersection of the lines of gratings is what will characterize the standard of Moiré (Bartl et al., 2001, Drerup, 1981, Dzielinski et al., 1990, Oster, 1988).

The phenomenon can also be generated when there is a small difference in the thickness and distance between the lines of the grating (or reticulum), also with the use of circular forms of the standards of Moiré.

Depending on the technique used, however, it is possible that the two gratings created for the generation of the Moiré phenomenon are not both in reality a physical object. This occurs with the method Shadow Moiré Technique (SMT), Figure 1, in which the shade of the projected grating on the analysis surface functions as the second grating (Breque et al., 2004, Oster, 1988). Likewise, it occurs in the Projection Moiré Technique (PMT), Figure 2, in which the first grating is projected on the analysis surface and the optic phenomenon is generated subsequently when the image is processed by software (Mínguez et al., 2007). Moreover, these techniques seem to be the two main ones for the evaluation of human body surfaces, which has also been pointed out by Lim, Kim and Chung (Lim et al., 1989).

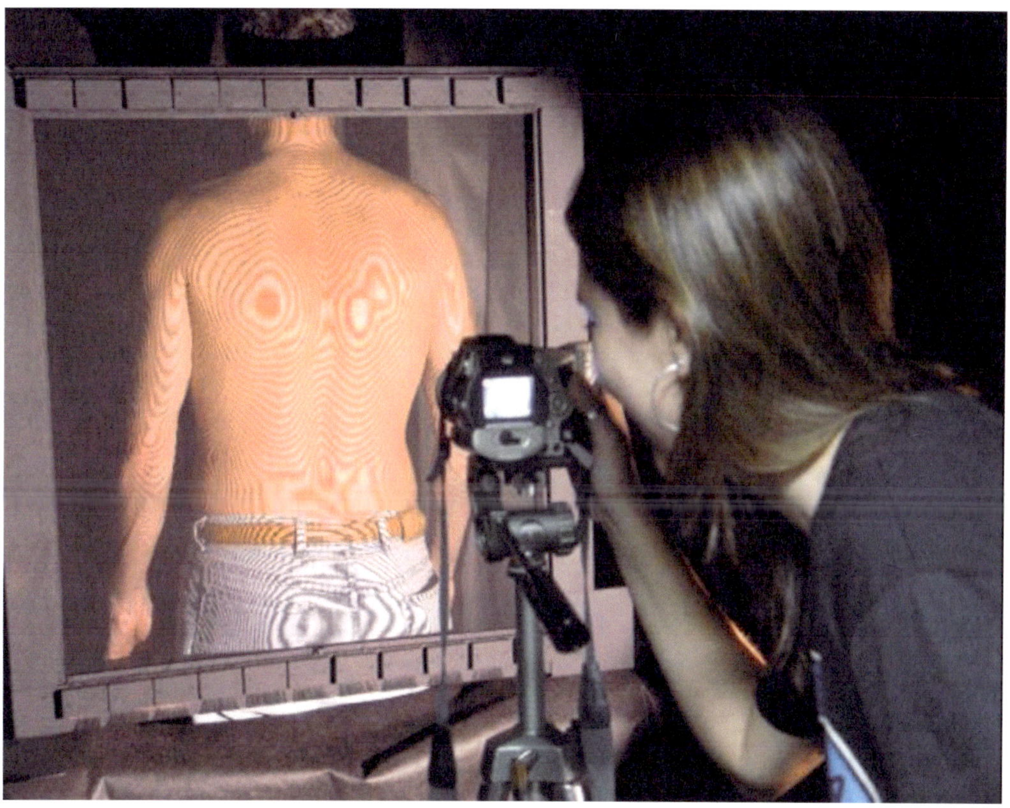

Fig. 1. Shadow Moiré Technique. *By the authors.*

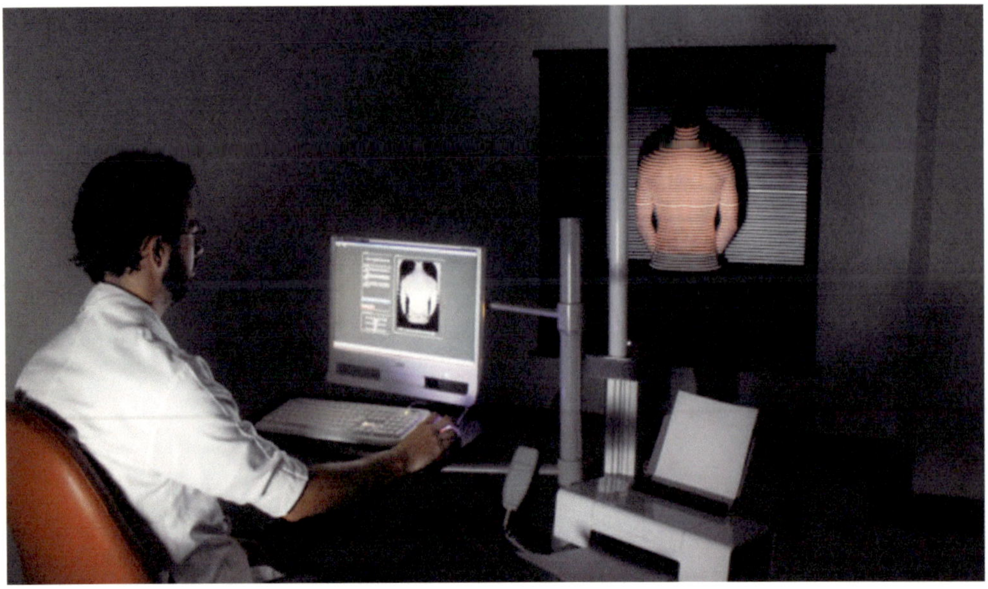

Fig. 2. Projection Moiré Technique. From: www.miotec.com.br.

Moiré can be used to study the topography of surfaces, therefore the fringes of Moiré form the lines of contour - or the levels of curves - of the surface of the object under analysis (Breque et al., 2004, Yeras et al., 2003).

The word Moiré comes from a French terms meaning *wet* or *waved* and is related to an imported silk from China in which the fabric itself gives this peculiar appearance to the cloth (Bartl et al., 2001, Sciammarella, 1982). In Brazil, the fabric of this same appearance is called *Tafetá* or *Chamalote*. In accordance with the Textile Glossary, supplied by Hering company (Hering, 2004), Chamalote, which is made from a mix of camel hair and silk gives the same impression of the "waved" effect (Moiré).

3.2 The Moiré techniques

The Moiré techniques are a set of procedures based on the physical phenomenon of Moiré (Lino & Fabbro, 2004). They are stereometric methods of three-dimensional analysis of an object from a bidimensional image (Drerup, 1981, Kim et al., 2001). The Moiré techniques are: Moiré in plane, Shadow Moiré, Projection Moiré, Interferometry Moiré, Microscopical Moiré, Holographic Moiré and Interference Moiré (Rössler et al., 2006, Yeras et al., 2003). These techniques differ by the way the phenomenon of Moiré is generated and further used in the topographical analyses.

In general, MT consists of a simple method and requires a camera, a light source and a grating. The images (topograms) are formed by the alternation of clear and dark fringes (Batouche & Benlamri, 1994, Batouche et al., 1996, Drerup, 1981, Kim et al., 2001), the dark ones being called fringes of Moiré (Rössler et al., 2006). The pattern created by these fringes on the surface of the object is used for further analysis.

The generation of the optic phenomenon will depend on the MT used. With SMT, for example, the shadow of the grating functions as the second grating (Breque et al., 2004,

Oster, 1988). In this case, the shadow of the object under analysis is deformed by the form of its own surface (Rössler et al., 2006).

Therefore, the physical principle of SMT is: a source of light P illuminates at an oblique angle on the grating G and produces then an image on the surface S. An observer, called O, (or a camera, C) is placed in front of the grating. The shadows formed on the surface (the object) are either seen by the observer or captured by a camera. The results will look like a topographic map, which results from the Moiré optic process (Turner-Smith, 1997).

The positioning of the camera and the light source can vary. For example, the light source can be above the camera and both lined up exactly in the same plane (Hamra & Volpon, 1995). Also, the light source can be located a little in front of the camera and closer to the grating (Yeras et al., 2003). Other alternative methodologies for the application of Moiré topography are: a) positioning of the light source and camera side by side and at the same level, but maintaining the oblique incidence of light on the grid (Castro, 2007, Hertz et al., 2005, Hertz, 2005, Porto et al., 2007); b) to use a mobile light source (Lim et al., 1989); c) to replace the camera with a video camera (Turner-Smith, 1997, Yeras et al., 2003).

A lack of standardization in the Moiré technique for the topographical analysis of the human body is perceived. Few studies mention the measurements of distance left between the material employed during the technique (camera, source of light, grating, individual), as well as other important characteristics, such as: details of the reticulum (Castro, 2007, Hamra & Volpon, 1995, Hertz et al., 2005, Hertz, 2005, Kilpeäinen et al., 1996) and the calibration procedures used (Mínguez et al., 2007). This raises a concern given that replicability of measurement is compromised by a lack of information. The difficulty of standardizing measurement procedures in TM generates a need for even greater reliability on procedure definitions.

Another relevant aspect of the studies reviewed is that the equipment used for MT is of unknown origin in the majority of cases, meaning that it may or may not have been developed by the laboratory conducting the research. Noteworthy are the studies (Castro, 2007, Hamra & Volpon, 1995, Hertz et al., 2005, Hertz, 2005, Porto, 2008) that used TMS and stated that the grids were developed by the respective research groups, having also provided information regarding the methodology applied. In relation to grid design, it is common to find that it is made of wood (Castro, 2007, Hertz, 2005, Porto, 2008). Considering the distortion that can occur with this type of material due to tension of the nylon threads, Adair (Adair et al., 1977) proposed that the grid should be made from aluminum instead. Takasaki (Takasaki, 1973) also suggested that the grid size used for analysis of the whole human body should be 1.8 x 1.8 x 0.9 m^3. For analysis of the trunk, studies have shown that a square grid of 600mm is satisfactory (Castro, 2007, Hertz et al., 2005, Hertz, 2005, Porto, 2008).

Even in those studies where the equipment manufacturer was mentioned, the characteristics of the material employed for the MT were not always explained, as in the study by Mínguez et al. (Mínguez et al., 2007), which evaluated postural deviations due to scoliosis of the vertebral column.

The experimental design of MT can vary from one study to the next, depending on the type of MT employed. When using SMT, for example, a mobile grating can be adopted (Dzielinski et al., 1990) as opposed to a fixed one (Castro, 2007, Hamra & Volpon, 1995,

Hertz et al., 2005, Hertz, 2005, Porto, 2008). The mobile grating can move horizontally in front of the object being studied.

In relation to the camera, the opening of the equipment must be sufficient to include in the field of vision both the grating and its shadow (Hamra & Volpon, 1995, Takasaki, 1973) and therefore, can make use of the camera optical zoom (Hertz, 2005, Porto, 2008). On the other hand, the shutter speed should preferably be less than 1/8 of a second to avoid the inevitable movement of the body. With such care, according to Takasaki (Takasaki, 1973), good contrast of the fringes can be ensured.

When looking at the light source it can be seen that the literature also does not present standard procedures for the application of TMS. Porto (Castro, 2007, Hertz et al., 2005, Porto, 2008) indicated using a 100W light bulb. Takasaki (Takasaki, 1973) suggested a 2-4kW Xenon lamp as being ideal, but notes that the 500W Iodine lamps have a good cost-benefit.

The Moiré topogram depends on the position of the object behind the grating. Therefore, it is essential to standardize the position of the object to be analysed (Drerup, 1981, Hamra & Volpon, 1995). This care may be justified also by measuring the deviations presented, as with the notion of depth proposed by Takasaki (Takasaki, 1970). There was no standardization in this aspect found in the literature. Adair (Adair et al., 1977) proposed a protocol in which the individual stands upright, feet together, with buttocks close to the screen and shoulders parallel to the grid. This schematic can camouflage the problem that the posture of the person is being "arranged" by the evaluator (although the results of their study were really satisfactory for the detection of scoliosis in school children). Alternatively, another study [6,16,19,30] proposed that the person being evaluated should be in the standing position, feet apart naturally, and body as close to the grid as possible without touching it. The lack of methodological standardization in the application of TM hinders a better understanding of the deformities of the trunk including generating misinterpretation of results (Patias et al., 2010). For this reason, the determination of the Cobb angle is still the gold standard for diagnosis of scoliosis (Kotwicki et al., 2009).

By reviewing the scientific literature, it is apparent that some of the MT techniques are more used than others for the analysis of the human body surface. The SMT appears to be the best for evaluating deviations of the vertebral column and/or of the trunk (Adler et al., 1984, Castro, 2007, Hertz et al., 2005, Hertz, 2005, Takasaki, 1970, Uetake et al., 1998), which can be explained by the fact that SMT was the first MT employed for the topographical evaluation of human body.

Other areas of the human body have also been studied through the use of SMT, such as the arc plantar (Hamra & Volpon, 1995, Yeras et al., 2003), lower limbs (Yeras et al., 2003) and the scapular region (Chalupová, 2001).

In recent years, the Projection Moiré Technique has appeared more frequently in the scientific literature, especially in relation to postural evaluations (Kim & al., 2004, Kim et al., 2001, Mínguez et al., 2007). This can mainly be explained by the current technological evolution in the area of image processing, which also allows the use of the MT in more delicate and complex topographic areas of the human body, such as some bones, using the Interferometry Moiré Technique (Wood et al., 2001).

3.3 Calibration of the equipment

The procedure of calibration of the MT refers to the analysis of the surface of an object with a known geometry in order to prevent direct marks on the surface under evaluation from being made (Ortiz & Patterson, 2005). Moreover, it is possible to reconstruct the geometry of a known object from the generated fringes and to calculate the standard error of the instrument, which will give the accuracy of the equipment used during the performance of the technique (Hertz, 2005).

The calibration procedure of the SMT is described for Hertz (Hertz, 2005). She used a white cone (height = 30mm) made in TECNIL (nylon), with some ring marks, each one every 5mm of depth of the object (total of six marks). The cone was fixed on a wooden structure and placed behind the grating (reticulum) at a distance of 10mm. The image was captured with an optic resolution of 96x96pp and the camera optic zoom of 2x. After analysis of the images, standard error of the instrument was calculated (SE = 0.05136). According to the author, the results showed to be acceptable for a significance level of 5%. It was verified, by the calibration procedure that the distance in between each fringe was equivalent to 4.9mm.

A typical calibration of apparatus used for PMT was described by Mínguez et al. (Mínguez et al., 2007). According to these authors, two images obtained from the projected grating on a plane surface (without the object of analysis) are captured in two different positions with distance of 400mm in between them. These images are called *front grating* and *back grating*. Subsequently, the individual to be evaluated is placed in front of the plane surface, acting himself as the *back grating* (note that the 400mm distance is sufficient to fit a person between the two projected gratings). The idea is that, after the generation of the fringes of Moiré on the surface of the body of the individual, the previous projected grating serves as the basis for the calculations of the topograms.

Some authors, however, prefer to use a reference object by the side of the one being evaluated in order to calibrate the distances between the fringes. This object can be rectangular with known measurements (Ortiz & Patterson, 2005) or any another object of known geometry.

3.4 Analysis of the topograms

The medical analysis of the Moiré images is based on the symmetry of the fringes of both sides in different regions of the body (Batouche & Benlamri, 1994), as represented in Figures 3 and 4. Therefore, it is predominantly classified as a qualitative analysis (Adler et al., 1984).

As much as the quantitative parameters are important in the diagnosis of body asymmetries, there is no denying that the visual inspection of images provides information absolutely relevant for the evaluator and useful in the decision making process that follows. For example, Adair (Adair et al., 1977) tracked scoliosis in 1,132 school children in Ottawa, Canada. Benefitting from the advantage of the easy use of TMS, the author was able to photograph 40 children per hour, both boys and girls. When evidence of asymmetries in the back were detected, the children's spines were X-rayed to confirm the suspicion of scoliosis. The results showed that TMS identified 94% of the positive cases diagnosed by X-ray.

The qualitative medical evaluation of the produced topograms, based on visual inspection of the images, can be an extremely tiring task, especially when evaluating postural

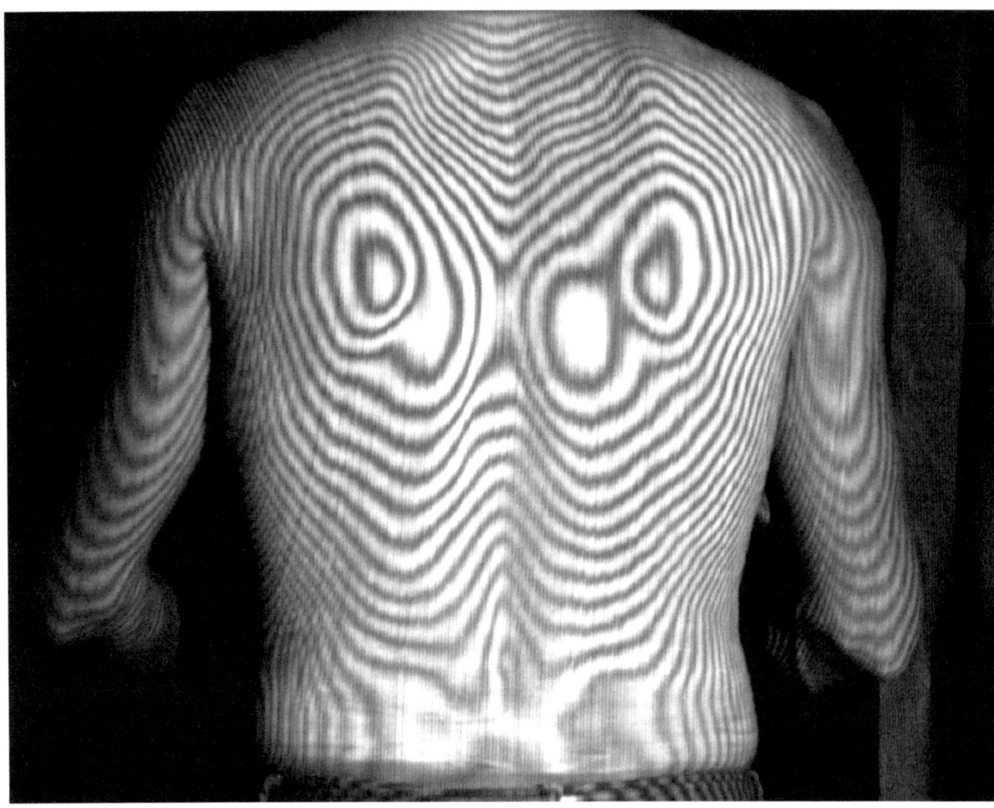

Fig. 3. Moiré topogram of an adult. *By the authors.*

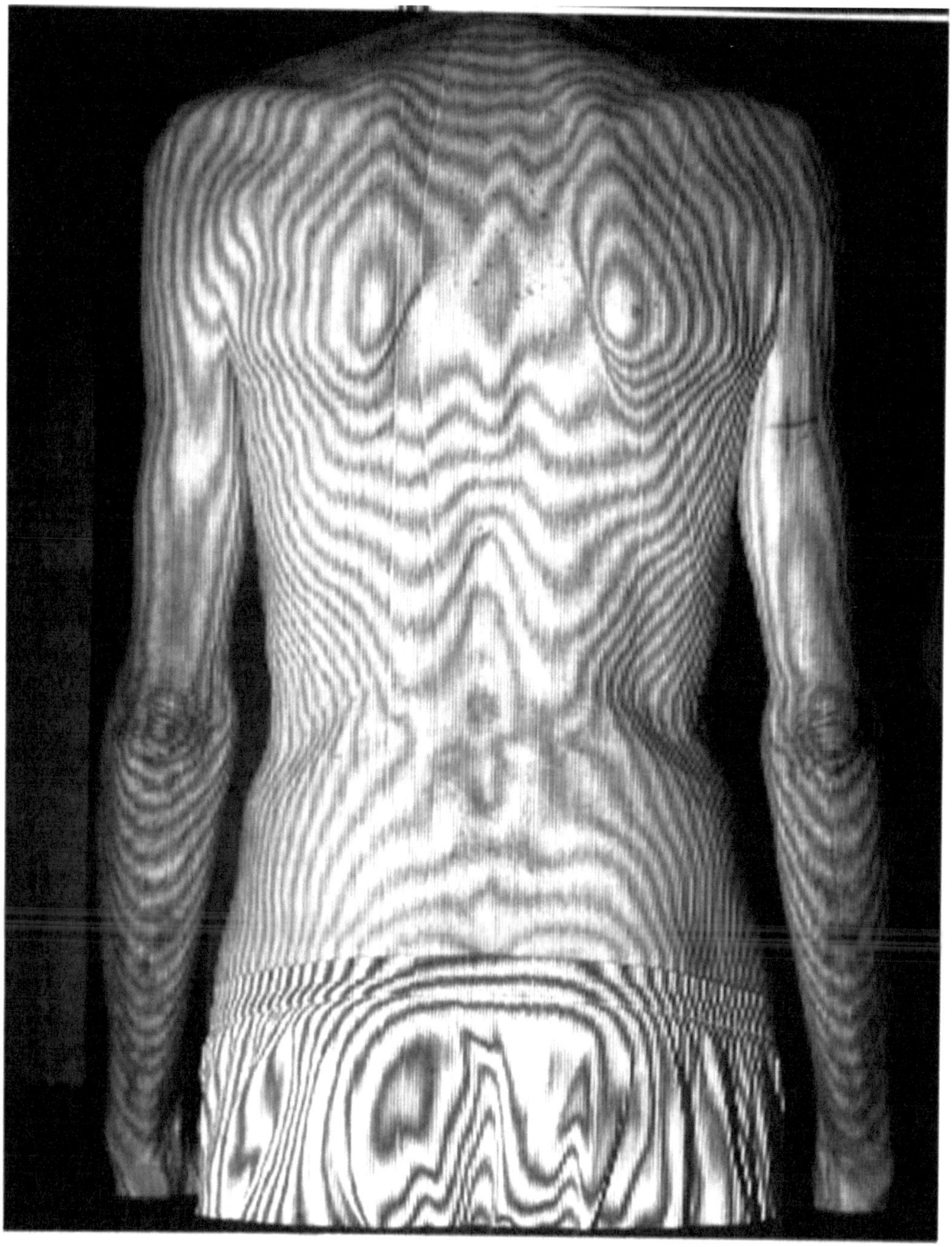

Fig. 4. Moiré topogram of an elderly person. *By the authors.*

deformities of a large number of people in a short period of time, as occurs in population studies (Porto, 2008) or when it is used to identify scoliosis in children at schools (Adler et al., 1984). Also, Kim et al. (Kim et al., 2001) and Kim et al. (Kim et al., 2006) believe that fatigue caused by the performance of many subjective evaluations can interfere with the judgment of the Moiré images. For this reason, these authors advocate the need for the automatization of the analysis procedure of the topograms captured from the back of individuals.

Having this in mind, Porto et al. (Porto, 2008), in a population study of postural evaluation of individuals of more than 60 years of age (Multidimensional Study of the Elderly Populations of Porto Alegre, Brazil), considered the use of a free software for analysis of the topograms. It did not detect deformities in the dorsal region of individuals automatically, but facilitated the evaluation by giving measurements of angular deviation and depth with more precision.

Photographs with 256 grey tones, ranging from 0 (black) to 255 (white), were captured on the back of each elderly individual. Porto et al. (Porto, 2008b) evaluated the lateral deviations of the thoracic column with the measurement of the joint angles formed (in degrees) and the characteristics of the concavities present, the unevenness of scapulas in the frontal plane with the measurement of angular deviations, in degrees, and hyperkyphosis thoracic. For this evaluation, the authors used a free software (Power Draw 2D Application Vector), which optimized the evaluation process of the images.

Previously, other authors (Castro, 2007, Hertz et al., 2005, Hertz, 2005) considered similar characteristics of the MT evaluation and tried to search for a numerical parameter for the evaluations of the volunteers. However, in these studies, they used more rudimentary instruments for the analysis of postural deviations, such as paper, pencil or pen and ruler.

The subject aspect of the MT is a limiting factor. According to Kim et al. (Kim et al., 2001), the numerical information of the asymmetry is useful in the evaluation of the deformity. Therefore, it is clear that the attempts of many authors in quantifying subjectively postural deviations are not the best option, although less expensive. These initiatives, however, show the concern of these scientists in improving this biomechanical evaluation. This might imply that an important limiting factor is the financial obstacle.

The automatization of the evaluation procedure for the Moiré images has many advantages, especially for the study of large number of people in short periods of time, when compared to the manual, visual and semi-automatic way. Kim et al. (Kim & al., 2004), for example, used a new technique of automatic detection of scoliosis during a study evaluating 1,200 topograms of young individuals. However, even with automatic detection of the fringes, there are serious problems related to ambiguous fringe patterns and to non-continuous fringes. According to Cline, Lorensen and Holik (Cline et al., 1984), non-continuous surfaces generate broken fringes which make subjective analysis very difficult. In this situation, errors of evaluation also occur when software is used to analyze topograms.

When evaluating the human body surface certain fringe patterns are perceived depending on the area studied. In this sense, according to Cline, Lorensen and Holik (Cline et al., 1984), the fringes become enclosed within the image plane when the surface is very inclined. This occurs, for example, in very thin individuals or those who present with thoracic kyphosis. Yet when the surfaces are very narrow, the breaks between the pixels prevent automatic construction of the image. Non-uniform surfaces with low reflectance might not generate clean fringe patterns. Other complex Moiré patterns that make the analysis of topograms difficult occur when individuals for evaluation are obese, according to Ruggerone and Austin (Ruggerone & Austin, 1986) and when they present with excess skin and hair.

3.5 Applications

The MT method has the advantages of being a non-invasive method and does not produce radiation, as occurs in X-ray exams (Ikeda & Terada, 1981, Yeras et al., 2003), does not require a highly trained professional for its application (Batouche & Benlamri, 1994, Ikeda & Terada, 1981, Yeras et al., 2003), allows the evaluation of many people in a short period of time (Ikeda & Terada, 1981, Yeras et al., 2003), is reproducible (Batouche & Benlamri, 1994, Ikeda & Terada, 1981), is low-cost (Batouche & Benlamri, 1994, Yeras et al., 2003), is able to substitute the use of an X-ray exam or to act as a complementary method in the diagnosis of disease (Hertz et al., 2005, Hertz, 2005, Yeras et al., 2003).

The MT method seems to be very efficient in the topographical analysis of an object that has irregular surfaces and that is not very rigid, such as a pile of sand, the surface of water or the human body (Takasaki, 1982). However, it is believed that MT is also a versatile method, being suitable for use for deflectometry and tension-deformation situations (Dzielinski et al., 1990).

The use of MT in the topographical analysis of the human body is possible because it is able to indirectly identify places with structural deformities under the skin through the form of the surface area (Chalupová, 2001). MT has, therefore, many possible applications and uses for health professionals in clinical evaluation of patients and for researchers and professors in their academic activities with students. These applications include: early detection of scoliosis (Pearsall et al., 1992, Takasaki, 1982, Yeras et al., 2003); the not-invasive reconstruction of the vertebral column based on the generated topograms (Dzielinski et al., 1990); the detection of other deformities of the vertebral column (hyperkyphosis, hyperlordosis, planar back, gibosity) in different planes (sagital, frontal and transverse) from only one image obtained from the back of an individual (Batouche & Benlamri, 1994, Castro, 2007, Hertz et al., 2005, Hertz, 2005); the evaluation of the foot sole (Hamra & Volpon, 1995, Yeras et al., 2003); the characterization of the palatal morphology (Kilpeäinen et al., 1996); the characterization of the form and the detection of abnormalities of the lower limbs (Yeras et al., 2003); the description of the scapular area and its symmetry in relation to the vertebral column and between both scapulas (Chalupová, 2001); the verification of the influence of sport activities in the morphology of the trunk (Uetake et al., 1998).

Japan was a pioneering country in the use of MT, and was first to use it for identifying scoliosis in school children. Currently, 11 city halls (of a total of 47, including Tokyo) use the SMT for this. According to Kim et al. (Kim et al., 2001), in 1977, the Japanese Minister of Education initiated a program for early identification of scoliosis in children and young individuals in Japanese schools. The detection of scoliosis in its early phase was done through physical evaluation, which is a non-reproducible and very subjective. Therefore, SMT became an alternative method, through the visualization of the asymmetry of the fringes of Moiré on the back of the individual, making it a very popular method.

Some researchers have applied SMT on a large-scale for the evaluation of postural deviations of children and young individuals, as did Adler, Csongradi and Bleck (Adler et al., 1984), Yeras, Peña and Junco (Yeras et al., 2003).

Adler, Csongradi and Bleck (Adler et al., 1984) evaluated 327 girls, in five of the eight public schools of Clara Saint, in California, United States, in order to identify early signs of scoliosis. The authors applied SMT and studied the asymmetry of the fringes, and also applied the clinical postural examination. Comparing the two methods, the authors found a low correlation (r=0.16), which they attributed to the method of Moiré employed in the evaluated schools.

Yeras, Peña and Junco (Yeras et al., 2003) evaluated 203 individuals between 10 and 15 years of age from a school in Havana, Cuba. The authors compared the evaluation of the fringes of SMT produced on the back of the individual and the same fringes that were recorded on a video. Moreover, they compared with the classical physical examination performed by doctors that include: complete physical examination, measurement of vertical alignment with the use of a pendulum and the flexion of the trunk for the detection of idiopathic scoliosis. The results showed that SMT was more precise than the physical examination and was very efficient in the detection of false-positives.

The MT method was also used to detect deformities of the trunk and column in the elderly, but the number of studies that applied this method in older individuals is minimal when compared to studies focusing on young individuals and children. The Aerospace Biomechanics Laboratory (NUBA, Microgravity Centre, School of Engineering, PUCRS, Brazil) together with the Institute of Geriatrics and Gerontology and the School of Physical Education of PUCRS evaluated the elderly population of a city in Rio Grande do Sul state, in a pioneering study (Porto, 2008).

The MT has presented a good correlation with the X-ray, becoming a reliable method for giving measurements, as shown by the studies of Daruwalla and Balasubramaniam (Daruwalla & Balasubramaniam, 1985), Ruggeroni and Austin(Ruggerone & Austin, 1986), and Kovac and Pecina (Kovac & Pecina, 1999).

3.6 Precautions

When an alternative method of medical evaluation is developed which prioritizes reduced costs, it is necessary that the new method proves to be a good substitute. Having this in mind, MT must have an excellent reproducibility when performed on the same patient many times. Statistically, the best way to validate a new method is by comparing it to the gold-standard one (Hulley et al., 2003).

Since publication in 1970 of the application of the Moiré phenomenon for human body surface analysis, some doubts have emerged regarding the ability to capture topograms with good fringe contrasts. These difficulties arise because of such factors as the size and depth of the surface not being able to show good fringe contrast (Takasaki, 1973).

There is a huge lack in the scientific literature of studies that have evaluated the accuracy of the MT when used on the human body. Daruwalla and Balasubramaniam (Daruwalla & Balasubramaniam, 1985) have evaluated the accuracy of MT applied on the back of young individuals and compared the results with the x-ray of each examined person. A total of 1,342 topograms of children from a school in Singapore were studied in 1982. The results of this study demonstrated that the accuracy of the curves was identified in 68% of thorax columns, in 54% of thorax-lumbar columns and in 15% of the lumbar region. The authors believe that the test that includes the flexion of the trunk provides more information and is a more economic method for large scale evaluation and that MT is a complementary method of diagnosis.

Standardization of the evaluation protocol and design of the experimental project must be pre-determined. This idea is corroborated by Ikeda and Terada (Ikeda & Terada, 1981). Drerup (Drerup, 1981) believes that a crucial aspect of the MT method is the position of the object, in this case the person. It is easy to notice in the scientific literature that there are more studies relating to MT application than those that focus on the accuracy of the method itself and the standardization of the measurements obtained.

One of the disadvantages of MT is that it is labor intensive when it comes to evaluation of the images. Some authors believe that the best solution would be the development of an automatic system for the analysis of the Moiré images (Batouche & Benlamri, 1994, Ikeda & Terada, 1981, Kim & al., 2004, Kim et al., 2001).

4. Conclusion

This chapter aimed to review aspects related to Moiré topography published in scientific journals from 1970 onwards, when this technique was first used for medical purposes. The method proved sufficiently versatile in its clinical applications and extremely useful as a complementary diagnostic technique. It is a time effective, low cost, user friendly method for evaluating body posture and deviations. It was noted, however, that there was a lack of studies in the literature reviewed evaluating the topography of the human body through MT, especially in the elderly population.

5. Acknowledgements

This study was partially supported by National Council for Scientific and Technological Development (CNPQ/ Brazil), Carlos Chagas Filho Research Foundation (FAPERJ) and Coordination for the Improvement of Higher Level Personnel - Doctor scholarship (PROSUP/ CAPES/ Brazil).

6. References

Adair, I. V., Van Wijk, M. C. & Armstrong, G. W. (1977). Moire topography in scoliosis screening. *Clin Orthop Relat Res*, Vol No. 129, (Nov-Dec), pp. 165-171, 0009-921X (Print)

Adler, NS, Csongradi, J & Bleck, EE. (1984). School screening for scoliosis - one experience in California using clinical examination and Moiré Photography. *West J Med*, Vol 141, No. 5, pp. 631-633,

Bardin, Laurence. (2000). *Content analysis* Edições 70, Lisbon, PT

Bartl, J, Fíra, R & Hain, M. (2001). Inspection of surface by the Moiré method. *Meas Sci Rev*, Vol 1, No. 1, pp. 29-32,

Batouche, M & Benlamri, R. (1994). A computer vision system for diagnosing scoliosis. IEEE International Conference on Pervasive Computing and Communications, Orlando, Florida,

Batouche, M, Benlamri, R & Kholladi, MK. (1996). A computer vision system for diagnosing scoliosis using Moiré images. *Comput Biol Med*, Vol 26, No. 4, pp. 339-353,

Breque, C, Dupre, J & Bremand, F. (2004). Calibration of a system of projection moiré for relief measuring: biomedical applications. *Opt Lasers Eng*, Vol 41, No. pp. 241-260,

Castro, SLS. (2007). A comparison of two postural assessment techniques in elderly of Porto Alegre and their level of physical activity [thesis]. Porto Alegre: Pontifical Catholic University (PUCRS)

Chalupová, M. (2001). Use of a biomechanical model of the scapula region for the identification of muscle disbalance. Vol No. Retrieved from <mms.tudelft.nl/dsg/intersg/Proceedings_2001_files/06_chalupova.pdf>

Cline, Harvey E., Lorensen, William E. & Holik, Andrew S. (1984). Automatic moire contouring. *Appl Opt*, Vol 23, No. 10 pp. 1454-1459,

Daruwalla, J. S. & Balasubramaniam, P. (1985). Moire topography in scoliosis. Its accuracy in detecting the site and size of the curve. *J Bone Joint Surg Br*, Vol 67, No. 2, (Mar), pp. 211-213, 0301-620X (Print)

Drerup, B. (1981). A procedure for the numerical analysis of Moiré topograms. *Photogramm*, Vol 36, No. pp. 41-49,

Dzielinski, A, Skoneczny, S, Zbikowski & Kuklinski, S. (1990). Cellular neural network application to Moiré pattern filtering. IEEE CNNA'90 Workshop, Budapest, Hungary,

Hamra, A & Volpon, JB. (1995). Fotopodometria "quantitativa" na avaliação do arco plantar longitudinal medial. *Rev Bras Ortop*, Vol 30, No. 8, pp. 609-614,

Hering. Glossary of textile industry. 2004. [captured in: Ago 23 2007]. Available in: http://www.previ.com.br/pls/portal/docs/PAGE/PG_PREVI/INVESTIMENTOS/2004GOVERNANCACORPORATIVA/20050414%20GLOSSARIO%20CONSELHEIROS/GLOSS%C3%81RIO%20TEXTIL.DOC

Hertz, H, Russomano, T, Porto, F, Gurgel, JL, Steiger, A, et al. (2005). Development of shadow Moiré technique as an alternative low-cost method for postural evaluation. *Scientia Medica*, Vol 15, No. pp. 235-242,

Hertz, HRG. (2005). Construction and calibration of the shadow moiré technique for postural analysis [thesis]. Porto Alegre: Pontifical Catholic University (PUCRS)

Hulley, SB, Newman, TB & Cummings, SR. (2003). Choosing the study subjects: specification, sampling and recruitment, In *Outlining the clinical research: an epidemiological approach*, Hulley, SB, Cummings, SR, Browner, WS, Grady, D, Hearst, N & Newman, TB, pp. (55-68), Artmed, Porto Alegre

Ikeda, T & Terada, H. (1981). Development of Moiré method with special reference to its application to biostereometrics. *Opt Laser Technol*, Vol No. pp. 302-306,

Kilpeäinen, PVJ, Laine-Alava, MT & Lammi, S. (1996). Palatal morphology and type clefting. *Cleft Palate Craniofac J*, Vol 33, No. 6, pp. 477-482,

Kim, H & al., et. (2004). Scoliosis detection based on difference of apexes position and angle on Moiré topographic images. *Int Congr Ser*, Vol No. pp. 1268:1294,

Kim, H, Tan, JK, Ishikawa, S, Khalid, M, Otsuka, Y, et al. (2006). Automatic judgment of spinal deformity based on back propagation on neural network. *IJICIC*, Vol 2, No. 6, pp. 1271-1279,

Kim, HS, Ishikawa, S, Ohtsuka, Y, Shimizu, H, Shinomiya, T, et al. (2001). Automatic scoliosis detection based on local centroids evaluation on Moiré topographic images of human backs. *IEEE Trans Med Imaging*, Vol 20, No. 12, pp. 1314-1320,

Kleiman, A. (1989). *Reading: teaching and research* Pontes, Campinas, São Paulo

Kotwicki, T., Negrini, S., Grivas, T. B., Rigo, M., Maruyama, T., et al. (2009). Methodology of evaluation of morphology of the spine and the trunk in idiopathic scoliosis and other spinal deformities - 6th SOSORT consensus paper. *Scoliosis*, Vol 4, No. pp. 26, 1748-7161 (Electronic) 1748-7161 (Linking)

Kovac, V. & Pecina, M. (1999). Moire topography in measurement of the sagittal curvatures of the spine. *Coll Antropol*, Vol 23, No. 1, (Jun), pp. 153-158, 0350-6134 (Print)

Lim, Jae Sun , Kim, Jongsu & Chung, Myung Sai (1989). Automatic shadow moire topography: a moving-light-source method. *Opt Lett*, Vol 14, No. 22 (November 15), pp. 1252-1253,

Lino, ACL & Fabbro, IMD. (2004). Fruit profilometry based on shadow Moiré techniques. *Ciênc Agrotec*, Vol 28, No. 1, pp. 119-125,

Mínguez, MF, Buendía, M, Cibrián, RM, Salvador, R, Laguía, M, et al. (2007). Quantifier variables of the back surface deformity obtained with a noninvasive structured light method: evaluation of their usefulness in idiopathic scoliosis diagnosis. *Eur Spine J*, Vol 16, No. pp. 73–82,

Ortiz, MH & Patterson, EA. (2005). Location and shape measurement using a portable fringe projection system. *Exp Mech*, Vol 45, No. 3, pp. 197-204,

Oster, G. (1988). Moiré pattern, In *Optics source book – Science reference series*, Parker, SP, pp. (379-381), McGraw-Hill, USA

Patias, Petros, Grivas, Theodoros B, Kaspiris, Angelos, Aggouris, Costas & Drakoutos, Evangelos. (2010). A review of the trunk surface metrics used as Scoliosis and other deformities evaluation indices. *Scoliosis*, Vol 5, No. 12, pp.

Pearsall, DJ, Reid, JG & Hedden, DM. (1992). Comparison of three noninvasive methods for measuring scoliosis. *Phys Ther*, Vol 72, No. 9, pp. 648-657,

Porto, Flávia. (2003). Journal of Biomechanics production between 2000 and 2001 concerning to issue "body balance" [thesis]. Rio de Janeiro: Rio de Janeiro State University (UERJ)

Porto, Flávia. (2008). Postural Assessment of the elderly of Porto Alegre-RS using the Shadow Moiré Technique [thesis]. Porto Alegre-RS: PUCRS

Porto, Flávia, Gurgel, Jonas Lírio, Sepúlveda, G, Gonçalves, Fabiano, Flores, Felipe Lima, et al. (2007). Postural evaluation of men aged between 60 and 65 years old of Porto Alegre-RS based on Shadow Moiré Technique. International Symposium on Biomechanics in Sports, Ouro Preto, Minas Gerais,

Rössler, T, Hrabovský, M & Pochmon, M. (2006). Moiré methods for measurement for displacement and topography. *Czech J Phys*, Vol 56, No. 2, pp. 101-216,

Ruggerone, M. & Austin, J. H. (1986). Moire topography in scoliosis. Correlations with vertebral lateral curvature as determined by radiography. *Phys Ther*, Vol 66, No. 7, (Jul), pp. 1072-1077, 0031-9023 (Print)

Sciammarella, CA. (1982). The Moiré method – a review. *Exp Mech*, Vol No. pp. 418-433,

Takasaki, H. (1973). Moire Topography. *Appl Opt*, Vol 12, No. 4, pp. 845-850,

Takasaki, H. (1970). Moiré Topography. *Appl Opt*, Vol 9, No. 6, pp. 1467-1472,

Takasaki, H. (1982). Moiré topography from its birth to practical application. *Opt Lasers Eng*, Vol 3, No. pp. 3-14,

Takasaki, H. (1976). Simultaneous all-around measurement of a living body by Moiré topography. Congress of the International Society of Photogrammetry, Helsinki,

Turner-Smith, AR. (1997). Structured light surface measurement techniques, In *Optical measurement methods in biomechanics*, Orr, JF & Shelton, JC, pp. (39-58), Chapman & Hall, Weinheim, Germany

Uetake, U, Ohtsuki, F, Tanaka, H & Shindo, M. (1998). The vertebral curvature of sportsmen. *J Sports Sci*, Vol 16, No. pp. 621-628,

Wood, J, Saha, S, Rao, R & Grillo, D. (2001). Investigation of non-homogenous strain distributions in bone using Moiré Interferometry. Vol No. Retrieved from <s/p>

Yeras, AM, Peña, RG & Junco, R. (2003). Moiré topography: alternative technique in health care. *Opt Lasers Eng*, Vol 40, No. pp. 105-116,

8

Three-Dimensional Assessment of the Scoliosis

Jean Legaye
University of Louvain, Mont-Godinne
Belgium

1. Introduction

Scoliosis is a twisting deformation of the spine, including all the related anatomical structures (bones, muscles, ligaments, organs). It is essentially three-dimensional, non reducible and progressive, opposite to "scoliotic attitudes" which are simple compensatory deviation in the frontal plane to lower leg asymmetry, or to secondary deformities corrected after resolving of the cause (infection, prolapsed intervertebral disc, osteoid osteoma, etc.). (Figure 1)

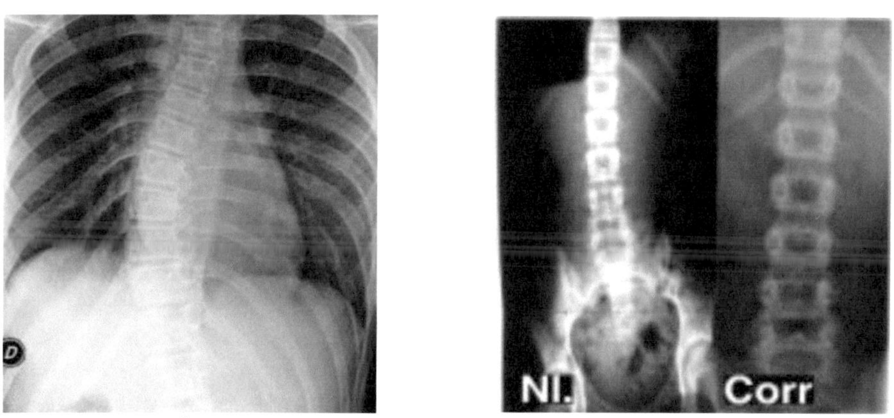

A. B.

Fig. 1. A. Real scoliotic deviation, with vertebral rotation and costal deformation. B. Scoliotic attitude without vertebral rotation and correction by rectification of the leg length asymmetry.

The spinal 3D distortions and mostly their esthetical repercussions are the main patient's complaints, leading to the diagnosis: the rib hump, the asymmetry of the shoulders or of the flanks. This was well known in the historic medicine (already by Hippocrates in the ancient Greece) (Vasiliadis 2009), and the therapeutics were acting to correct these tree-dimensional distortions by traction and derotating bands. (Figure 2)

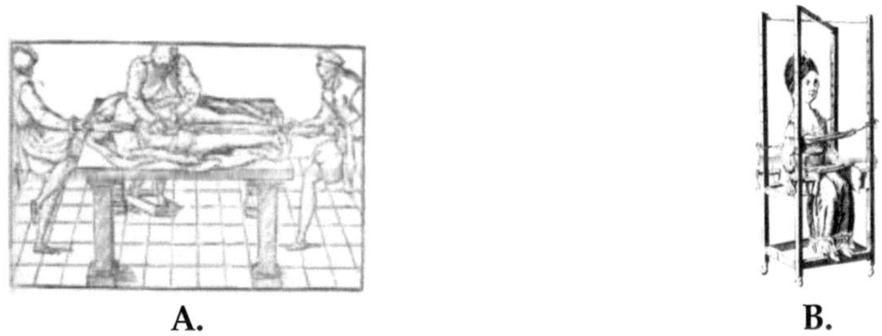

Fig. 2. 3D historic corrections of scoliotic deformation by axial traction and derotating maneuvers (A.) or bands (B.).

Nevertheless, this tree-dimensional appearance was perverted by the use of the radiographic projections. Considering scoliosis only as a frontal deformation had a negative impact on the therapeutic processes, especially surgery.

The assessment of the spine in 3D through reconstruction models is so of first importance for the diagnosis, the follow-up and the treatment of the scoliosis.

2. The anatomical 3D deformities

3D models of reconstruction of the spine provide a virtual representation of the overall organization of the vertebrae distorted in diverse ways by distinctive distortions affecting the spine, the pelvis, the rib cage, the ligaments and the muscles. Such individual anatomical deformations are not apprehended nor by the imaging techniques nor by the 3D reconstructions. Only the knowledge of the evolution of the vertebral deformities allows an individualized analysis of the global 3D virtual representations and their use for a diagnostic, a prognostic or a therapeutic procedure.

2.1 From the "normal" to the scoliosis

Asymmetry is systematic in all individuals. A common significant trunk asymmetry was described in juveniles, which is changing into the adolescent pattern at a later age for boys than in girls. (Grivas 2006, 2008) Boulay (2006) described a systematic total asymmetry involving the right and the left pelvis. It follows a spiral path always in the same way for all the individuals: in the upper part, the iliac blades rotate clockwise; in the lower part, the pubic symphysis rotates anticlockwise. Nevertheless, such asymmetry is not source of spinal distortions, even if a twist occurs in the pelvis during the walk. (Figure 3)

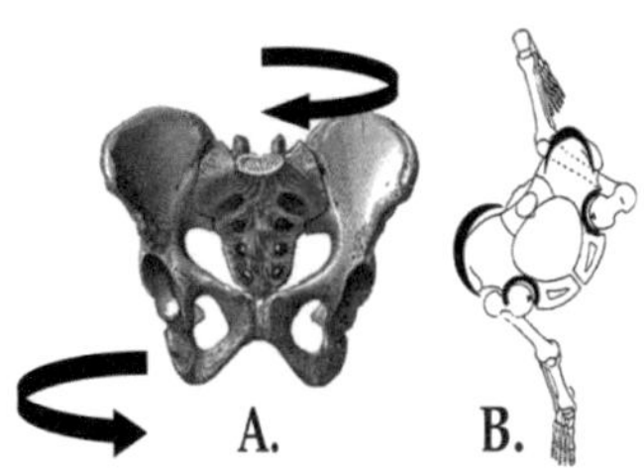

Fig. 3. Systematic morphological asymmetry of the pelvis (A.) and its repercussion on the walk (B.) occurring in all normal subjects.

Moreover, distorted vertebrae in congenital scoliosis, acting as local deforming corners, don't induce surrounding deformities once they are well balanced. (Figure 4 A.) Otherwise, the spinal curvatures of neurological or muscular origin occur in particular area and are typical by their long extension (Figure 4 B.) and often in the contrary side than the "idiopathic" scoliosis or the degenerative scoliosis of the elderly. (Figure 4 C. D.)

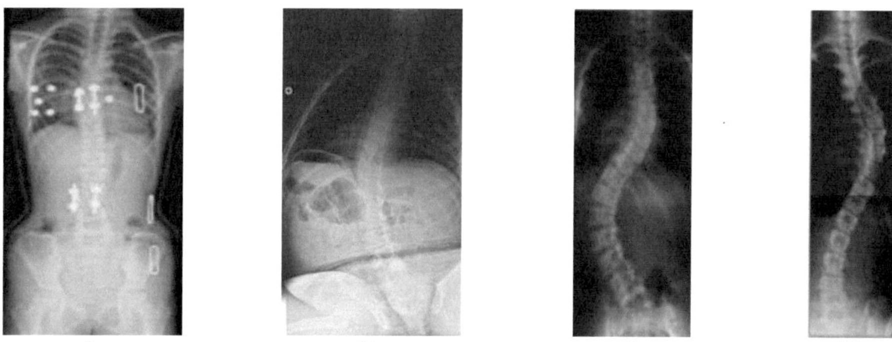

A. B. C. D.

Fig. 4. A. Congenital scoliosis with double asymmetric vertebra stabilised and well balanced, without other associated deformations - B. Long curve of a neuro-muscular scoliosis – Left lumbar (C.) and right thoracic (D.) idiopathic scoliosis.

Such developmental scoliosis are essentially three-dimensional and their progression is so explicable once the distorting process is initialized. In the animals, they occur only in bipedal species, as experimentally by Machida (1994) and Lafortune (2007) in the pinealectomized chicken. (Figure 5)

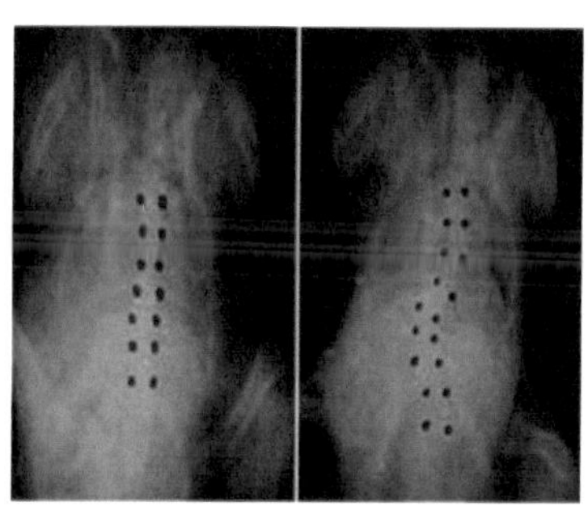

Fig. 5. Radiography of normal and scoliotic pinealectomized chicken.

Some anatomical particularities are encountered in scoliotic cases, as the asymmetric morphology of the facet joints (lumbar at one side, thoracic at the other side) at the lumbo-thoracic level, but they are insufficient to explain the origin of the disease.

Grivas (2002) assumed that the deformity of the thorax develops first and then the deformity of the spine follows. He emphasised the role of the diurnal variation and the asymmetric water distribution in the discs and the subsequent alteration of the mechanical environment of the adjacent vertebral growth plates, especially in the apex of the curve. (Grivas 2006c, 2008c) The deformation of the apical intervertebral disc seems so to be an important contributory factor in the progression of a scoliotic curve. (Will 2009)

2.2 The structural curve and the deformed vertebra

Contrary to other deformations (as the scoliotic attitudes or the curves induced by diseases as infection, tumour or disc protrusion), the true idiopathic scoliosis is characterized by a structured area, i.e. stiff and not reducible, which the vertebrae are gradually irremediably distorted. So, the scoliosis becomes more and more structured.

Vertebral deformity consists in a vertebral body asymmetry, a deformation of the articular processes, a torsion of the entire vertebra involving the discs, the ligaments and the other related structures as the ribs. (Figure 6)

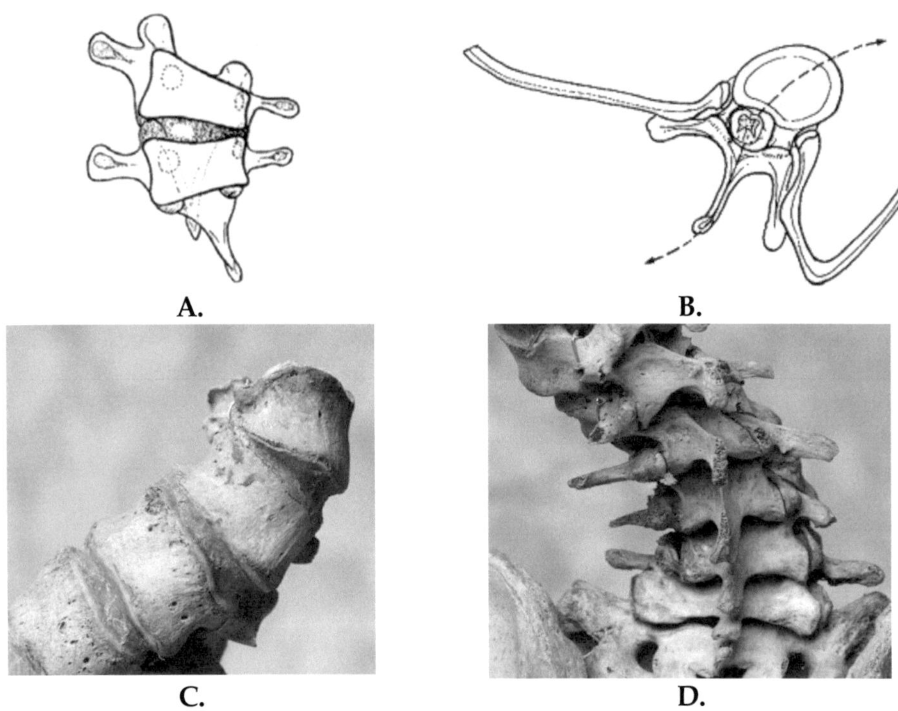

Fig. 6. Structural deformation of the scoliotic vertebrae. A. Cuneiform deformation of the vertebral body. B. Transversal torsion phenomenon of the entire vertebra involving the ribs. C. Torsion of the vertebral body and discal structures. C. Asymmetric deformation of the posterior articular and arch.

This structured deformation of the vertebra is so three dimensional and irreversible, defining the really structural principal curvature in case of multiple curves. On the contrary, the secondary or compensatory curves do not exhibit this anatomical irreversibility and are correctible, even partially.

It is noticeable that the entire spine is organized to lead ultimately to a horizontal gaze. These patterns of adaptation are three-dimensional and allow understanding the distorting process.

2.3 The key vertebrae

A scoliotic curvature is classically defined by its apical vertebra and its limits, or junctional, vertebra. (Figure 7) The rotation is maximal at the apical vertebra and near insignificant at the ends of curvature.

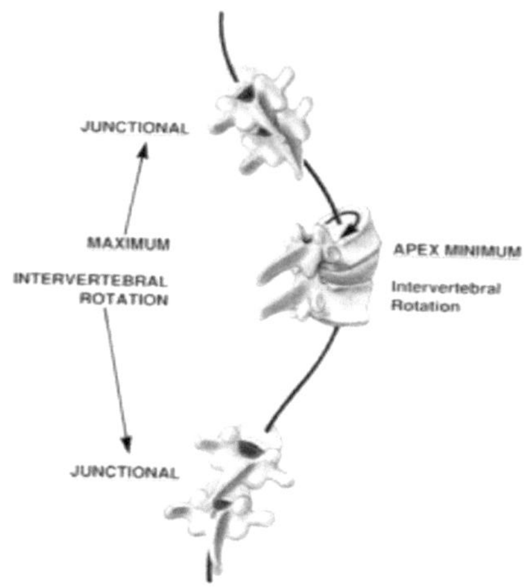

Fig. 7. The junctional and apical vertebrae of a scoliotic curve.

These definitions allow defining the topography of the curves and the classifications of the scoliosis, proposed in the literature to improve in the therapeutics, mostly surgical.

2.4 The classifications of the structural scoliosis

The classical classification simply describes the topography of the structural curve (lumbar, thoraco-lumbar, thoracic, double curve).

King's scoliosis classification is similar and defines 5 types of idiopathic scoliosis, whereby the severity of a case is based on the following parameters:

- Cobb angle on x-ray image
- Determination of "flexibility index" on bending radiographs

King's classification was proposed to establish the limits of the fusion in surgical procedures. (King 1983)

The disadvantages is that it doesn't not included the sagittal plane in the evaluation and don't consider the scoliosis with two or three major curves.

In 2001, Lenke introduced a new classification system for idiopathic scoliosis which is much more complex. It is based on survey spine radiographs in 2 planes, as well as right and left side bending radiographs with the following parameters: localization, degree and flexibility

- The curve apex is defined as follows for localization purposes:
  - Upper thoracic localization: curve apex between T2 and T6
  - Thoracic localization: curve apex between T6 and inter-vertebral disc T11/12
  - Thoraco-lumbar localization: curve apex between T12 and L1

- Lumbar localization: curve apex between inter-vertebral disc L1/2 and L4

- The determination of the flexibility of the curve is assessed either based on the residual curve in the bending radiograph or the extent of kyphosis. A curve is defined as structural if the bending Cobb angle exceeds 25° or the kyphosis angle exceeds 20°.

2.5 The Satagnara's plane of maximal curvature

However, these definitions are based on the radiographic 2D projections of the curves, regardless of their three-dimensional condition. Already in 1965, Stagnara defined the "plane of choice" of the curvatures, or plane of maximal curvature. (Figure 8 A.) Indeed, a curve may remain unchanged but rotating within the body. This will result in a feeling of increase or decrease of the curve in its radiographic lateral and antero-posterior (AP) 2D projection. Moreover, such structural curves are frequently stiffened by vertebral spontaneous fusions. (Figure 8 B)

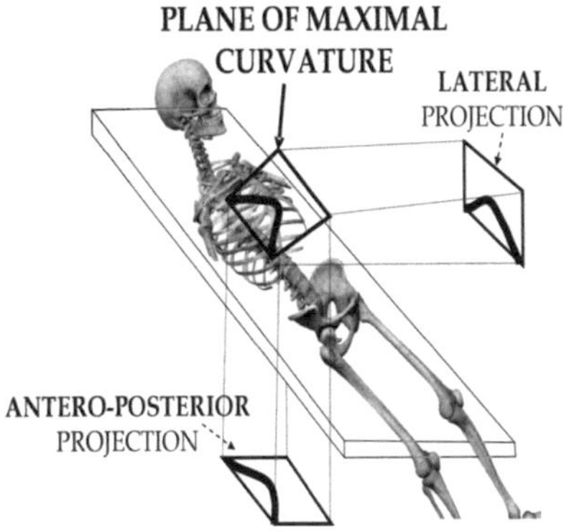

A.

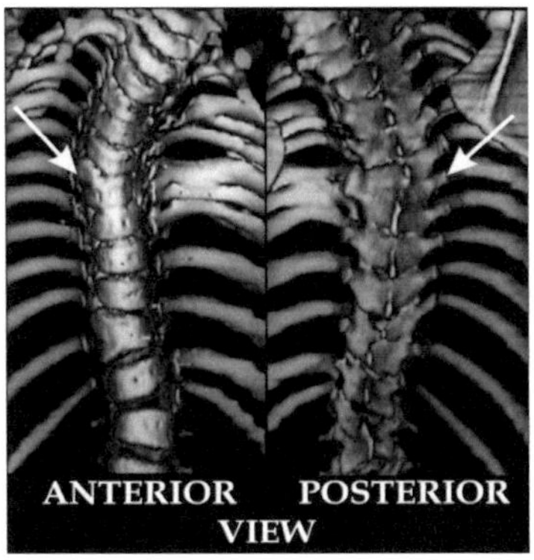

B.

Fig. 8. A. The plane of maximal curvature and it lateral and AP projection. B. The stiff area of a curve by spontaneous fusion of the apical vertebral bodies and posterior arch.

This rotational effect is to be distinguished from a real aggravation. This requires defining three-dimensionally the "plane of choice" of the curvature, the area of stiffness or of suppleness, the inter-vertebral mobility. It emphasizes the necessity of a 3D appraisal of the spine for a real evaluation of the scoliosis. The anatomy of the scoliosis is so to be conceived on two levels: firstly as a mobilization between the vertebrae related to loading forces, secondly as structural deformations of the discs, the ligaments and the bony structures induced by unbalanced loads and corrective compensation. It is the purpose of the three-dimensional reconstruction models of the spine to explain and to quantify these 3D distortions of the scoliosis for a better diagnostic and prognostic evaluation, for an adjustment of the corrective processes by corsets or for the surgical planning.

2.6 The reference system

The reference system is universally used and was proposed by Stoke in the Scoliosis Research Society in 1994. It describes the planes and axis reference systems, for the whole body (global system), for regional (as the spine, the scoliotic curves…) or local structures (as a vertebra). (Figure 9) This reference system was so defined: the X axis follows the gravity line, the Y- and Z-axes point toward respectively left and cephalad directions. The origins of the axes of global or local systems were defined according to the involved anatomical structures. The orientation of X, Y and Z axis are identical for all axis systems.

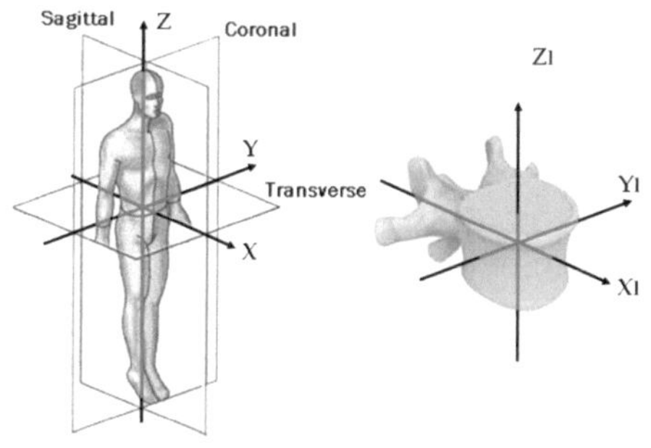

A. B.

Fig. 9. The referential planes and axes in A. the global referential system (X, Y, Z) and in B. the local vertebral system (Xl, Yl, Zl).

2.7 The vertebral rotation

The vertebral rotation is to be distinguished from intrinsic spinal anatomical torsion, even they are progressively entangled.

2.7.1 The apparent rotation

Several techniques were proposed for the measurement of the vertebral rotation, using the radiographic projections of the spinal structures. It is the "apparent rotation".

First techniques used the relative projection of the spinous process into the vertebral body shadow. Nevertheless, it involves the structured torsion of the vertebrae.

Most accurate techniques estimate the relationship between the shadows of the pedicles and the edges of the vertebral body. (Nash & Moe 1969) (Figure 10)

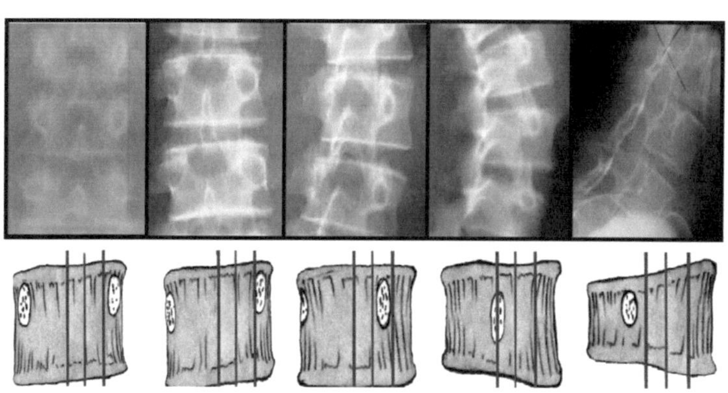

Fig. 10. Projection of the shadows of the pedicles into the vertebral bodies according to the increasing axial rotation.

Several authors proposed a variety of geometrical formulae using diverse anatomical vertebral structures projected in AP radiographs to develop a quantitative measurement of axial rotation, implicitly referred to the global referential system (Drerup 1984). Perdriolle (1987) propose a device named "torsiometer" allowing an easy measurement on AP radiographs. (Figure 11)

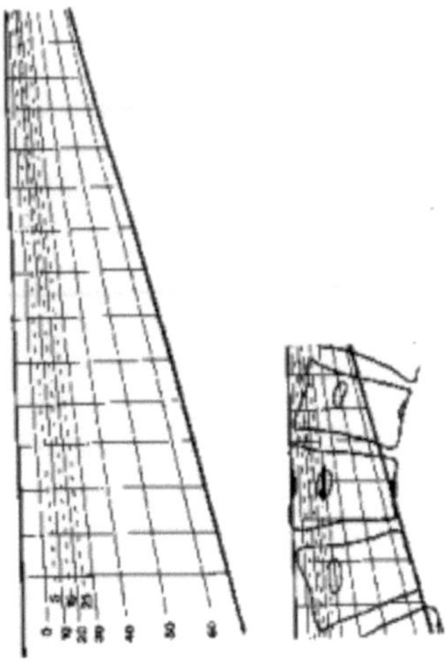
A. B.

Fig. 11. A. The Perdriolle's torsiometer. B. Measurement of the rotation with the torsiometer using the edges of the vertebral body and the most visible pedicular shadow.

The use of CT scan and MRI was proposed for measurement of rotation, but radiography is still the more commonly used method. (Lam 2008)

2.7.2 The induced rotation

The induced rotation depends of the 3D tilts of vertebra in its local vertebral referential system. Its direction is definite by the order in which these tilts occur: the absolute rotations produced by tilting an object in its sagittal plane and then in its frontal plane, and vice versa, are similar but in opposite directions. (Figure 12 A) A formula describes this rotation:

$$\text{Sin}\ (\textit{induced rotation}) = \frac{\sin(\textit{frontal tilt})x\sin(\textit{lateral tilt})}{1+\cos(\textit{frontal tilt})x\cos(\textit{lateral tilt})}$$

where the lateral and frontal tilts are expressed in the local reference system and the "induced rotation" in the global system. (Hecquet 1998)

The position of each vertebra in a scoliotic curve changes at the same time in both frontal and sagittal planes, thus producing an "induced rotation" which is greater at the junctional (or end) vertebra.

Once more, the orientation of the radiographic rays introduces an artifact on the classical rotation measurement techniques like Perdriolle's one. (Figure 12 B) This figure represents the projected view of the same curvature, but the impact of the X-rays is different: both intensity and side of the projected curve changes, as well as the apparent rotation. Otherwise, the measurement of the successive induced rotations from the bottom of the curvature does not change. The induced rotation is a really 3D measurement, while the usual radiographic techniques are 2D measurements with artefacts. It allows also explaining the paradox of true scoliosis with rib hump induced by the curvature while the apparent rotation is zero: this is also due to the artefact induced by the incidence of the X-rays on the 2D projection. (Figure 12 C)

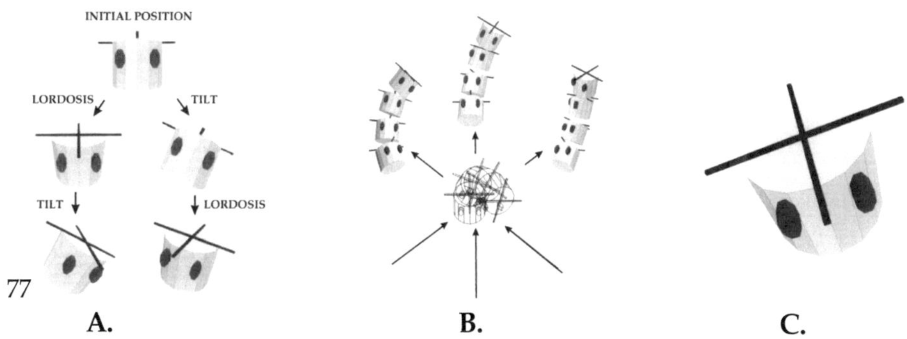

Fig. 12. A. Induced rotation by successive lordotic and lateral tilts of a vertebra depending of the order of local tilts. B. Projections according different impacts of X-Rays showing different 2D parameter of the same curve. C. Real induced rotation for which the apparent rotation is zero using the 2D measurements techniques.

2.8 Rotation and torsion

Rotation is characteristic of the scoliosis. In a normal movement of a disco-vertebral unit, the 3D rotations are associated (flexion-extension, lateral bending and rotation), related to the orientation of the posterior articular processes. The axis of motion is mobile according to the movement but confined at the posterior third of the disc (centrode). The local combination of an antero-posterior with a lateral tilting induces a 3D "induced rotation". These 3D rotations are reversible according to the disco-ligamentar flexibility. *Torsion* is the intrinsic twisting deformation of the vertebrae induced by the asymmetrical bone growth. These anatomical distortions are irreversible: it characterizes the structural deformation. (Figure 13) Tedious CT measurement methods were described (Doi 2011)

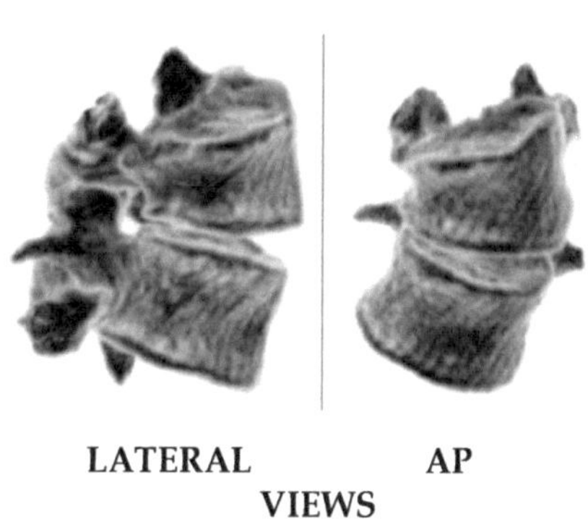

Fig. 13. Irreversible axial torsion of the vertebrae in structural scoliotic curve.

2.9 The 3D bodily scoliosis

Both rotation and torsion have repercussion on the adjacent spinal structures, as well on their own sagittal and lateral displacement inside the body. So are created the 3D deformations characterizing the aesthetic disturbances leading the patient to consult and allowing diagnosing the scoliosis by its 3d repercussions. (Figure 14)

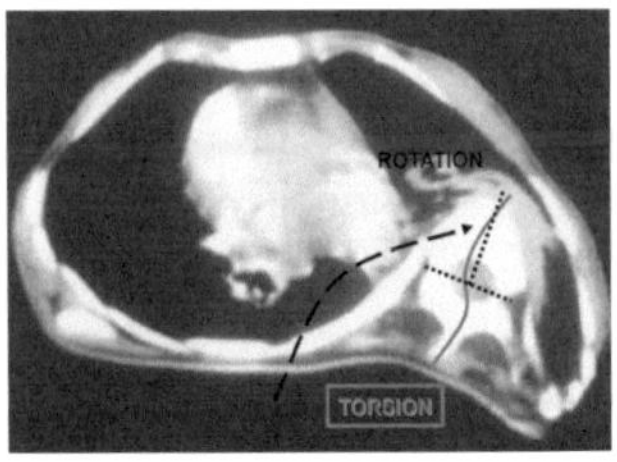

Fig. 14. CT scan of a thoracic curve induced by vertebral torsion, rotation and displacement involving the bony structures (vertebrae, ribs) and the organs (heart, lung, muscles). These 3D phenomenons occur all together. The flexible and reversible rotation predominates in the early development of the scoliosis in growing ages. The three-dimensional clinical analysis aims to quantify these events from imaging spinal reconstruction techniques. Assessment of the scoliosis using 3D models has a prognostic value and aims to increase the correction of therapeutic techniques, conferring to the 3D analysis of the spine an essential role.

3. The techniques for 3D reconstructions

3.1 CT Scan and MRI 3D reconstructions

CT scan and MRI could be used to assess the spine in 3D. Nevertheless, they are performed in lying position, not allowing assessing the balance in standing position. CT scan of MRI has only interest for a precise morphological description of malformations, tumours or infection inducing scoliosis. In congenital scoliosis, such 3D technique determine the individual morphology of unsegmented fused area or deformed parts of vertebrae, and the associated malformations, as for the ribs. (Figure 15)

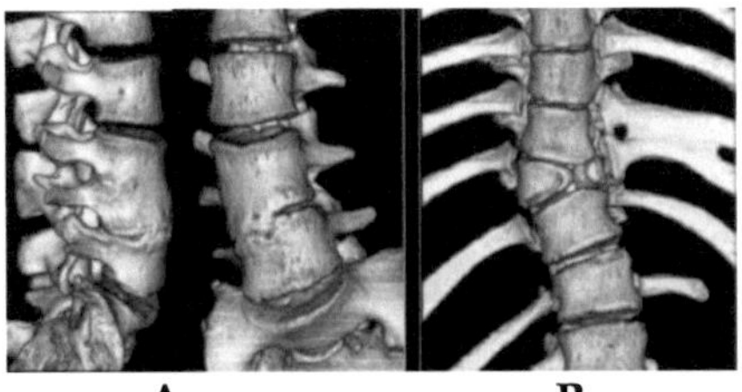

A. B.

Fig. 15. 3D reconstruction by CT scan of congenital scoliosis: A. Unsegmented area between two vertebrae by loss of segmentation. B. asymmetrical vertebral bodies and fusion of ribs.

3.2 The radiographic techniques

3D reconstruction techniques allow a virtual assessment of the spine. Classically, such 3D reconstructions are performed from multi-planar (usually orthogonal) standing radiographies. (Figure 16)

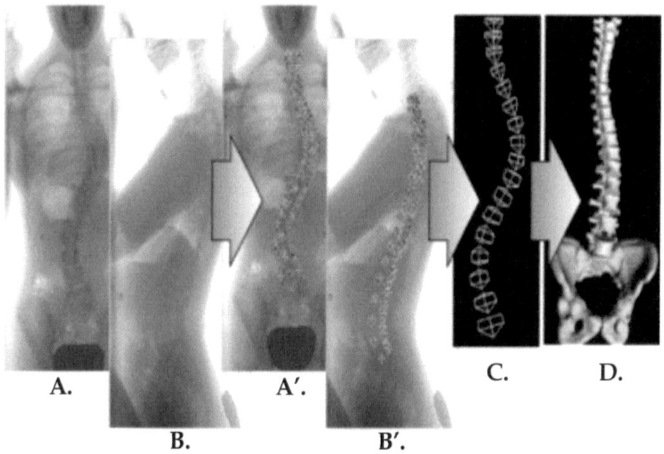

Fig. 16. "Standard" main steps of 3D modelling process of the vertebral structures: (A. B.) radiographic orthogonal AP (A.) and lateral (B.) views
(A′. B′.) manual identification of six anatomical landmarks per vertebra,
(C.) "standard" 3D reconstruction of the anatomical landmarks,
(D.) visualization of the geometric model

Various techniques are proposed:

- *the stereo radiographic techniques*: they use 4 to 25 anatomical points for a vertebra to reconstruct the 3D spinal structures. The *non stereo-corresponding techniques* use algorithms developed from the knowledge a priori of the anatomy. (Mitton 2000, Mitulescu 2001) The anatomical vertebral landmarks are either "corresponding anatomical points" (identifiable both in frontal and lateral views), either "not corresponding points" (identifiable only on one of the radiographic view). (Figure 17)

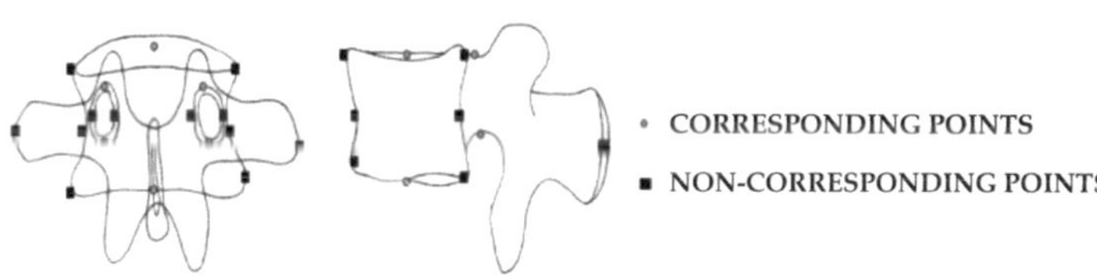

Fig. 17. Corresponding and non corresponding points on an AP and lateral radiographic shadows of a vertebra for a stereo-graphic 3D reconstruction technique.

However, it is relatively long to implement and therefore not used in everyday clinical practice. Moreover, its precision is related to the ability of the observer to identify the anatomical structures on the radiographs (especially difficult in upper thoracic area, or in case of major deformity).

- *The semi-automatic statistical techniques* are faster to use. Reconstructions are performed from some not anatomically corresponding points (the corners of the vertebral bodies) related to a morphological database by interpolation and optimalization. It supposes a priori knowledge of the structure of the objects and of their deformation. (Pomero 2004) The 3D representations can eventually be individually adjusted during handling according to the X-ray imaging for better reliability. (Blanchard 2008, Dumas 2008)

Then, a customization process improves the visual appearance of the bony reconstruction. (Figure 18)

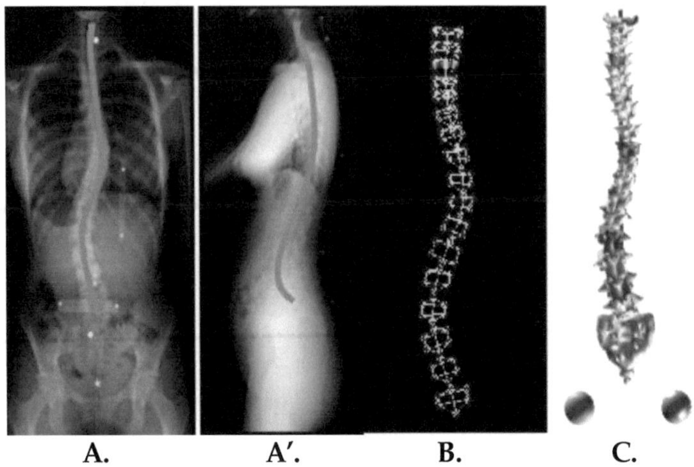

Fig. 18. Statistical method for 3D spine reconstruction: spinal "spline" determined on the AP (A.) and lateral (A'.) radiological view. B. 3D reconstruction linked to a statistical database. C. Customization of the vertebrae.

The accuracy of these techniques, tested on models, was similar to the precision of manual stereo-radiographic techniques: 1 degree for lateral and sagittal tilts and 3 degrees for the axial rotation of each vertebra. (Labelle 1995, Dumas 2004)

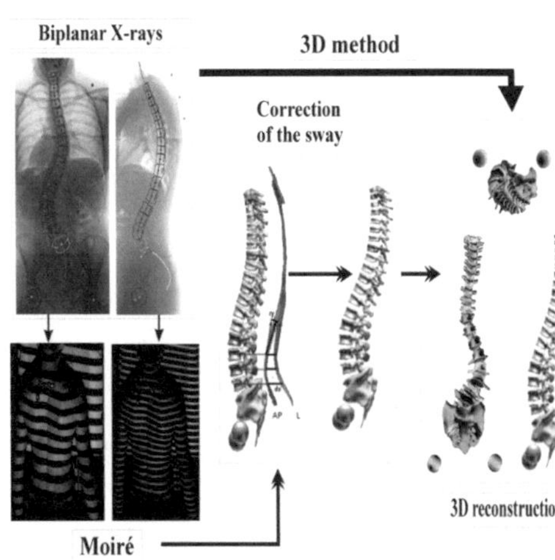

Fig. 19. 3D reconstruction with hybrid X-ray / Moiré imaging for a scoliotic patient: the trunk deformation due to the sway of the subject between the exposures was detected by the Moiré imaging - the correction factors assessed by the Moiré method was then applied to the 3D reconstruction for an optimal accuracy.

However, the mobilization or the sway of the subject between the two X-rays or during their completion is a source of artefact, and so of inaccuracy. Such a tilt of 10 degrees between AP and lateral radiographic exposure is usual. (Bellefleur 2002) To correct this source of lack of precision, the use of an optical assessment of the skin surface of the back (morphometry by Moiré technique) simultaneously to the X-rays has been proposed. (Legaye 2009) A common calibration tool unifies the two referential systems for automatic corrective procedure. So the precision was 1.3 mm for the 3D location of the vertebrae and 1.5 degrees for the tilts and rotation. For a sway greater than 10 degrees, the improvement persists, but a risk of lack of accuracy exists and is detected by the method. (Figure 19)

A recent imaging system (EOS) allows simultaneous lateral and antero-posterior radiographic views of the whole body in standing position, including the lower limbs and notably reducing the irradiation from 8 to 10 times. (Dubousset 2008) The classical radiographic 3D techniques are usable, but it doesn't avoid the consequence of a moving of the subject during the procedure

3.3 The optical surface topography techniques

3.3.1 Interest of 3D trunk evaluation by non invasive techniques

Although scoliosis is characterized by a 3D deviation of the spine, its results clinically in a deformation responsible for geometric and morphologic changes of the trunk and rib cage witch lead to initial complaints. (Nault 2002) The trunk symmetry is what it is seen and praised by the child, not the radiograph itself which is traditionally used by the physician. Moreover, the cosmetic improvement of the trunk after any treatment is of paramount importance for the child under treatment and his family. (Figure 20)

For the medical physician also, trunk analysis can help to document the external asymmetry associated with different types of spinal curves in scoliosis as well as the cosmetic improvement obtained after surgical interventions. (Pazos 2007).

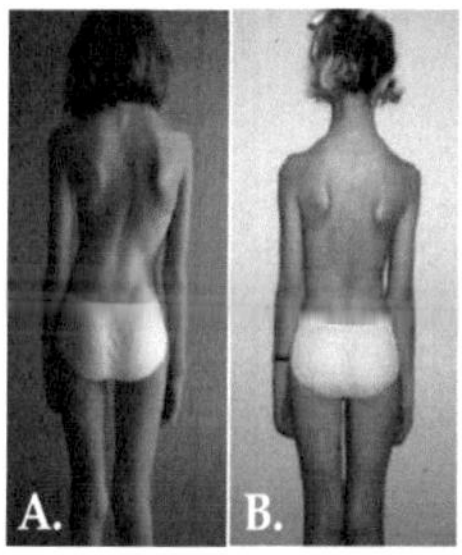

Fig. 20. Pre (A.) and post-operative (B.) back shape of a scoliotic case.

Otherwise, school screening was proposed for an early diagnosis of scoliosis and to improve the results by early treatments. But such screening, and eventual subsequent follow-up, should need multiples X-rays. Unfortunately, cumulative X-rays were reported increasing the risk of future cancers, particularly of the breast in girls. (Denton 1992) Therefore, the use of optical techniques was proposed for such screening.

Such optical techniques for the assessment of the skin surface topography of the back assume that the trunk deformities reflect the underlying bone deformations. Specific parameters were proposed, some specific, some analogous to those measured on radiographs but not similar because both techniques evaluate different structures (the bony spine for the X-ray techniques, the skin surface for the optical techniques).

3.3.2 Optical techniques

Optical systems have been developed as non-invasive imaging techniques. Such systems are the Moiré-fringe mapping, the structured light techniques or Integrated Shape Imaging System (ISIS) (Turner-Smith 1984, 1988, Weisz 1988, Theologis 1997, Berryman 2008), 360° scanning devices (Poncet 2000) and stereo-photogrammetric systems (Frobin 1983). Laser techniques were also developed for corset manufacturing, but not for clinical use.

3.3.3 The "Moiré fringe" technique

Moiré-fringes procedures are most often used for 3D assessment of the back morphology. Moiré is an optical contrast effect changing with the deformation of an object. The moiré is created by dark and light lines resulting from the superposition and interference of two networks of light (generally a set of parallel lines). This can be used to analyze the deformation of an object. (Figure 21)

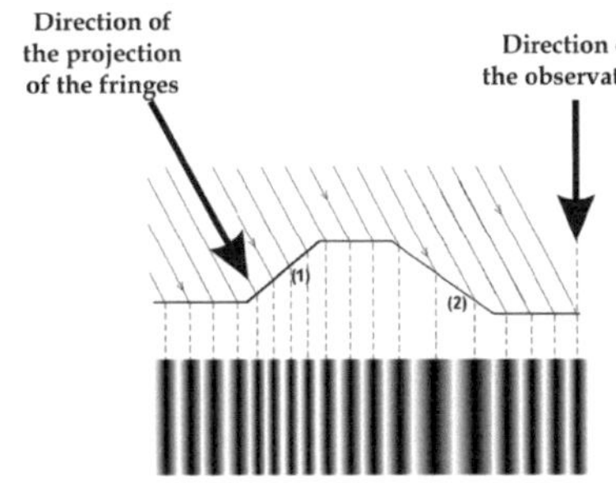

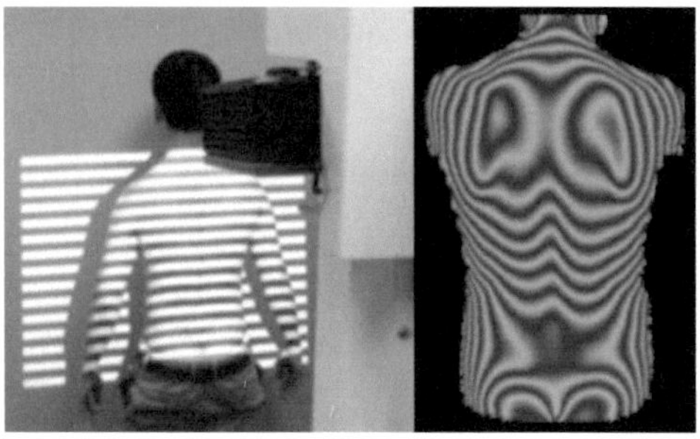

A. B. C.

Fig. 21. A. The theoretical principle of the Moiré-fringe. B. Its use for the back surface analysis. C. The imaging of the back surface relief.

The moiré topography was abundantly described for the analysis of the back shape in scoliosis. (Sahlstrand 1986, Breque 2004, Turner-Smith 1984, 1988, Weisz 1988, Theologis 1997, Berryman 2008).

In structural scoliosis, the 3D deformation of the spine is assumed to influence directly and proportionally the morphology of the back. Indeed, back asymmetries are mainly caused by the vertebral rotations. Also, rib hump was reported as the key parameter to detect and to follow the evolution a scoliotic deformation. It has also been reported that patients with double curves have significantly less trunk deformity (both in the transverse and coronal plane) than patients with thoracic and thoraco-lumbar curves of similar Cobb size. Goldberg assumed that assimilation between corresponding optical and radiological parameters is unsuitable because both methods focus on different aspects of the deformity. Nevertheless, the 3D presentation accompanied by numerical data produced by surface topography systems offers a more complete perspective of the deformed back surface and enables a more thorough analysis of the patient's deformity pattern. (Goldberg 2001).

3.3.3.1 3D optical parameters

3D parameters are available for the back shape analysis. Some describe the global deformation of the skin surface, as the rib hump, some appraise the spinous process line (the relief's of the spine between the prominent C7 process at the top, and a point plumb the inter-gluteal fold at the bottom). Sagittal view help to assess the balance and the top view estimates the global spinous process line. (Figure 22)

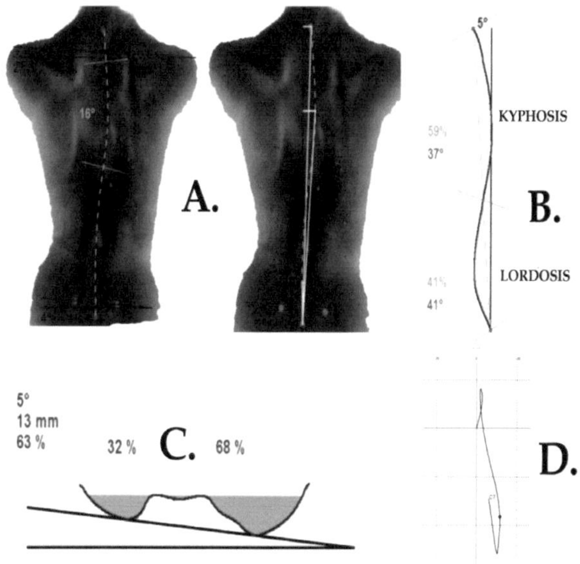

Fig. 22. Some Optical 3D parameters: A. Frontal parameters: spinous line angle and arrows, asymmetry of the shoulders; B. Sagittal parameters: global axis, lordosis, kyphosis; C. Transversal parameters: rib hump in standing position (in mm, degrees and %); D. The top view of the spinous line.

3.3.3.2 Reliability of the optical techniques

It has become apparent from many reports that, although there is a significant correlation between clinical deformity and radiographic measurement, the standard deviation is so high that it is not possible to reliably predict the degree of curvature from only the surface topography in any given patient. (Bunnell 2005)

Nevertheless, 3D Surface topography is mostly useful for scoliosis screening and follow-up in the growth period. Its sensitivity is 90%, its negative predictive value is 90% for curve progression detection. It is reproducible in intra and inter-operators. It can be used to space out and trigger X-ray controls with a mild risk of false negative.

Accurate follow-up is easy, repeatedly, as the technique is absolutely safe, using only the light and not potentially iatrogenic ionizing rays. Imaging is also easily understandable. It raised awareness of the deformation and motivates to the therapeutic process. Moreover, it is closer to the perception of the distortion by the patient, being mainly concerned with the aesthetics 3D deformities induced by the scoliosis rather than the radiological distortion of the spine. (Pazos 2007, Denton 1992, Weisz 1988, Theologis 1997, Sahlstrand 1986)

4. The three-dimensional conception of the spine

Assessing of the scoliosis in its correct 3D reality corrects the artefacts resulting from the two-dimensional X-ray projections. (Graf 1983) By example, the rotation of a rigid vertebral area will be seen on the 2D view as an increase or decrease of the Cobb angle, while the 3D analysis, especially by the top view, will detect the stiffness of this segment and its global rotation. Contrarily, a real correction in a supple area will be better assessed because taking into account the global 3D evolution, especially concerning the inter-vertebral tri-axial rotations.

Similarly, analysis of inter-vertebral rotations will highlight a segmental increasing of instability in the event of a change in the induced rotation. A potential evolution is detected in a forward-looking and therefore treated preventively.

5. The 3D reconstructions parameters

The perception of the spatial position of the vertebrae and their rotations and torsions led to the development of computerized 3D reconstructions of the spine, ideally adjusted of the sway of the patient between the achievements of the AP and lateral imaging.

The standard usual 2D radiographic parameters remain measurable on the 3D reconstructions, including those involving the femoral heads, but upgraded by its specific three-dimensional component. Additional purely 3D parameters have been proposed, particularly the "3D curve area" and the "top view" of the spine.

5.1 The 3D curve area

The spinal curvatures include themselves in flat surfaces. In normal subjects, these areas contain the lordosis and kyphosis, and are essentially sagittal. In case of scoliosis, the areas are disturbed or some are induced by the scoliotic deformation, influenced by the spinal rotations. These plans including the curvatures are easily detected by the 3D reconstruction software. (Figure 23)

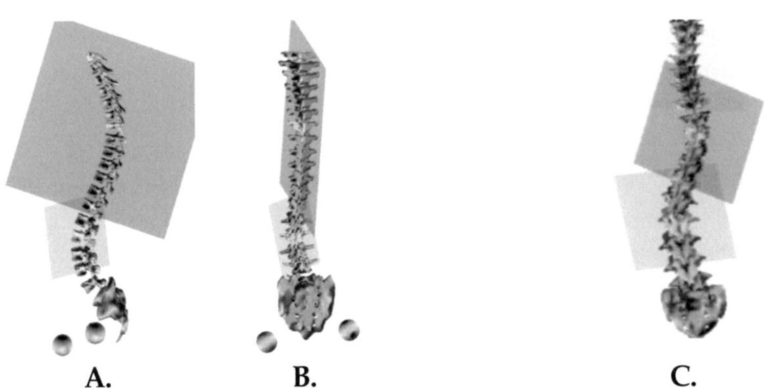

Fig. 23. 3D modification of the lordosis and kyphosis planes (normally strictly sagittal) induced by a lumbar scoliosis in 3D reconstruction lateral (A.) and AP (B.) view. C. Supplementary planes induced by the more marked scoliotic curves.

The extent and 3D orientation of these surface areas including the curves allow assessing worsening or correction of scoliosis, treatment processes, and provide guidance. By comparing successive examinations, a meaningful assessment of the rigidity or flexibility of spinal segments is achievable, as an accurate assessment of its evolution in the 3D conception. The same purpose is available by the optical morphometric technique, using the 3D shape of the spinous process line reflecting the underlying bony spine, the rotation of the body segment (rib hump) reflecting the underlying vertebral rotation.

5.2 The top view

Thanks to computerized spinal analysis, the top view was developed that displays the spine as if the observer were above and looking down on the patient. It is provided by the 3D reconstruction techniques, whatever its origin (X-ray or optical) with more or less sophisticated imaging representations. (Figure 24)

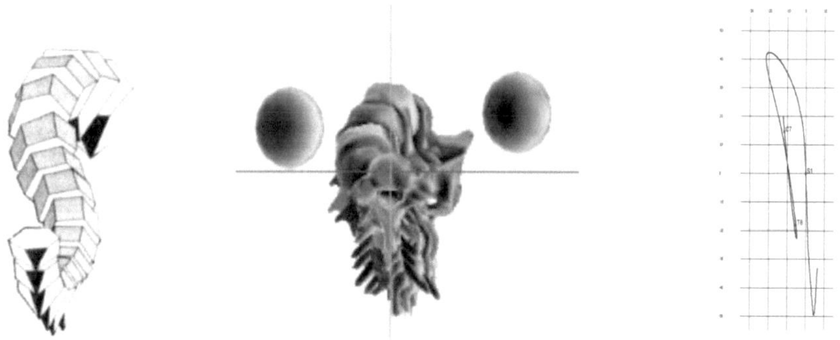

A. B. C.

Fig. 24. Top views from radiographs (A. cubic patterns- B. schematized vertebrae) and C. optical acquisitions (3.2.3.1).

Most software allows to "unstuck" the successive vertebrae to access a personalized view of the 3D rotations and positions of each vertebra into the global spine. Nevertheless, the intrinsic vertebral twist is not represented. (Kohashi 1996)

This top view is essentially three-dimensional. It allows to appreciate the scoliotic deformity as a whole: the importance of the deformation by the tilt from the top of the curve, the plane in which it is included (its extension and 3D orientation), the intensity of the vertebral rotation and the overall tilt. Its evolution is determined really three-dimensionally. It results in a moving of the top of curvature relatively to its limit vertebrae, an accentuation of the global rotation of the curvature, an extension to the adjacent levels. (Figure 25)

In addition to the 3D detection of progression or destabilization of a scoliotic curve, the top view makes it possible to understand its mechanism. This better understanding of the individual progression of a scoliosis allows a personalized adaptation of therapeutic action, whether by physical therapy, brace or surgery. The apical vertebra of a lumbar scoliosis moves laterally to the left and backwards with a counter-clockwise rotation (Figure 26 A.), while the apical vertebra of a progressive thoracic scoliosis moves laterally to the right and forwards with a clockwise rotation (Figure 26 B.).

1.

2.

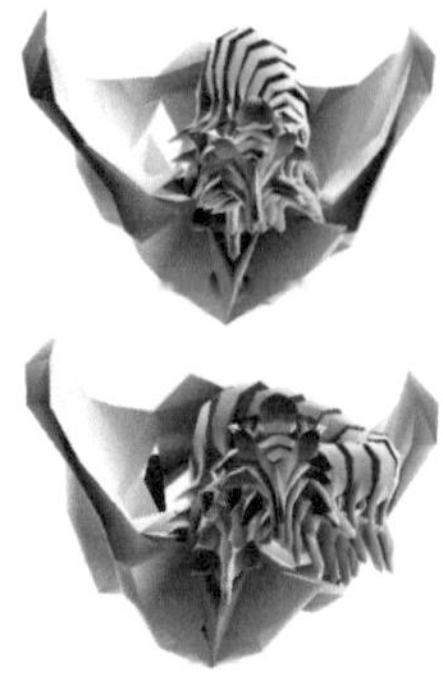

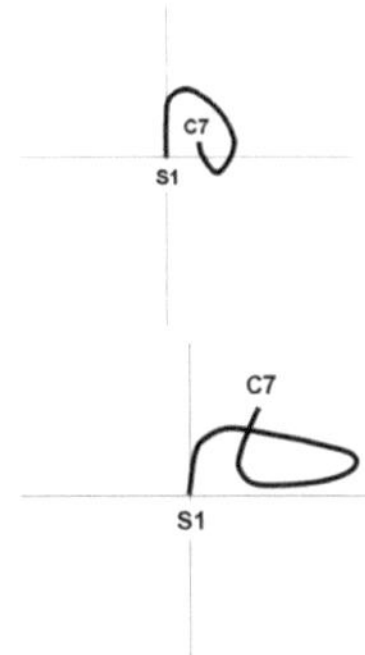

A. B.

Fig. 25. Top view of a progressive scoliosis (1. Original state. 2. final evolution) in vertebral schematic (A.) and filiform (B) representation: increased frontal diameter of the curve - decreased antero-posterior diameter (traducing the change in the orientation of the plan including the curvature) – increased lateral shift of the top of the curve (expressing the increasing of the curve) - loss of the lordotic area (by extension of the thoracic curve in the lumbar area) – forwards global tilt of C7.

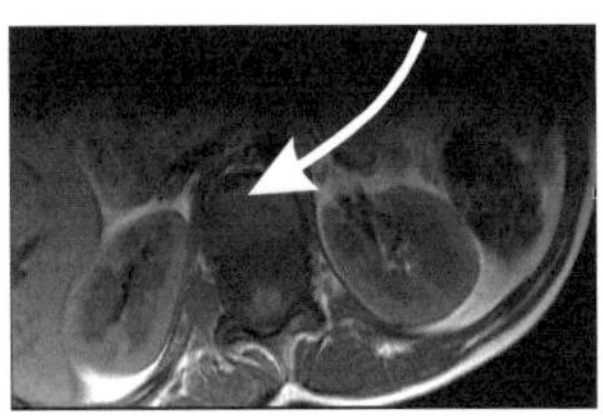

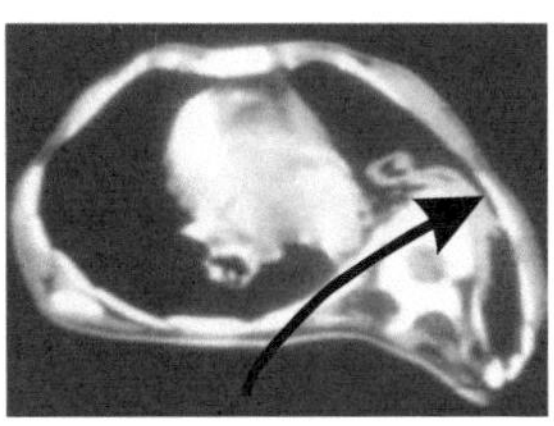

A. B.

Fig. 26. Transversal moving of the apical vertebra of a lumbar scoliosis (A.) and of a thoracic scoliosis (B.)

6. Functional evaluation

It is important for the physician to assess the balance of a scoliosis, both in the frontal as in the sagittal plane, to assess its potential instability, and how to avoid it. In the frontal plane, the "overhangs" between various levels (mostly from C7 to the sacrum) are easily measurable. (Figure 27 A.) In the sagittal plane, the individualized assessment of the balance of the lumbo-pelvic complex was well defined by Duval-Beaupère (1998). All anatomical (Pelvic Incidence) and positional spinal pelvic parameters as well as the evaluation of the respect of the harmony of their relations between parameters can be automatically calculated. (Figure 27 B.)

Morphological analysis of the pelvi-spinal balance was established from the study of the loads of the gravity at each level of the spine and the pelvis in standing position. Therefore, Duval-Beaupère developed an experimental gamma-ray scanner allowing locating of the gravity, coupled with a 3d reconstruction system: the barycentremetry. (Duval-Beaupère 1992) (Figure 28 A.) It has been observed that the gravity applies in the entire spine into a vertical cylinder of 1 cm diameter, usually located slightly forward of t9, crossing the spine at the thoraco-lumbar junction to place backward the lumbar spine and behind the femoral

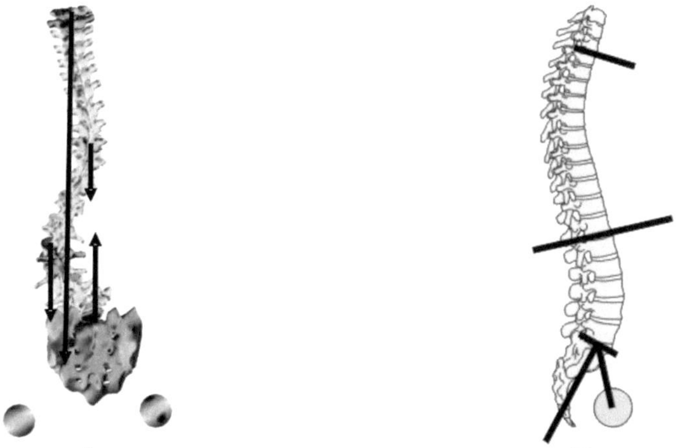

A. B.

Fig. 27. Frontal (A.) and sagittal (B.) balance analysis.

heads, being centred in the frontal plane. Were thus determined the 3D lever arms of the gravity determining the evolution of spinal deformities.From these several observations, a predictive equation of the position of the gravity loads was established, using morphological, positional and anthropometrical parameters: the simili-barycentremetry. (Legaye 2008) (Figure 28 B.) It allows so a functional personalized 3D evaluation of the balance and a functional assessment of individual. Asymmetries of these solicitations allow defining the 3D mechanical characteristics of a scoliotic deformation and establishing a prognosis of eventual increasing. Such assessment allows also adjusting the therapeutic goals to avoid such predicable accentuation of the curves and deterioration of the balance.

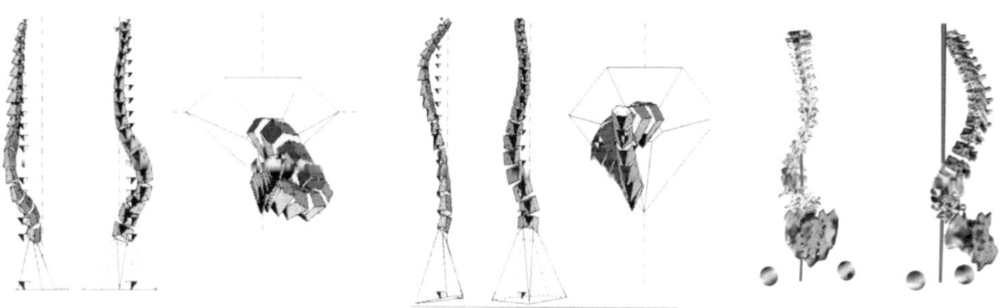

A.1. A.2. B.

Fig. 28. Functional analysis of the gravity loads: A. Barycentremetry of a lumbar scoliosis (A.1.) and of a thoracic scoliosis (A.2.) - B. Simili-barycentremetry.

7. 3D implications for the treatment of scoliosis

The 3D concept of scoliosis allows, using reconstruction software's, a better diagnosis and an appropriate individual evaluation of potential increasing of the curve(s): anatomical in curve angular progression, extension in adjacent area, 3D mobilization a stiff area thanks to supple levels. It implies a 3D assessment of those areas of rigidity and flexibility, and their 3D orientation. This new knowledge, not accessible by 2D imaging, has also given rise to conceptual treatment, whether medical or surgical.

7.1 Physiotherapy

Physiotherapy techniques are based on stretching in myotensif, or total work. When properly applied and well done, they offer good results. These techniques target mobility of the spine, better muscle flexibility for efficient movement, a reprogramming of neuromuscular postural adjustment. The analytical muscular correction needs to be three-dimensional, as well as the adaptation of sports (including swimming).

7.2 The corsets

Most of the time, the different types of corsets don't take into account the individual biomechanical properties of each patient's spine. Actually, it is essential to better understand the effect of the loads applied on the trunk and on the spine, and a 3D geometrical modelisation of these components is essential. The design and adaptation of individual braces or corsets are to be designed according to a 3D imaging of the spine and the skinny shape. Their effectiveness will be increased for optimal correction of the curves taking into account their three-dimensional component. The balance will also be maintained or restored. Such individual most appropriate corsets will also be better tolerated.

7.2.1 Manufacturing of corsets

Optical methods have been developed to simplify and optimize the manufacturing of corsets. These techniques virtually reproduce the contours of the subject's body, integrated into the 3D reconstruction of the spine. From there, the operator improves the corset by adequate 3D positioning of the pressure points. This also limits the use of body cast, though some consider the body cast as a prerequisite. From custom imaging the spine, corsets have been developed to optimize the correction even by active detorsion, some using the flexibility of some area and elastic traction in stiff area for a 3D correction.

7.3 The surgery

7.3.1 2D surgery

When scoliosis was considered only as a 2D frontal deviation, the correction consisted essentially of an axial vertical tension conducting to "dollar" montages (as Harrington's technique, 1962), leading to almost flat backs, without correction of rotations (nor so of the rib humps).

7.3.2 3D surgery

The rotational misalignment expressed by the rib hump has been the most difficult part of the deformity to correct. Effectively realigning vertebrae that have rotated out of position – a process called derotation – is an area of great interest in scoliosis correction surgery. In recent years, surgeons have sought new ways to maximize curve correction three-dimensionally. This means addressing the curve in all three "planes" of the deformity. Correcting vertebral rotation requires considering the axial aspect of the spine, or the cross-sectional top view.

It is up to Cotrel and Dubousset for using 3D conception of scoliosis to develop a technique also acting in 3D by a rotation effect of a pre-moulded rod, mainly using hooks to act on the bone structures. (Cotrel 1988, Lee 2004) (Figure 29 A.) The use of pedicle screws allowed a better action on the vertebrae, especially for the derotation, using instrumentation on segments rather than on the entire spine. Techniques of segmental corrections by in situ modelling of the rods have been developed (using hooks, screws or sub-laminar devices). (Figure 29 B.) This allows not only untwisting the vertebrae, but at the same time reducing the rib hump, since the ribs associated to the deformity are attached to the vertebrae being derotated.

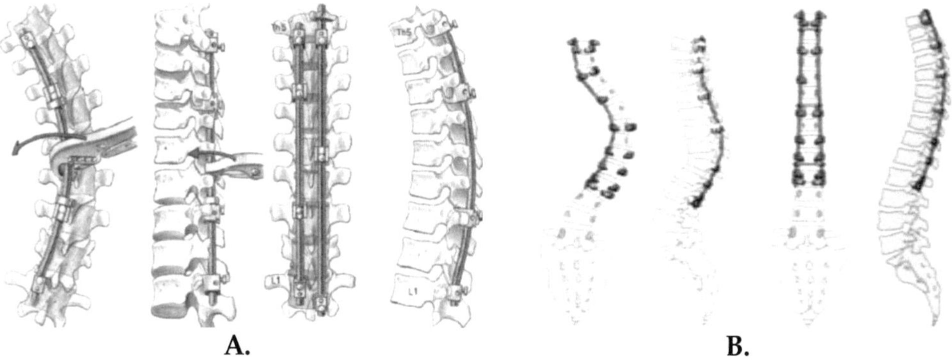

A. B.

Fig. 29. Surgical techniques. A. Cotrel-Dubousset: rood rotating technique – B. In situ rood modelling technique.

These moving of the fixations points must be adapted according to the 3D position of the vertebra (rotation and translation). (Dumas 2003, Steib 2004) Otherwise, it could lead to a increasing of the rotation rather than a correction. (Figure 30)

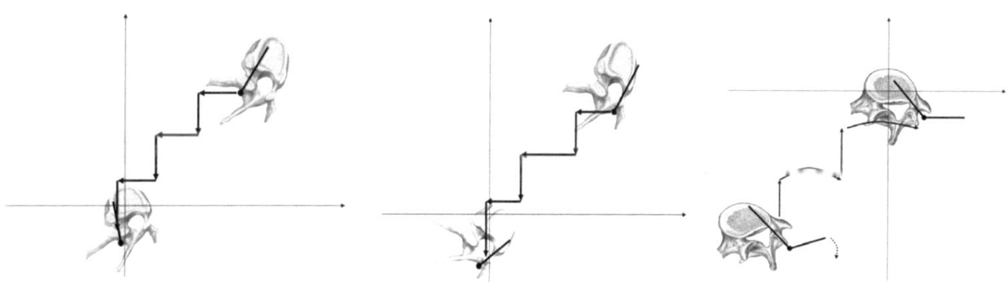

A. A′. B.

Fig. 30. Derotation technique for thoracic (A.) and lumbar (B.) scoliosis: A. Correct sequence on the screw in the concave side. A′. Accentuation of the rotation if acting on the convex side. B. Correction in the lumbar level by postero-anterior and local axial derotating forces.

So, for surgery, the 3D analysis is essential for planning and achieving the procedures. The 3D corrective principles are essential, distinct in the thoracic and lumbar area. Ignoring these principles can limit the corrections, and even increase the rotations or attempt unnecessary corrections of rigid segments instead of performing an action at their flexible extremities. Using of actual devices allows such 3D corrections, restoring optimal balance.

Nevertheless, the correction of the deformed ribs is not related to the vertebral correction related to the stiffness of the ribs. But this affects the aesthetic result.

7.3.3 The rib hump

If a patient has a significant rib hump that's expected to remain even after fusion surgery, a procedure called "thoraco-plasty" also may be performed, either along with the fusion or at a later date. It consists in sections of the ribs that form the hump which are surgically removed to shorten the ribs and reduce their prominence. (Figure 31) The benefits can include an improved appearance and pain relief.

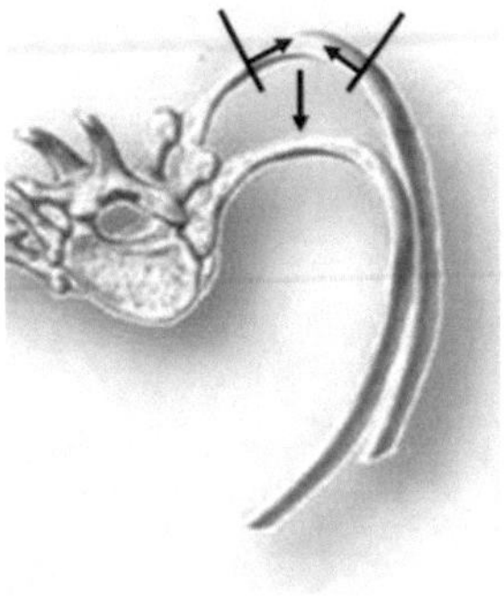

Fig. 31. Thoraco-plasty for correction of the rib-hump.

8. Usefulness of the 3D in diagnosis and treatment of scoliosis

Having a three-dimensional representation of the spine can result in a more accurate diagnosis, a more specific treatment, and less time in scoliosis surgery. The surgeon can improve the treatment of scoliosis by a better understanding of the deformity and perform an appropriate personalized procedure. An advantage of 3D reconstructions is that they identify defects that 2-D images do not. The preoperatively 3D analysis of a scoliotic deformity allows refine the limits for fusion and improve corrections by acting on the flexible zones surrounding stiff areas.

Therefore, 3D corrective techniques, both medical and surgical, are abundantly reported improving the corrections of the curves and restoring the balances. Subjective patient's outcomes are also better. Several studies have demonstrated the better significant relationship between results and 3D clinical parameters than for 2D evaluation.

9. Limits and perspectives

The 3D analysis is still only rarely used in daily practice because of the time required for certain reconstruction techniques. The development of automated and user-friendly methods will help the clinician in performing such procedures.

However, most 3D reconstructions have the disadvantage of not taking into account either the ribs or the rib cage and few of them include the lower limbs (or even the femurs), so essential for the analysis of the sagittal balance. Simultaneous use of optical morphometry allows already connecting the bony spine to the back shape.

The future aim is to access to individual inter-vertebral motilities for a more precise preoperative planning and also correction using dynamic systems to maintain spine mobility and avoid destabilisation of the adjacent levels occurring in case of fusion.

Moreover, the combined use of various 3D techniques (reconstructions of the bony spine, back shape morphology, dynamic tests, gravity loads on the spine, ...) will provide an individualized functional assessment of the spine and of the balances. (Figure 32)

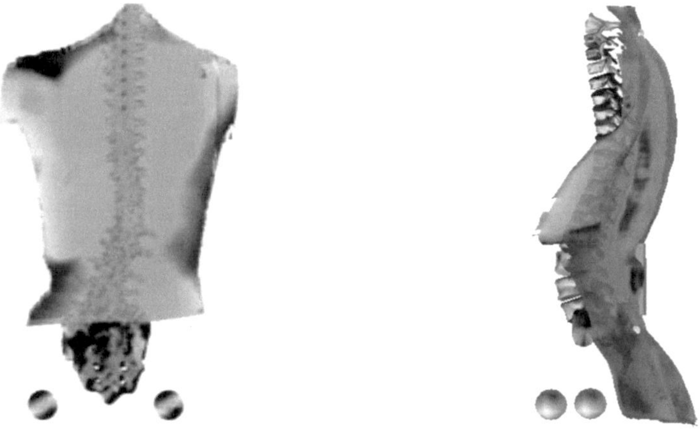

Fig. 32. 3D reconstruction of the bony structures from optical analysis of the back shape.

10. References

Vasiliadis, ES. ; Grivas, TB. & Kaspiris A. (2009). Historical overview of spinal deformities in ancient Greece. *Scoliosis*, Vol. 25, pp. 4:6

Grivas, TB. et al. (2006). Study of trunk asymmetry in normal children and adolescents. *Scoliosis*, Vol. 1, pp. 19

Grivas, TB. et al. (2008). Back trunk morphology in 3301 children aged 3-9 years old. *Stud Health Technol Inform.*, Vol. 140:, pp. 29-32

Boulay, C. et al. (2006). Three-dimensional study of pelvic asymmetry on anatomical specimens and its clinical perspectives. *J Anat*, Vol. 208, Issue 1, pp. 21-33

Machida, M. et al. (1994). Pathogenesis of idiopathic scoliosis: SEPs in chicken with experimentally induced scoliosis and in patients with idiopathic scoliosis. *J Pediatr Orthop*, Vol. 14, Issue 3, pp. 329-35

Lafortune, P. et al. (2007). Biomechanical simulations of the scoliotic deformation process in the pinealectomized chicken: a preliminary study. *Scoliosis*, Vol. 2, pp. 16

Grivas, TB. et al. (2002). The Double Rib Contour Sign (DRCS) in lateral spinal radiographs: aetiologic implications for scoliosis. *Stud Health Technol Inform*, Vol. 88, pp. 38-43

Grivas, TB. et al. (2006). Intervertebral disc biomechanics in the pathogenesis of idiopathic scoliosis. *Stud Health Technol Inform*, Vol. 123, pp. 80-3

Grivas, TB. et al. (2008). The role of the intervertebral disc in correction of scoliotic curves. A theoretical model of idiopathic scoliosis pathogenesis. *Stud Health Technol Inform*, Vol. 140, pp. 33-6

Will, RE. et al. (2009). Cobb angle progression in adolescent scoliosis begins at the intervertebral disc. *Spine*, Vol. 34, Issue 25, pp. 2782-6

King, HA.; Moe, JH. & Winter, RB. (1983). Adolescent idiopathic scoliosis: a new classification to determine extent of spinal arthrodesis. *J Bone Joint Surg* Am , Vol. 65, Issue 9, pp. 1302-13

Lenke, LG.; et al. (2001). The selection of fusion levels in thoracic idiopathic scoliosis. *J Bone Joint Surg Am*, Vol. 83-A, Issue 8, pp.1169-81

Stagnara, P.; Fauchet, R. & du Peloux, J. (1965). The plan of choice for the radiologic examination of kyphoscolioses. *Rev Chir Orthop Reparatrice Appar Mot*, Vol. 51, Issue 6, pp. 517-24

Nash, CL. & Moe, J H. (1969). A Study of Vertebral Rotation. *J. Bone and Joint Surg. Am* ., Vol. 51-A, pp. 223-9

Patias, P. et al. (2010). A review of the trunk surface metrics used as Scoliosis and other deformities evaluation indices. *Scoliosis*, Vol. 5, pp. 12

Stokes, IA. (1994). Three-dimensional terminology of spinal deformities. A report presented to the Scoliosis Research Society by the Scoliosis Research Society Working Group a 3D terminology of spinal deformity. *Spine*, Vol. 19, pp. 236-248

Drerup, B. (1984). Principles of measurement of vertebral rotation from frontal projections of the pedicles. *J Biomechanics*, Vol. 17, pp. 932-5

Perdriolle, R. & Vidal J. (1987). Morphology of scoliosis: three-dimensional evolution. *Orthopaedics*, Vol. 10, Issue 6, pp. 909-15

Lam, GC. et al. (2008). Vertebral rotation measurement: a summary and comparison of common radiographic and CT methods. *Scoliosis*, Vol. 3, pp. 16

Hecquet, J.; Legaye, J. & Duval-Beaupère, G. (1998). Access to a three-dimensional measure of vertebral axial rotation. *Eur Spine J*, Vol. 7, Issue 3, pp. 206-11

Doi, T. et al. (2011) A new method for measuring torsional deformity in scoliosis. *Scoliosis*, Vol. 6, pp. 7

Mitton, D. et al. (2000). 3D reconstruction method from biplanar radiography using non-stereocorresponding points and elastic deformable meshes. *Med Biol Eng Compu*, Vol. 38, pp. 133-9

Mitulescu, A. et al. (2011). Validation of the non-stereo corresponding points stereoradiographic 3D reconstruction technique. *Med Biol Eng Comput*, Vol. 39, Issue 2, pp. 152-8

Pomero, V. et l. (2004). Fast accurate stereoradiographic 3D-reconstruction of the spine using a combined geometric and statistic model. *Clin Biomech*, Vol. 19, pp. 240-7

Blanchard, B. & Elbaroudi, F. (2008). Imaging process for a computerized three-dimensional reconstruction from two-dimensional radiographic images; device implementation. Patent WO 2008/012479 (A1). France: Axs Ingenierie (Fr)

Dumas, R. et al. (2008). A semi-automated method using interpolation and optimisation for the 3D reconstruction of the spine by bi-planar radiography: a precision and accuracy study. *Med Bio Eng Comput*, Vol. 46, pp. 85-92

Labelle, H. et al. (1995). Variability of geometric measurements from three-dimensional reconstructions of scoliotic spines and rib cages. *Eur Spine J*, Vol. 4, pp. 88-94

Dumas, R. et al. (2004). Validation of relative 3D orientation of vertebrae reconstructed by bi-planar radiography. *Medical Engineering and physics*, Vol. 26, pp. 415-22.

Bellefleur, C. et al. (2002). Evaluation of the efficiency of patient stabilization devices for 3D X-ray reconstruction of the spine and rib cage. *Stud Health Technol Inform (IOS Press)* Vol. 88, pp. 127-31

Legaye, J. et al. (2009). Correction for patient sway in radiographic biplanar imaging for three-dimensional reconstruction of the spine: in vitro study of a new method. *Acta Radiol*, Vol. 50, Issue 7, pp. 781-90

Dubousset, J. et al. (2008). Skeletal and spinal imaging with EOS system. *Arch Pediatr.*, Vol. 15, Issue 5, pp. 665-6

Nault, ML. et al. (2002). Relations between standing stability and body posture parameters in adolescent idiopathic scoliosis. *Spine,* Vol. 27, Issue 17, pp. 1911-17

Pazos, V. et l. (2007). Reliability of trunk shape measurements based on 3-D surface Reconstructions. *Eur Spine* , Vol. 16, Issue 11, pp. 1882-91

Denton, T.; Randall, F. & Deinlein, D. (1992) The use of instant Moiré Photographs to reduce exposure from scoliosis radiographs. *Spine,* Vol. 17, Issue 5, pp. 509-12

Turner-Smith, A. & Harris, JD. (1984). ISIS - An automated shape measurement and analysis System. *In Proc of 3rd Int Symposium on Surface Topography and Spinal Deformity,*. Edited by Harris JD, Turner-Smith AR. Oxford, Gustav Fischer, Verlag;. ISBN 3-437-10962-6 Sept. 27-28, pp. 31-28

Turner-Smith, A. (1988). A television/computer three-dimensional surface shape measurement system. *J Biomech,* Vol. 21, Issue 6, pp. 515-29

Weisz, I. et al. (1988). ISIS scanning: a useful assessment technique in the management of scoliosis. *Spine*, Vol. 13, Issue 4, pp. 405-8

Theologis, T. et al. (1997). Early Detection of Progression in Adolescent Idiopathic Scoliosis by Measurement of Changes in Back Shape With the Integrated Shape Imaging System Scanner. *Spine,* Vol. 22, Issue 11, pp. 1223-7

Berryman, F. et al. (2008). A new system for measuring 3D back shape in scoliosis. *Eur Spine J,* Vol. 17, pp. 663-72

Poncet, P. et al. (2000). Reconstruction of laser-scanned 3D torso topography and stereo-radiographical spine and rib-cage geometry in scoliosis. *Comp Meth Biomech Biomed* Eng, Vol. 4, pp. 59-75

Frobin, W. & Hierholzer, E. (1983). Automatic Measurement of body surfaces using rasterstereograph. *Photogrammetric Engineering and Remote Sensing,* Vol. 49, Issue 3, pp. 377-84

Sahlstrand, T. (1986). The clinical value of Moiré Topography in the management of scoliosis. *Spine,* Vol. 11, Issue 5, pp. 409-417

Breque, C.; Dupre, JC. & Bremand, F. (2004) Calibration of a system of projection moiré for relief measuring: biomechanical applications. *Optics and Lasers in engineering,* Vol. 41, pp. 241-60

Goldberg, CJ. et al. (2001). Surface topography, Cobb angles, and cosmetic change in scoliosis. *Spine,* Vol. 26, Issue 4, pp. 55-63

Bunnell, WP. (2005). Selective screening for scoliosis. *Clin Orthop Relat Res,* Vol. 434, pp. 40-5

Graf, H.; Hecquet, J. & Dubousset, J. (1983). 3-dimensional approach to spinal deformities: application to the study of the prognosis of pediatric scoliosis. *Rev Chir Orthop,* Vol. 69, pp. 407–16

Kohashi, Y.; Oga, M. & Sugioka, Y. (1996) A new method using top view of the spine to predict the progression of curves in idiopathic scoliosis during growth. *Spine,* Vol. 21, pp. 212-17

Duval-Beaupère, G. et al. (1998). Pelvic incidence: a fundamental parameter for three-dimensional regulation of spinal sagittal curves. *Eur Spine J,* Vol. 7, pp. 99-103

Duval-Beaupère, G.; Schmidt, C. & Cosson, P. (1992). A Barycentremetric study of the sagittal shape of spine and pelvis: the conditions required for an economic standing position. *Ann Biomed Eng,* Vol. 20, Issue 4, pp. 451-62

Legaye, J. & Duval-Beaupere, G. (2008) Gravitational forces and sagittal shape of the spine. Clinical estimation of their relations. *Int Orthop.*, Vol. 32, Issue 6, pp. 809-16

Harrington, P. (1962) Treatment of scoliosis. Correction and internal fixation by spine instrumentation. *J Bone Joint Surg*, Vol. 44-A, pp. 591–610

Cotrel,Y.; Dubousset, J. & Guillaumat, M. (1988) New universal instrumentation in spinal surgery. *Clin Orthop* , Vol. 227, pp. 10–23

Lee, SM.; Suk, SI. & Ching, ER. (2004). Direct vertebral rotation: a new technique of three-dimensional deformity correction with segmental pedicle screw fixation in adolescent idiopathic scoliosis. *Spine,* Vol. 29, pp. 343-9

Steib, JP.; Dumas, R. & Mitton, D. (2004) Surgical correction of scoliosis by in situ contouring: a detorsion analysis. *Spine,* Vol. 29, pp. 193-9

Dumas, R. et al. (2003) Three-dimensional quantitative segmental analysis of scoliosis corrected by the in situ contouring technique. *Spine,* Vol. 28, pp. 1158-62

Fassier, A. et al. (2007) Preliminary study of the relation between the external surface of the trunk and the internal structure of the spine in the scoliosis of the child. *Rev Chir Orthop,* Vol 93, pp. 396-7

9

Emerging Technology and Analytical Techniques for the Clinical Assessment of Scoliosis

Karl F. Zabjek and Reinhard Zeller
Department of Physical Therapy, University of Toronto
The Hospital for Sick Children
Canada

1. Introduction

Paediatric spinal deformities are the most prevalent musculoskeletal conditions observed in children and youth. Idiopathic Scoliosis (IS), a sub-class of these spinal deformities is commonly recognized by a lateral curvature of the spine that is of unknown cause and has the greatest risk of progression during periods of rapid growth and development.[1,2,3] The emergence of our contemporary perspective that this lateral curvature and axial rotation of the spine [4] is also accompanied by significant spatial disorientation of the spine and thoracic cage, [5,6] has motivated clinicians and scientists to develop new models of assessment for the purpose of guiding clinical decisions, orthopaedic interventions, and the evaluation of clinical outcomes.

Historically, the clinical management of IS has posed a significant challenge to the orthopaedic community. In part, this challenge arises from the complex inter-relationship between skeletal growth, deformity, vertebral spatial orientation, mechanical loading, and the neuromuscular mechanisms that control stability of the spine.[8,9] The advent of modern day clinical and diagnostic imaging tools has provided an opportunity to describe, and characterize the breadth of deformity and spatial disorganisation of the spine across children and youth who are living with IS. In particular, three-dimensional imaging techniques have provided unique insight into the complexity and severity of vertebral deformity, and the complex translation and rotation of individual vertebral elements and the spine.[5,6,9,10,11] In parallel, clinical observational tools [12,13] and optoelectronic techniques [14,15,16] have enhanced our knowledge related to the extent of trunk surface deformity and spatial disorientation of the pelvis, thoracic cage, and shoulders[12-16]. Emerging technological developments have provided a unique opportunity to enhance our contemporary understanding of IS, and provide information that may compliment current models of clinical assessment.

The overall aim of this chapter is to provide an overview of current clinical models of assessment for scoliosis, and bring to attention new approaches that may provide opportunity to enhance fundamental knowledge and compliment clinical models of assessment. The specific aims are: 1) review the theoretical construct of posture; 2) identify the clinical terms and frames of reference that are commonly adopted to describe the posture of children and youth with IS; 3) identify and discuss the potential of emerging techniques that may enhance current clinical models of assessment.

2. Contemporary models of assessment for Idiopathic Scoliosis

The standard clinical model of assessment for children and youth who are evaluated for IS typically involves a review of family history, a neuromuscular exam, observation of posture and mobility and a radiological evaluation of the spine. This clinical model founds the diagnosis for IS, and guides the clinical decisions that are fundamental to the clinical management of the spinal deformity.

Although a subtle curvature of the spine and spatial disorientation of the pelvis, thorax and shoulders are observed quite frequently in children and youth (2-38 %) [17,18], a clinical diagnosis of IS is not communicated until there is of unknown cause, an emergence of axial and lateral deviation of the spine that exceeds 10 ° [4]. The frontal plane radiograph has historically served as the primary diagnostic clinical tool. The severity of spinal curvature may be measured using the technique often referred to as the angle of Cobb[19]. This angle is the angle between two-end vertebras that define the limits of a spinal curve [20]. The estimation of the amplitude of vertebral rotation has been performed using a variety of techniques [21,22]. The most common is the approach developed by Perdirolle & Vidal (1985) that utilises the Torsion meter [22]. When placed on a Posterior-Anterior radiograph this meter utilises the outer edges of the vertebra, and the longitudinal axis of the pedicles to measure vertebral rotation [22]. The Risser sign, is an additional measure that may be obtained from a frontal plane radiograph and is an index of maturity rated on a scale of 0-5. This index refers to the amount of ossification of the iliac epiphyses that is closely synchronized with the development of the vertebral growth plates [23]. This process of ossification may take 2-3 years, with completion around 14 years for girls, and 16 years for boys.

The risk of progression of the curvature of the spine is associated with a number of factors. These factors include the severity of the initial curve [1,24], age [24], menarche [1,24], skeletal maturity [1,24,25] and gender of the patient [24,25]. The risk of progression has been found to be greatest in children and youth who have a moderate or severe curvature of the spine and significant potential to grow. Lonstein & Carlson 1984, found that with a spinal curvature between 20-29°, and a Risser sign of 0, 1 or an age of 12 years, the risk of progression is 68% and 61% respectively. Whereas a patient with a Risser sign of 2, 3 or 4, or an age of 15 years, the risk of progression decreased considerably and was estimated to be 1.6% and 4% respectively [1].

Evidence from computational [26] and animal models [8] have supported the hypothesis that asymmetric loading of the spinal elements influences the development of vertebral deformities, and consequently progression of the spinal curve [7]. These models are in agreement with emerging evidence from biomechanical and neurophysiologic measures that suggest dysfunction of the neuromuscular system may be an additional factor and indicator of progression risk in IS. This evidence is drawn from studies that have demonstrated increased asymmetry in paraspinal muscle activity [27,28,29], altered sensory weighting [30], and postural control [31]. Of these studies, only a few have focused on identifying the predictive ability of neuromuscular measures [27,28,29]. For example, in patients who have IS, the presence of asymmetrical activation of the paraspinal muscles when standing quietly upright has been found to have a 68 % probability of progression, which increases to 80 % when combined with growth velocity [28]. Further work by this group also related paraspinal muscle activity with radiological measures of the spine in progressive and non-progressive IS, revealing an association with increased kyphosis and axial rotation of the spine prior to onset of progression [29]. This body of work has provided initial empirical evidence that associates altered paraspinal muscle activity with the progression of the spinal curvature. Our own studies have revealed that dysfunction in postural control may be evident in children with a spinal curvature as small as 15°, and that asymmetric positioning of the Centre of Mass (COM) in relation to the spine and sacrum may predispose children and youth to progression of their spinal curvature [32]. The findings from this recent work aligns itself with emergent hypothesis that have related neuromuscular dysfunction/dyscontrol, vertebral loading, vertebral deformity and further progression of the curvature of the spine [7]. This conceptual and empirical foundation provides rational for the development of complimentary approaches to the clinical assessment of *Posture* and *Mobility* in a clinical setting.

3. Conceptual construct, terms of reference and measurement of Posture and Mobility

3.1 Conceptual constructs of Posture and Mobility

The conceptual constructs of *Posture* and *Mobility* are central to the clinical evaluation of a child or youth diagnosed with IS. The former concept relates to the position and orientation of individual body segments (Postural Alignment) and the central nervous system control of these segments for the purpose of stability and orientation (Postural Control) [33]. The latter, is a broader term that introduces an element of movement that is afforded by individual joints, multi-articulate structures such as the spine and thorax, and results in relative motion between segments and of the body in relation to the external environment. The application of anatomical frames of reference, terminology and metrics that quantify these constructs are embodied within modern day clinical practice. This is evidenced by the emergence of observational tools, quantitative measurement devices and medical imaging techniques that serve a role in early screening, diagnosis, monitoring and clinical decisions.

3.2 Postural Alignment and Postural Control

Fundamental to the conceptual construct of *Posture* are the elements of *Postural Alignment* and *Postural Control*.[33] Although in clinical and research environments these elements are most often evaluated independently of one another, they are inherently interdependent, and not exclusive. *Postural alignment* is most accurately defined as the position and orientation of body segments in relation to each other and the external environment [33]. This alignment is a reflection of the overall organisation of the musculoskeletal system, and is influenced by underlying bone morphology, joint composition and structure, muscle length, strength and size. The central nervous system inherently controls the alignment of the body for the primary purpose of stability and orientation against gravity and to perform movement [33]. This is accomplished through the integration and interpretation of sensory information, the development of muscle tone to counter the mechanical effects of gravity when sitting and standing, and the generation of context appropriate anticipatory and reactive neuromuscular synergies in response to internal and/or external threats to stability [33]. It is this underlying central contribution to the maintenance of the position and orientation of the body that unifies the concepts of *Postural alignment* and *Postural control*.

3.3 Anatomical terms, and frames of reference for the description of Postural Alignment

Fundamental to the description of a child's posture who is living with a spinal deformity is the adoption of consistent anatomical terms of reference. These terms of reference found the communication of clinical observations that guide treatment decisions and assist in the evaluation of clinical outcomes. Our contemporary perspective of pediatric spinal deformities recognizes that scoliosis is a three-dimensional curvature of the spine [4-6] and has evolved to include deformity and spatial disorientation of adjacent skeletal structures such as the pelvis, thorax and shoulder's [14,15,34]. (See Figure 1) The complexity and severity of these deformities have necessitated the adoption of terms and frames of reference that are specific to the field of paediatric spinal deformities.

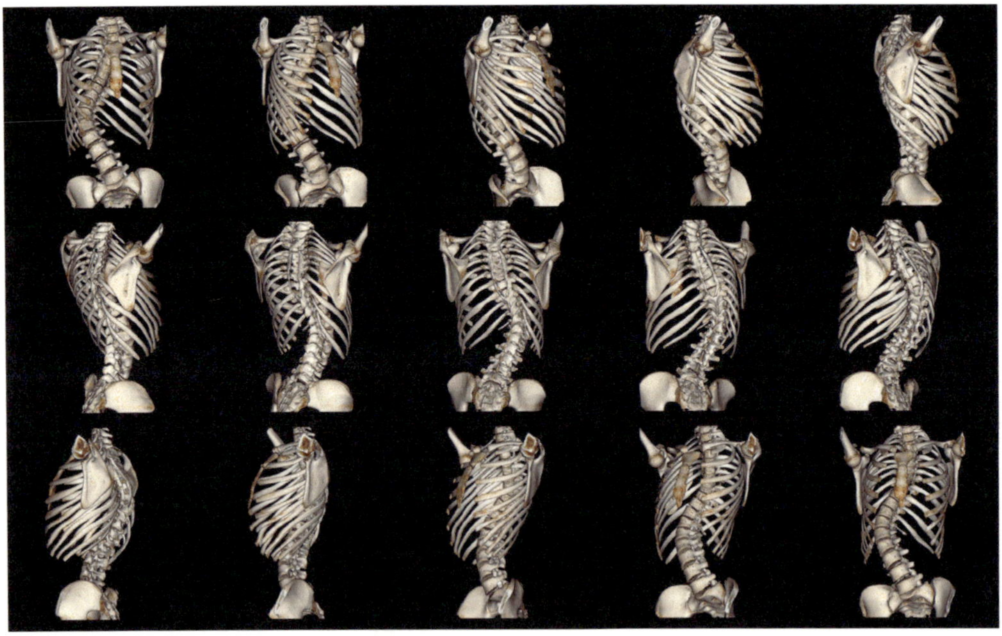

Fig. 1. Three dimensional rendering of scoliosis.

3.3.1 Anatomical terms and frames of reference

The cardinal planes of reference are commonly adopted by clinicians and scientists within the fields of orthopaedics, anatomy, biomechanics and rehabilitation. The three cardinal planes of reference include the Sagittal, Frontal (Coronal) and Transverse (Axial) planes and axis. The Sagittal plane is a vertical plane that passes through the body from front to back, the Frontal plane is a vertical plane that passes through the body from right to left, and the transverse plane is a horizontal plane that divides the body in an upper and lower section. Each of these planes has an axis which lies perpendicular to this plane. The position, orientation and motion of the body within a cardinal plane, or about an axis may then be described. The terms of flexion, extension, abduction, adduction, rotation, tilt, circumduction, protraction, retraction, elevation, depression, inversion, eversion, are universally accepted descriptors of segment position and motion [35]. In clinical settings, these terms are often used to effectively describe the posture and gait of a wide spectrum of orthopaedic, and neurological conditions.

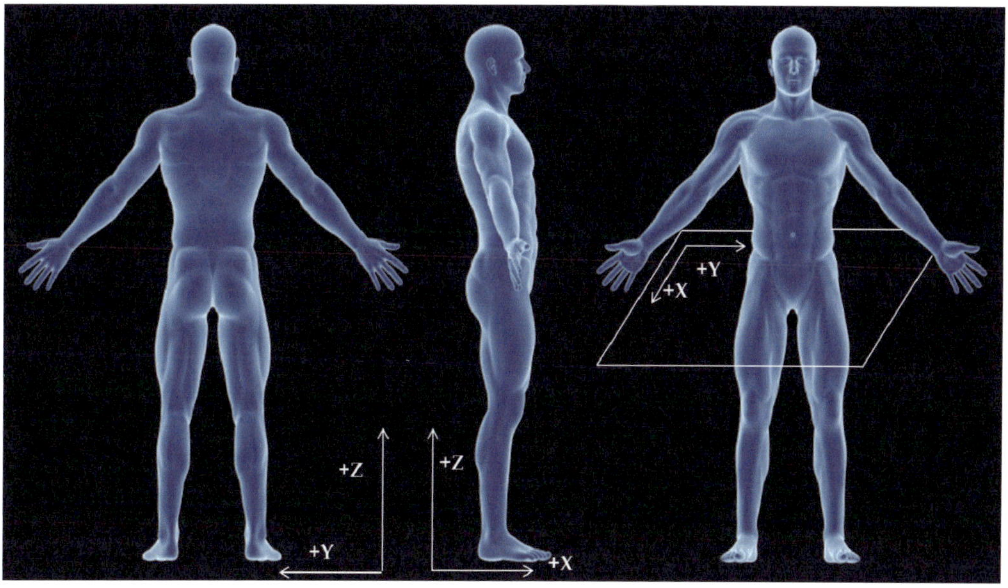

Fig. 2. Anatomical planes of reference, and cartesian co-ordinate system.

3.3.2 Cartesian co-ordinate systems

The cartesian co-ordinate system provides the basis to quantify the position and orientation of the pelvis, thorax, scapula and spine. This 3-Dimensional co-ordinate system consists of an origin (0,0,0) and three perpendicular axis (x,y,z) projecting from this origin and defines three planes (x,y; y,z; x,z). (See Figure 2)The position of a point in this co-ordinate system may then be described in relation to these three axis (x,y,z). The location of this co-ordinate system in relation to the body, and individual skeletal structures will provide a frame of reference to describe and quantify posture. A global co-ordinate system is commonly adopted to describe the position and orientation of the body in relation to the external environment. This system is defined by alignment of the cartesian co-ordinate system with the cardinal planes of reference, where the x-axis lies within the sagittal plane and perpendicular to the frontal plane, the y-axis lies within the frontal plane and perpendicular to the sagittal plane, and the z-axis lies within both the frontal/sagittal planes and is aligned with the gravity. The appropriate alignment of this axis system with the cardinal planes of reference, and in particular with gravity is critical. In contrast to a global co-ordinate system, a local co-ordinate system will align the cartesian co-ordinates in relation to individual skeletal structures. The SRS 3D Terminology work group has proposed that a local reference system may be adopted to describe a) vertebral deformity; b) regional curvatures of the spine; c) the spine. This approach will then provide the capacity to quantify deformity and spatial orientation of the individual vertebra, the spine and the adjacent skeletal structures [20]. The adoption of a cartesian co-ordinate system that is in alignment with the global cardinal planes of reference, and the local frames of reference has served as the basis for a number of tools to quantify the 3 dimensional alignment and spatial orientation of the spine and adjacent skeletal structures.

3.3.3 Terms of reference for the clinical description of Idiopathic Scoliosis

In recognition that a comprehensive description of the complex deformity and disorientation of the spine and adjacent skeletal structures extends beyond the scope of these standard anatomical terms, collective work has assembled detailed terminology to describe spinal deformity [20,36,37]. These work groups have provided terms of reference that describes deformity, alignment and shape of the spine, and the alignment (position/orientation) of individual vertebra and adjacent skeletal structures such as the pelvis, thorax and scapula. Interested readers are further directed to the Scoliosis Research Society documentation related to 3-D Terminology, Biomechanics Documentation, and Revised Glossary of Terms, and in addition to the 6th SOSORT consensus paper, and recent review of trunk surface metrics [20,36,-38].

Shape and alignment of the Spine

With the emergence of modern day diagnostic imaging techniques our understanding of the complexity of the three dimensional curvature of the spine, and the inherent variability observed across children and youth with scoliosis has grown extensively [39]. The development of terms of reference to describe these complex spinal curves has also occurred in parallel.[20,37,38] The Scoliosis Research Society Working group proposed three dimensional terminology to describe scoliosis [20], and has recently been updated by the Working Group on 3D Classification [38]. The terminology proposed by this working group has historically been applied in reference to a bi-planar radiograph (frontal, and lateral) and more recently 3D reconstructions of the spine. Within this context, spine alignment is generally described in relation to the central sacral line, which is defined as a vertical line that traverses the centre of the sacrum [38]. This line of reference provides a reference to identify the most laterally positioned vertebrae, or apical vertebrae. In relation to the apical vertebra, the first vertebra with the greatest tilt of the superior surface towards the concavity of the curve is termed the 'Cephalad end vertebra', and the first vertebra with the inferior surface tilted maximally towards the concavity of the curve is termed the 'Caudad end vertebra'.[20,38] The definition of the apical, cephalada and caudad vertebra define curvature, with the term 'major' commonly referring to the largest curvature, and the term 'minor' refers to the curve with the smallest curvature. Under certain circumstances the terms 'compensatory curve' implies a non-structural minor curve that is located above or below the major curve.[20,38] The location and side of the apical vertebra then provides the basis to define the general class of curvature as either Cervical, Cervical-Thoracic, Thoracic, Thoracolumbar, Lumbar, and Lumbar, Thoracolumbar, Lumbar and Lumbar Sacral (See Table 2).[20,38] This terminology has founded clinical decisions related to the prescription of conservative treatment approaches and surgical intervention, and the evaluation of clinical outcomes.

Scoliosis Type	Location of Apical Vertebra
Cervical	C1 vertebra - C6-C7 Disc
Cervical-Thoracic	C7, T1 vertebra or intervening Disc space
Thoracic	T2 vertebra - T11-T12
Thoracolumbar	T12, L1 vertebra - T12-L1 Disc
Lumbar	L1-L2 disc - L4-L5 Disc
LumboSacral	L5 vertebra or below

Table 2. Scoliosis Research Society classification of scoliosis according to level of apex. [38]

This work group has also defined sagittal alignment of the spine [38]. The overall sagittal spinal balance (or alignment) has traditionally referred to the location of the body of the C7 verteba to the superior posterior aspect of the sacrum. The spine also has four notable curves that correspond to the cervical (C1-C7), thoracic (T1-T12), lumbar (L1-L5), and sacral regions. The curvature associated with each region is commonly described by the concavity or convexity when viewed in the posterior-anterior direction. In an able bodied adult, the former is referred to as Kyphosis typically observed in the Thoracic and Sacral regions, and the later Lordosis typically observed in the Cervical and Lumbar regions [35,38]. Across children and youth diagnosed with scoliosis, it is recognized that there is considerable variability in the amplitude and direction of the spinal curvature observed in the sagittal plane [38,40,41].

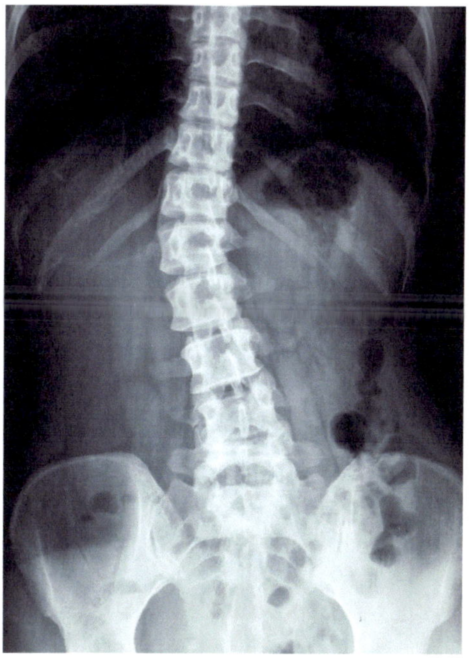

Fig. 3. Frontal plane radiograph of a spine.

Position and Orientation of Adjacent Skeletal Structures (Pelvis, Thorax, Shoulders)

The documentation of the position and orientation of the pelvis, thorax and shoulders has often been performed in a clinical setting utilizing observational, quantitative and radiographic approaches. The position and orientation of these segments have traditionally been referred to in relation to the cardinal planes of reference.

Pelvis

The terms and measures that have been adopted to describe the position and orientation of the pelvis are quite extensive, and specific to the sacrum, iliac bones and pelvis [34,36,38,42-45]. The anatomical landmarks that provide the point of reference to describe the pelvis include: Anterior-Superior Iliac Spines (ASIS), Posterior-Superior Iliac Spines (PSIS), Superior Lateral Border of the Iliac Crests, and the Sacral Plateau [34,36,38,42-45]. These landmarks have served to measure pelvic position and orientation radiologically [38] and with optoelectronic and digitization techniques [34,42-45]. The premise of this choice of landmarks is founded on the desire to distinguish the spatial disposition of the pelvis from the relative alignment of the right and left iliac bones. Figure 4 provides a perspective of the pelvis from the Frontal, Sagittal, and Transverse planes. The global orientation of the pelvis is generally defined by the angle of a line that is drawn between these landmarks and horizontal [34,42-46]. The angle of the pelvis in the sagittal plane is typically defined by a line between ipsilateral ASIS and PSIS (Figure 4: D3). The rotation of the pelvis in the transverse plane is calculated by a line drawn between the contralateral ASIS, PSIS, and Superior Lateral Border of the Iliac Bones (Figure 4: D4). Adopting the same landmarks, the tilt of the pelvis in the frontal plane is also calculated (Figure 4: D1,D2) [42-46]. These angles provide the basis to define global orientation of the pelvis [42-46], with the difference between angles serving to define the relative orientation between right and left iliac bones [42-43].

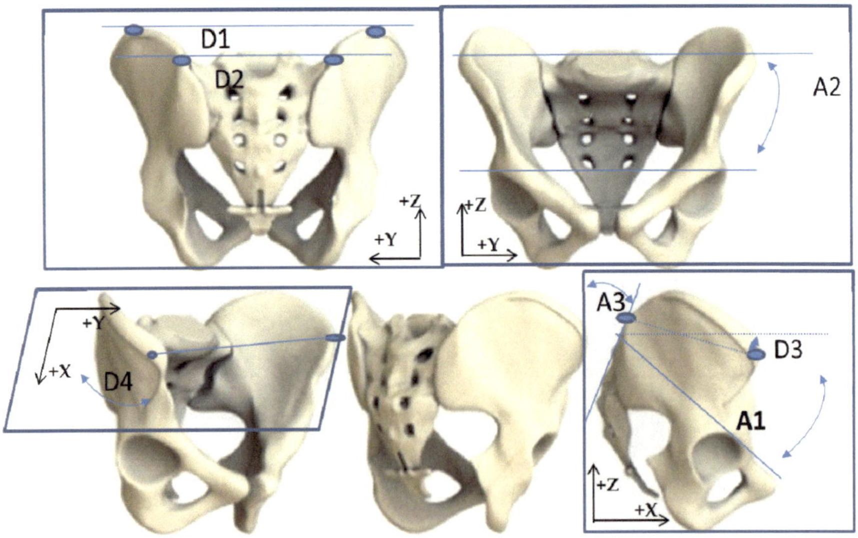

Fig. 4. Frontal, Sagittal and Transverse perspectives of the pelvis.

The Scoliosis Research Society working group, has proposed a standardized list of terms that may describe these angular measures [38]. Specifically, orientation of the sacrum and pelvis in the frontal plane are described as obliquity and orientation in relation to the sagittal plane is referred to as inclination. Pelvic obliquity is suggested by the SRS to be measured by the angle of a line between the iliac crests in relation to horizontal (Figure 4: D1), and the Sacral obliquity is measured by the angle between a line drawn across the superior border of the sacrum, and the right and left femoral heads (Figure 4: A2) [38]. The posterior surface of the Sacrum serves to define Sacral Inclination in relation to vertical (Figure 4: A3), and pelvic inclination is defined by a line drawn from the superior aspect of the sacrum to the superior aspect of the pubis (Figure 4: A1) [38].

Thorax

The rotation of the thorax has commonly been measured in the transverse plane with the patient in an anteriorly flexed position [12,13]. In this position, the region of the spine with the greatest vertical protrusion, or commonly referred to as prominence is chosen as the location to measure the Angle of Trunk Inclination. The Angle of Trunk Inclination is then measured through the angle defined by the surface of the protruding thorax and the horizontal [12,38].

Shoulders and Scapula

The orientation of the shoulders and scapula have most often been measured through the use of the non-invasive optoelectronic and digitization techniques [34,42-46]. The motivation to measure scapular orientation is founded on the understanding that a rotation of the thoracic cage, will affect scapular orientation due to the positioning of the scapula over the thorax, and the inherent articulation between the scapula, clavicle and sternum [34,42-46]. Within this context, tilt and rotation of the shoulders is defined by a line that is drawn between the right and left scapula and the associated angle in relation to the transverse and frontal planes. The rotation of the scapula has been suggested to include both a measure of the superior rotation (angulation) and inferior rotation (angulation). This is defined by a line that is drawn between the right and left acromions, and/or a line drawn between the inferior border of the right and left scapula and the angulation of these two lines in relation to the transverse (rotation) and frontal planes (tilt). These measures may be expressed in relation to the global reference system, or relative to a pelvis reference system [34,42-46].

3.4 Clinical application for terms of reference and metrics

The anatomical terms, frames of reference and metrics developed by the orthopaedic community has afforded a unique opportunity to characterize the complexity of the 3D deformity of the spinal curvature and evaluate clinical outcomes associated with conservative and surgical management of IS. Although, the extent of application of radiological and non-invasive techniques for these purposes extends beyond the scope of the present chapter, it is notable to briefly discuss the relationships between the underlying skeletal alignment of the spine and the spatial disorientation of the thoracic cage, pelvis and shoulders observed clinically.

Investigation of the clinical utility of the application of metrics to the spatial disorientation of the thoracic cage, pelvis and shoulders has been the focus of numerous studies [12-18,42-47]. Within the context of this work, a significant interest is devoted to quantifying the relationship between surface metrics and the underlying alignment of the spine [12,47]. A weak to strong correlation between back surface metrics has been reported [12,47,58], with evidence of stronger associations through application of advanced analytical techniques such as neural networks and regression models that are specific to frontal and sagitall spinal alignment [13,54-57]. These observations have founded considerable interest to explore their utility in school screening programs [49-51], and clinically for the purpose of optimizing the number of x-rays [13,54-56]. There is an increased understanding that the limitations that exist with the application of these surface metrics are associated with inherent variability across children that are associated with growth [48], location of the deformity [34] and treatment [52]. Notably, recent work has highlighted a stronger correlation between surface metrics and spinal curvature in older children vs younger children [48]. In addition, significant differences were noted in spatial orientation of the pelvis, and spatial orientation of the shoulders, and shoulder blades when individuals are categorized by the side and location of the apical vertebra [34]. This work revealed that predominant spatial deformity in the frontal plane at the pelvis is greater in curves with an apex in the thoracolumbar region, and conversly in the transverse plane for the shoulders/scapula for the curves with an apex in the thoracic region. This knowledge founds the motivation to expand current models that aim to predict the degree of spinal curvature, and also further explore the clinical utility of surface deformity measures to evaluate the outcomes associated with treatment.

4. Emerging and complimentary measures of Posture and Mobility

4.1 What is the motivation to expand current models of Posture and Mobility assessment?

Historically, the assessment of a child and youth with a spinal deformity has focused on the observation and measurement of skeletal deformity and spatial disorientation of the spine. It is evident, that significant attention has been devoted to the development of imaging techniques, and clinical tools within this regard. It is clear that contemporary models of assessment found the clinical diagnosis and treatment decisions for spinal deformities. With the exception of the Adam's forward bending test [12,13], the upright static standing posture has served as the frame of reference for clinical characterization of spinal deformity. However, there are emerging criticisms that question the relevance of one measure of spinal deformity such as the Cobb angle as one of the primary indicators of surgical outcomes [36]. In part, this criticism is founded on the recognition that the spatial deformity of the spine extends beyond the characterization provided by one summary measure, inconsistencies in surgical decision making [59] and is paralleled by evidence that it does not correlate with perceptions of appearance by parents and patients [60].

Emerging hypothesis related to association between neuromuscular dyscontrol, vertebral deformity, asymmetric vertebral loading, growth, and complimentary empirical evidence has provided a foundation for the expansion of current clinical models of assessment. Our current understanding of the frequency and duration of the actual time that children spend in this position is limited. Furthermore, it is postulated that children and youth spend considerable amounts of time seated either at school or at home. Studies that have investigated the sitting postures of children at school have revealed that children may spend 85 % - 97 % of their time relatively stationary or static, and 28-45 % of the time in forward flexion with only a small proportion of the time dynamically moving their trunk [61-62]. This predisposition to fixed static postures over extended durations may exert unhealthy loads on the passive elements of the spine. These findings are confounded by the recognition that school furniture design is often mismatched to the anthropometric dimensions of the children, and a change in workstation design ultimately affects muscle activity [63]. The relevance of these studies is appreciated when it is recognized that adolescents with IS adopt different postures in the sitting position when compared to standing [64]. These differences have been noted to favour asymmetric loading of the spine as noted by an increased lateral shift of the thoracic vertebrae in relation to the sacrum [64]. Similarly in adults, sitting postures have been noted to vary from standing and are accompanied by increased loads on the lumbar spine segments [65]. Increased loading of the passive spinal elements has also been observed to occur at smaller angles of flexion during slouched sitting and is attributed to decreased activity of the erector spinae muscles [66].

It is apparent that factors affecting the load distribution on the spine over an extended period of time will affect spinal stability. Common behaviours such as sitting, standing, walking, ascending/descending stairs all vary with respect to the adopted postures and the level of muscle activation that is employed to counter the external accelerations applied on the body. However, there is a limited understanding of the frequency and duration of the asymmetric postures that are assumed on a daily basis, and the nature of the neuromuscular recruitment strategies that are involved. It has been hypothesized that these latter strategies will have the greatest contribution to the loads placed on the spine [7]. It is therefore hypothesized that an augmented understanding of the mechanisms and risk factors associated with the early progression of IS, may be obtained through coupling radiological measures of spinal deformity with measures of neuromuscular function obtained across a range of activities that are representative of the physical demands experienced during everyday life. This body of works brings to light the need to explore new models of assessment that encompass the broader constructs of postural control, and mobility.

4.2 Contemporary perspectives of Postural Control and Idiopathic Scoliosis

The central nervous system regulation of the position and orientation of the body for the purpose of regulating posture and movement is often defined as *Postural Control.* Insights into how the central nervous system controls posture has traditionally focused on the measurement of displacement of the centre of mass (COM) in relation to the base of support. Stability of the body is thus a reflection of how effective the CNS is in maintaining the COM within the base of support under circumstances that destabilize the body.

The COM of the entire body represents a weighted average of COM position of each individual body segment in space, and evidently is affected by the underlying skeletal structure, mass distribution of body segments and the central nervous system strategies that integrate sensory information and regulate muscle tension [67]. It is the tension generated by individual muscles that produce a moment of force (torque) about a joint that is responsible for the stabilization of the body against gravitational loads. Contemporary approaches to understanding how the CNS controls posture have focused on modelling the body in an upright standing position as an inverted pendulum. Fundamental to this model is the recognition that CNS control may be presented by the displacement of the Centre of Pressure (COP). The COP represents the net location of the ground reaction forces located under the base of support (feet), and is a reflection of the net effect of the stabilizing torques generated by the body. Within the concept of the inverted pendulum model, the horizontal acceleration of the COM is strongly correlated with the difference between the COP and

COM (COP-COM) [68]. The application of this model to the study of upright standing balance control has suggested that A/P control of standing is primarily related to the ankle plantar/dorsi flexors, and M/L control is related to the hip abductors/adductors [68-70]. Although this model has informed about fundamental strategies involved in global postural control, there has been limited application of this model to the field of spinal deformities. In particular, relatively few studies have examined how the postural control of children and youth with IS may be compromised, and in particular direct associations with the risk of curve progression.

The overall postural stability of children with IS has been examined through characterization of COP displacement, during quiet standing with the eyes open [71-79] and under altered sensory conditions [72]. Children and youth with IS were found to have a greater displacement of the COP than able bodied children [73,77,78]. However, this is in contrast to other studies that have either found no differences, or decreased sway. Alghouh, the majority of studies examined postural stability in children and youth with a similar amplitude in the spinal curvature, they did not differentiate the type of curve. Gauchard et al., (2001) revealed that overall sway of children and youth with IS was greater in lumbar curvatures, and smallest in double curves [74]. This body of work reveals the complexity of understanding how postural control is affected in children and youth with IS. In part, the current model's of postural control do not differentiate stability of the trunk and spine from overall stability of the body. Traditional measures of standing balance as reflected by the COP under the feet are the net effect of all of the segmental torques generated by the body [67]. Therefore, there is the potential for significant advancements to be made with the enhancement of these models to consider the segmental control of the spine and trunk.

4.3 Emerging approaches for the modelling of the Centre of Mass

Obtaining an accurate estimation of the position and the displacement of the COM has been the focus of numerous studies. These studies have directly measured the position of the COM and moment of inertia in cadavers [80] and on live subjects, through a variety of techniques that includes stereophotogrammetry [81] cross-sectional modelling of body segments [82], and medical imaging techniques [83]. Of these techniques the cadaver studies were principally performed on adults and the remainder on adult subjects with the exception of the cross-sectional elliptical approach employed by Jensen (1989), who studied children and adolescents [84]. The research by Jensen (1989) revealed that during growth and development there is a decrease in the COM proportion of the head and an increase in the COM proportion of the arms and legs. The positions of the COM relative to the proximal joint centres also shifted proximally in the upper legs forearms and arms [84].

Techniques have been proposed to estimate the COM and overcome the difficulties of anatomical landmark detection, and the estimation of anthropometric variables (segment COM and moment of inertia). These techniques involve estimating the position of the COM based on measurements obtained from a force plate. The techniques generally include 1) a filtering technique of the COP [85], 2) Newtonian mechanics based equations [86], 3) filtering technique combined with a mathematical relationship between the COP and COM [87], 4) double integration of the horizontal ground reaction forces [88,89]. These techniques have been developed and initially applied to estimate the displacement of the COM in adult subjects in a quiet standing position [85,87,89]. Recently in a simulation study, Lenzi et al.,

(2003) compared the technique of Caron et al., (1997), Zatsiorsky & King (1998), and Shimba (1984), with a link segment model based on anthropometric parameters obtained from Winter (1990) [67,87,88-91]. Through changing the body segment parameters and evaluating each model in simulated quiet standing, ankle sway, hip sway and the sit to stand task the sensitivity of each technique was tested. The technique by Zatsiorsky & King (1998) was found to be unaffected by changes in body segment parameters, unlike the link segment model which was most sensitive to changes in body segment parameters across conditions [90]. This independence to anthropometric parameters provides a possibility of overcoming the limited source of anthropometric data available for IS patients and healthy adolescents. Recent work that has applied this approach to quantify the position of the COM in children and youth with scoliosis, has revealed notable and significant differences between the two approaches. Importantly, an anthropometric model will overestimate the anterior position of the COM in relation to the Sacrum up to 16 mm, and 3.8 mm in the medial-lateral direction. Similarly, the variability of the COM over time was found to be greater in scoliosis patients than non-scoliosis [32]. The observed differences between models may in part be contributed to the variability in the spatial deformation of the pelvis, trunk and spine often observed in children in youth with scoliosis. It is hypothesized that traditional anthropometric models are not sensitive to these deformities, and thus lack precision in accurately tracking the position and displacement of the COM when standing. This issue is also exhibited when dynamic activities are examined such as lateral trunk bending. Figure 5 presents the COM estimated from a forceplate (COMfp) [32,88] and that estimated from a standard link segment kinematic model [32]. Initial comparison of the COM trajectory using both techniques reveals similar spatial and temporal characteristics. However, importantly, the kinematic model over-estimates COM trajectory at the end range of a movement (ie., full anterior-flexion, full lateral flexion).

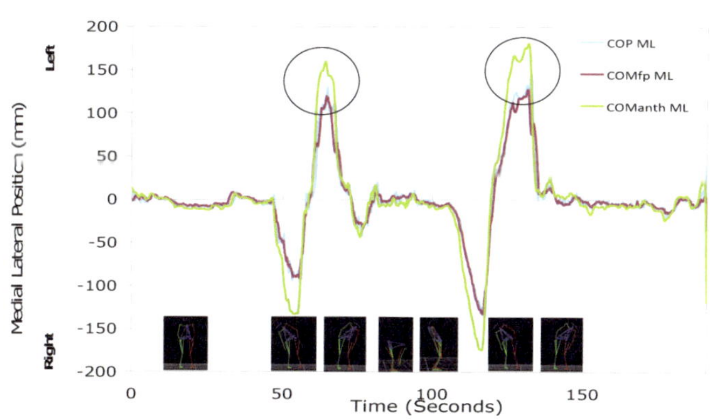

Fig. 5. Medial-Lateral position of the Centre of Pressure, (COP), Centre of Mass, (COM) estimated from a traditional 3D motion capture system and anthropometric model (COManth) [32], a forceplate based approach (COMfp)[32,88].

4.4 Emergent technologies that may afford new insight into Posture and Mobility

Recent advancements in portable technology have increased the feasibility of obtaining neuromuscular and quantitative measurements of movement while an individual is engaged in activities of everyday life. The potential of instruments such as an accelerometer, or a gyroscope to provide indications of the type of activity that is performed has received increasing attention [92-94]. This body of work has focused on the application and evaluation of machine learning techniques [92,93], discrete wavelet transforms [93], and binary decision trees that categorize activities according to rest or activity (falls, walking, transition, postural orientation) [95]. These classification techniques provide the foundation to identify activity patterns, and differentiate both the frequency and duration of each activity throughout the day. Additional research within this area has focused on characterizing in greater detail the nature of the activities, with particular emphasis placed on the extraction of features related to the quality and quantity of walking [96], segmental accelerations [97,98], transitions in positioning and orientation [99], and trunk posture [100-106]. Within this context, there has been a limited focus of the application of this technology for the measurement of trunk postures in children and youth with Scoliosis. Initial work by Bazzarelli et al., 2002 [105], and Lou et al., 2002 demonstrated the potential of an accelerometer based, trunk mounted sensor to measure trunk posture, and provide postural feedback during the performance of daily activities [105,106]. Recent work by Wong & Wong 2008, focused on a three accelerometer system that positioned the sensors on the pelvis (Sacrum), mid-thorax (T12) and high thorax (T1/T2). In comparison to a standard motion capture system, this approach demonstrated a strong correlation, and root mean square differences of less than 3.1° and 2.1° in the sagittal and coronal planes respectively [103]. Further application of this type of device provided an opportunity to quantify the frequency distribution of the range of postures that are assumed on a daily basis [103]. These two studies have clearly demonstrated the potential utility of a trunk mounted sensor network to measure posture during activities of daily life, and the alteration of the postures assumed with the provision of daily feedback [103-106]. It is clear from this body of work that the premise of a body mounted sensor network that integrates tri-axial accelerometers and gyroscopes has the potential to provide information related to the type, frequency and duration of daily activities, as well as specific information related to the segmental body postures and movement. Notably, there is limited work that has focused on the further development and application of this technology to the study of spinal deformities, and the exploration of the clinical potential to inform about treatment outcomes.

5. Conclusion

Contemporary perspectives acknowledge that scoliosis is a complex musculoskeletal condition that is characterized by spatial disorientation of the spine and thoracic cage. The emergence of novel three dimensional imaging, optoeletronic, and ambulatory monitoring tools provides clinicians and researchers an unprecedented opportunity to accurately characterize the spatial deformation of the spine and thorax, skeletal deformity, and monitor segment postural alignment in the clinic, at home and in the community. With further development and application, these tools may provide the foundation for the development of new clinical models of assessment and evaluation of outcomes related to treatment.

6. References

[1] Lonstein JE, & Carlson, JM (1984) The prediction of curve progression in untreated idiopathic scoliosis during growth. J Bone Joint Surg Am. 66:1061-71.

[2] Little DG, Song KM, Katz D, & Herring JA (2000) Relationship of peak height velocity to other maturity indicators in idiopathic scoliosis in girls. J Bone Joint Surg Am. 82:685-93.
[3] Risser JC (1958) The Iliac apophysis; an invaluable sign in the management of scoliosis. Clin Orthop Relat Res. 4:111-9.
[4] Kane WJ (1977) Scoliosis prevalence: a call for a statement of terms. Clin Orthop Relat Res.126:43-6.
[5] Stokes IA, Bigalow LC, Moreland MS (1987) Three-dimensional spinal curvature in idiopathic scoliosis. J Orthop Res. 5(1):102-13.
[6] Stokes IA, Dansereau J, Moreland MS (1989) Rib cage asymmetry in idiopathic scoliosis. J Orthop Res. 7(4):599-606.
[7] Stokes IA, Burwell RG, Dangerfield PH (2006) Biomechanical spinal growth modulation and progressive adolescent scoliosis - a test of the 'vicious cycle' pathogenetic hypothesis: Summary of an electronic focus group debate of the IBSE. Scoliosis. 1:16.
[8] Stokes IA, Spence H, Aronsson DD, Kilmer N (1996) Mechanical modulation of vertebral body growth. Implications for scoliosis progression. Spine. 21(10):1162-7.
[9] Dansereau J, Stokes IA. (1988) Measurements of the three-dimensional shape of the rib cage. J Biomech. 21(11):893-901.
[10] Ilharreborde B, Steffen JS, Nectoux E, Vital JM, Mazda K, Skalli W, Obeid I (2011) Angle measurement reproducibility using EOS three-dimensional reconstructions in adolescent idiopathic scoliosis treated by posterior instrumentation. Spine. 36(20):E1306-13.
[11] Villemure I, Aubin CE, Grimard G, Dansereau J, Labelle H (2002) Evolution of 3D deformities in adolescents with progressive idiopathic scoliosis. Stud Health Technol Inform. 91:54-8.
[12] Cote P, Kreitz BG, Cassidy JD, Dzus AK, Martel J (1998) A study of the diagnostic accuracy and reliability of the Scoliometer and Adam's forward bend test. Spine. 23, 796-802.
[13] Griffet J, Leroux MA, Badeaux J, Coillard C, Zabjek KF, Rivard CH (2000) Relationship between gibbosity and Cobb angle during treatment of idiopathic scoliosis with the SpineCor brace. Eur Spine J. 9:516-22.
[14] Goldberg CJ, Kaliszer M, Moore DP, Fogarty EE, Dowling FE (2001) Surface topography, Cobb angles, and cosmetic change in scoliosis. Spine. 26:E55-63.
[15] Inami K, Suzuki N, Ono T, Yamashita Y, Kohno K, Morisue H (1999) Analysis of Posterior Trunk Symmetry Index (POTSI) in Scoliosis. In: IAF. Stokes (Ed), Part 2. Research into Spinal Deformities. 2:85-88.
[16] Jaremko JL, Poncet P, Ronsky J, Harder J, Dansereau J, Labelle H, Zernicke RF (2002). Indices of torso asymmetry related to spinal deformity in scoliosis. Clin Biomech. 17:559-68.
[17] Vercauteren M, Van Beneden M, Verplaetse R, Croene P, Uyttendaele D, Verdonk R (1982) Trunk asymmetries in a Belgian school population. Spine. 7:555-62.
[18] Nissinen M, Heliovaara M, Tallroth K, Poussa M (1989) Trunk asymmetry and scoliosis. Anthropometric measurements in prepuberal school children. Acta Paediatrica Scandinavica,78:747-53.
[19] Cobb JR (1948) Outline for the study of scoliosis. American Academy of Orthopedic Surgeons. 7:261-75.

[20] Stokes IAF (1994) Scoliosis Research Society Working Group on 3-d terminology of spinal deformity: Three-dimensional terminology of spinal deformity. Spine. 19:236-248.
[21] Ho EK, Upadhyay SS, Chan FL, Hsu LC, Leong JC (1993) New methods of measuring vertebral rotation from computed tomographic scans. An intraobserver and interobserver study on girls with scoliosis. Spine. 18:1173-7.
[22] Perdriolle R, Vidal J (1985) Thoracic idiopathic scoliosis curve evolution and prognosis. Spine. 10:785-91.
[23] Risser JC (1958) The Iliac apophysis; an invaluable sign in the management of scoliosis. Clin Orthop Relat Res. 4:111-9.
[24] Bunnell WP (1986) The natural history of idiopathic scoliosis before skeletal maturity. Spine. 11:773-6.
[25] Peterson LE, Nachemson AL (1995) Prediction of progression of the curve in girls who have adolescent idiopathic scoliosis of moderate severity. Logistic regression analysis based on data from The Brace Study of the Scoliosis Research Society. J Bone Joint Surg AM,77:823-7.
[26] Stokes I, Gardner-Morse M (2002) The role of muscles and effects of load on growth. Stud Health Technol Inform. 91:314-7.
[27] Cheung J, Halbertsma JP, Veldhuizen AG, Sluiter WJ, Maurits NM, Cool JC, van Horn JR (2005) A preliminary study on electromyographic analysis of the paraspinal musculature in idiopathic scoliosis. Eur Spine J. 14(2):130-7.
[28] Cheung J, Veldhuizen AG, Halbertsma JP, Maurits NM, Sluiter WJ, Cool JC, Van Horn JR (2004) The relation between electromyography and growth velocity of the spine in the evaluation of curve progression in idiopathic scoliosis. Spine. 29(9):1011-6.
[29] Cheung J, Veldhuizen AG, Halberts JP, Sluiter WJ, Van Horn JR (2006) Geometric and electromyographic assessments in the evaluation of curve progression in idiopathic scoliosis. Spine. 31(3):322-9.
[30] Simoneau M, Mercier P, Blouin J, Allard P, Teasdale N (2006) Altered sensory-weighting mechanisms is observed in adolescents with idiopathic scoliosis. BMC Neurosci. 7:68.
[31] Nault ML, Allard P, Hinse S, Le Blanc R, Caron O, Labelle H, Sadeghi H (2002) Relations between standing stability and body posture parameters in adolescent idiopathic scoliosis. Spine. 27(17):1911-7.
[32] Zabjek KF, Coillard C, Rivard CH, Prince F (2008) Estimation of the centre of mass for the study of postural control in Idiopathic Scoliosis patients: a comparison of two techniques. Eur Spine J. 17(3):355-60.
[33] Shumway-Cook A, Wollacott MH (2000). Motor Control: Theory and Practical Applications. Toronto: Lippincott, Williams & Wilkins.
[34] Zabjek KF, Leroux MA, Coillard C, Prince F, Rivard CH (2008) Postural characteristics of adolescents with idiopathic scoliosis. J Pediatr Orthop. 28(2):218-24.
[35] Moore KL. (1985) Clinically Oriented Anatomy (2nd Edition). Baltimore, Williams & Wilkins.
[36] Kotwicki T, Negrini S, Grivas TB, Rigo M, Maruyama T, Durmala J, Zaina F (2009) Members of the international Society on Scoliosis Orthopaedic and Rehabilitation Treatment (SOSORT). Scoliosis. 4:26.
[37] Grivas TB, de Mauroy JC, Négrini S, Kotwicki T, Zaina F, Wynne JH, Stokes IA, Knott P, Pizzetti P, Rigo M, Villagrasa M, Weiss HR, Maruyama T (2010) SOSORT

members. Terminology - glossary including acronyms and quotations in use for the conservative spinal deformities treatment: 8th SOSORT consensus paper. Scoliosis. 2;5:23.

[38] Lenke L, & Terminology Committee (2000). Research Society Terminology Committee and Working Group on Spinal Classification Revised Glossary of Terms. http://www.srs.org/professionals/glossary/SRS_revised_glossary_of_terms.htm

[39] Carpineta L, Labelle H (2003) Evidence of three-dimensional variability in scoliotic curves. Clin Orthop Relat Res. (412):139-48.

[40] Sangole AP, Aubin CE, Labelle H, Stokes IA, Lenke LG, Jackson R, Newton P (2009) Three-dimensional classification of thoracic scoliotic curves. Spine. 34(1):91-9.

[41] Duong L, Mac-Thiong JM, Cheriet F, Labelle H (2009) Three-dimensional subclassification of Lenke type 1 scoliotic curves. J Spinal Disord Tech. 22(2):135-43.

[42] Zabjek KF, Leroux MA, Coillard C, Martinez X, Griffet J, Simard G, Rivard CH (2001) Acute postural adaptations induced by a shoe lift in idiopathic scoliosis patients. Eur Spine J. 10(2):107-13.

[43] Beaudoin L, Zabjek KF, Leroux MA, Coillard C, Rivard CH (1999) Acute systematic and variable postural adaptations induced by an orthopaedic shoe lift in control subjects. Eur Spine J. 8(1):40-5.

[44] De la Huerta F, Leroux MA, Zabjek KF, Coillard C, Rivard CH (1998) [Stereovideographic evaluation of the postural geometry of healthy and scoliotic patients]. Ann Chir. 52(8):776-83.

[45] Nguyen VH, Leroux MA, Badeaux J, Zabjek K, Coillard C, Rivard CH (1998) Classification of left thoracolumbar scoliosis according to its radiologic morphology and its postural geometry]. Ann Chir. 52(8):752-60.

[46] Zabjek KF, Simard G, Leroux MA, Coillard C, Rivard CH (1999) Comparison of the reliability of two 3D acquisition systems used for the study of anthropometric and postural parameters]. Ann Chir. 53(8):751-60.

[47] Stokes IA, Armstrong JG, Moreland MS (1988) Spinal deformity and back surface asymmetry in idiopathic scoliosis. J. Orthop. Res. 6, 129-37.

[48] Grivas TB, Vasiliadis ES, Mihas C, Savvidou O (2007) The effect of growth on the correlation between the spinal and rib cage deformity: implications on idiopathic scoliosis pathogenesis. Scoliosis. 2:11.

[49] Grivas TB, Vasiliadis E, Savvidou OD, Triantafyllopoulos G (2008) What a school screening program could contribute in clinical research of idiopathic scoliosis aetiology. Disabil Rehabil. 30(10):752-62.

[50] Grivas TB, Wade MH, Negrini S, O'Brien JP, Maruyama T, Hawes MC, Rigo M, Weiss HR, Kotwicki T, Vasiliadis ES, Sulam LN, Neuhous T (2007) SOSORT consensus paper: school screening for scoliosis. Where are we today? Scoliosis. 26;2:17

[51] Grivas TB, Koukos K, Koukou UI, Maziotou C, Polyzois BD (2002) The incidence of idiopathic scoliosis in Greece--analyais of domestic school screening programs. Stud Health Technol Inform 91:71-5.

[52] Kotwicki T, Kinel E, Stryla W, Szulc A (2007) Discrepancy in clinical versus radiological parameters describing deformity due to brace treatment for moderate idiopathic scoliosis. Scoliosis 2:18.

[53] Krawczyński A, Kotwicki T, Szulc A, Samborski W (2006) Clinical and radiological assessment of vertebral rotation in idiopathic scoliosis. Ortop Traumatol Rehabil 8(6):602-7.

[54] Leroux MA, Zabjek K, Simard G, Coillard C, Rivard CH (2002) Estimated kyphosis and lordosis changes at follow-up in patients with idiopathic scoliosis. J Pediatr Orthop. 22(1):73-9.

[55] Leroux MA, Zabjek K, Simard G, Badeaux J, Coillard C, Rivard CH (2000) A noninvasive anthropometric technique for measuring kyphosis and lordosis: an application for idiopathic scoliosis. Spine. 25(13):1689-94.

[56] Jaremko JL, Poncet P, Ronsky J, Harder J, Dansereau J, Labelle H, Zernicke RF (2002) Genetic algorithm-neural network estimation of cobb angle from torso asymmetry in scoliosis. J Biomech Eng. 124(5):496-503.

[57] Jaremko J, Delorme S, Dansereau J, Labelle H, Ronsky J, Poncet P, Harder J, Dewar R, Zernicke RF (2000) Use of Neural Networks to Correlate Spine and Rib Deformity in Scoliosis. Comput Methods Biomech Biomed Engin. 3(3):203-213.

[58] Pearsall DJ, Reid JG, Hedden DM (1992) Comparison of three noninvasive methods for measuring scoliosis. Physical Therapy. 72:648-57.

[59] Donaldson S, Stephens D, Howard A, Alman B, Narayanan U, Wright JG (2007) Surgical decision making in adolescent idiopathic scoliosis. Spine. 32(14):1526-32.

[60] Smith PL, Donaldson S, Hedden D, Alman B, Howard A, Stephens D, Wright JG (2006) Parents' and patients' perceptions of postoperative appearance in adolescent idiopathic scoliosis. Spine. 2006 31(20):2367-74.

[61] Cardon G, De Clercq D, De Bourdeaudhuij I, Breithecker D (2004) Sitting habits in elementary schoolchildren: a traditional versus a "Moving school". Patient Educ Couns. 54(2):133-42.

[62] Geldhof E, Cardon G, De Bourdeaudhuij I, De Clercq D (2006) Back posture education in elementary schoolchildren: a 2-year follow-up study. Eur Spine J. 16(6):841-50.

[63] Parcells C, Stommel M, Hubbard RP (1999) Mismatch of classroom furniture and student body dimensions: empirical findings and health implications J Adolesc Health. 24(4):265-73.

[64] Gram MC, Hasan Z (1999) The spinal curve in standing and sitting postures in children with idiopathic scoliosis. Spine. 24(2):169-77.

[65] Callaghan JP, McGill SM (2001) Low back joint loading and kinematics during standing and unsupported sitting. Ergonomics. 44(3):280-94.

[66] Callaghan JP, Dunk NM (2002) Examination of the flexion relaxation phenomenon in erector spinae muscles during short duration slumped sitting. Clin Biomech. 17(5):353-60.

[67] Winter DA (1990) Biomechanics and motor control of human movement. 2nd edition. Toronto: Wiley-Interscience Publication.

[68] Winter DA, Patla AE, Ishac M, Gage WH (2003) Motor mechanisms of balance during quiet standing. J Electromyogr Kinesiol. 13(1):49-56.

[69] Winter DA, Prince F, Stergio P, Powell C (1993) Medial-lateral and anterior-posterior motor responses associated with centre of pressure changes in quiet standing. Neuroscience Research Communications,12:141-148.

[70] Winter DA, Prince F, Frank JS, Powell C, Zabjek KF (1996) Unified theory regarding A/P and M/L balance in quiet stance. J Neurophysiol 75:2334-43.

[71] Adler N, Bleck EE, Rinsky LA, Young W (1986) Balance reactions and eye-hand coordination in idiopathic scoliosis. J Orthopaedic Res. 4:102-7.

[72] Byl NN, Gray JM (1993) Complex balance reactions in different sensory conditions: adolescents with and without idiopathic scoliosis. J Orthopaedic R. 11:215-27.

[73] Chen PQ, Wang JL, Tsuang YH, Liao TL, Huang PI, Hang YS (1998). The postural stability control and gait pattern of idiopathic scoliosis adolescents. Clin Biomech, 13:S52-S58.
[74] Gauchard GC, Lascombes P, Kuhnast M, Perrin PP (2001) Influence of different types of progressive idiopathic scoliosis on static and dynamic postural control. Spine. 26:1052-8.
[75] Gregoric M, Pecak F, Trontelj JV, Dimitrijevic MR (1981) Postural control in scoliosis. A statokinesimetric study in patients with scoliosis due to neuromuscular disorders and in patients with idiopathic scoliosis. Acta Orthop Scand. 52:59-63.
[76] Lidstrom J, Friberg S, Lindstrom L, Sahlstrand T (1988) Postural control in siblings to scoliosis patients and scoliosis patients. Spine. 13:1070-4.
[77] Nault ML, Allard P, Hinse S, Le Blanc R, Caron O, Labelle H, Sadeghi H (2002) Relations between standing stability and body posture parameters in adolescent idiopathic scoliosis. Spine. 27:1911-7.
[78] Sahlstrand T, Lidstrom J (1980) Equilibrium factors as predictors of the prognosis in adolescent idiopathic scoliosis. Clin Orthop Relat Res.152:232-6.
[79] Sahlstrand T, Ortengren R, Nachemson A (1978) Postural equilibrium in adolescent idiopathic scoliosis. Acta Orthop Scand. 49:354-65.
[80] Dempster WT, Gaughran GRL (1967) Properties of body segments based on size and weight. Am J Anat. 120:33-54.
[81] Zatsiorsky V, Seluyanov V (1983) The mass and Inertia characteristics of the main segments of the human body. In: Matsui H, Kobayashi K (Eds.), International Series on Biomechanics, Volume 4B. Proceedings of the Eight International Congress of Biomechanics (pp. 1152-1159). Champaign, Illinois: Human Kinetics Publishers.
[82] Jensen RK (1986) Body segment mass, radius and radius of gyration proportions of children. J Biomech. 19:359-368.
[83] Pearsall DJ, Reid JG, Livingston LA (1996) Segmental inertial parameters of the human trunk as determined from computed tomography. Ann Biomed Eng. 24:198-210.
[84] Jensen RK (1989) Changes in segment inertia proportions between 4 and 20 years. J Biomech. 22:529-536.
[85] Benda BJ, Riley PO, Krebs DE (1994) Biomechanical relationship between the center of gravity and center of pressure during standing. IEEE Trans Rehabil Eng. 2:3-10.
[86] Morasso PG, Spada G, Capra R (1999) Computing the COM from the COP in postural sway movements. Hum Mov Sci 18:759-767.
[87] Caron O, Faure B, Breniere Y (1997) Estimating the center of gravity of the body on the basis of the center of pressure in standing posture. *J Biomech* 30:1169-71.
[88] Zatsiorsky VM, King DL (1998) An algorithm for determining gravity line location from posturographic recordings. J Biomech. 31:161-4.
[89] King DL, Zatsiorsky VM (1997) Extracting gravity line displacement from stabilographic recordings. Gait Posture. 6:27-38.
[90] Lenzi D, Cappello A, Chiari L (2003). Influence of body segment parameters and modeling assumptions on the estimate of center of mass trajectory. J Biomech. 36:1335-41.
[91] Shimba T (1984) An estimation of center of gravity from force plateform data. J Biomech. 17:53:60.

[92] Allen FR, Ambikairajah E, Lovell NH, Celler BG (2006) Classification of a known sequence of motions and postures from accelerometry data using adapted Gaussian mixture models. Physiol Meas. 27:935-51.
[93] Mannini A, Sabatini AM (2011) Accelerometry-based classification of human activities using Markov modeling. Comput Intell Neurosci. 2011:647858.
[94] Aloqlah M, Lahiji RR, Loparo KA, Mehregany M (2010) A headband for classifying human postures. Conf Proc IEEE Eng Med Biol Soc. 2010:382-5.
[95] Mathie MJ, Celler BG, Lovell NH, Coster AC (2004) Classification of basic daily movements using a triaxial accelerometer. Med Biol Eng Comput. 42(5):679-87.
[96] Prajapati SK, Gage WH, Brooks D, Black SE, McIlroy WE (2011) A novel approach to ambulatory monitoring: investigation into the quantity and control of everyday walking in patients with subacute stroke. Neurorehabil Neural Repair. 25(1):6-14.
[97] Zijlstra W, Hof AL (2003) Assessment of spatio-temporal gait parameters from trunk accelerations during human walking. Gait Posture. 18:1-10.
[98] Murakami N, Okada S, Nakamura T, Saito N (2011) Analysis of pelvic movement in the elderly during walking using a posture monitoring system equipped with a triaxial accelerometer and a gyroscope. J Biomech. 44(9):1788-92. Epub 2011 May 4.
[99] Bidargaddi N, Klingbeil L, Sarela A, Boyle J, Cheung V, Yelland C, Karunanithi M, Gray L (2007) Wavelet based approach for posture transition estimation using a waist worn accelerometer. Conf Proc IEEE Eng Med Biol Soc. 2007:1884-7.
[100] Oliver M, Schofield GM, Badland HM, Shepherd J (2010) Utility of accelerometer thresholds for classifying sitting in office workers. Prev Med. 51(5):357-60.
[101] Ishigaki N, Kimura T, Usui Y, Aoki K, Narita N, Shimizu M, Hara K, Ogihara N, Nakamura K, Kato H, Ohira M, Yokokawa Y, Miyoshi K (2011) Analysis of pelvic movement in the elderly during walking using a posture monitoring system equipped with a triaxial accelerometer and a gyroscope. J Biomech. 44(9):1788-92.
[102] McDonald RL, Wilson GN, Molloy A, Franck LS (2011) Feasibility of three electronic instruments in studying the benefits of adaptive seating. Disabil Rehabil Assist Technol. 6(6):483-90.
[103] Wong WY, Wong MS (2008) Trunk posture monitoring with inertial sensors. Eur Spine J. 17(5):743-53.
[104] Wong WY, Wong MS (2008) Detecting spinal posture change in sitting positions with tri-axial accelerometers. Gait Posture. 27(1):168-71.
[105] Bazzarelli M, Durdle N, Lou E, Raso J, Hill D (2002) A wearable networked embedded system for the treatment of scoliosis. Stud Health Technol Inform. 91:383-6.
[106] Lou E, Raso J, Hill D, Durdle N, Moreau M (2002) Spine-Straight device for the treatment of kyphosis. Stud Health Technol Inform. 91:401-4.

10

Predicting Curve Progression in Adolescent Idiopathic Scoliosis - An Outline of Different Indicators of Growth

Iris Busscher and Albert G. Veldhuizen
University Medical Center Groningen
The Netherlands

1. Introduction

Successful treatment of adolescent idiopathic scoliosis (AIS) remains a complex challenge for the orthopaedic surgeon. For a good planning of the conservative or surgical treatment it is essential to understand the prognosis of the deformity. The timing of treatment is mainly dependent on the timing of the progression of the scoliotic curve.

Earlier research has shown that curve progression is primarily related to periods of rapid skeletal growth of the patient during puberty[1,2]. In order to predict the timing of curve progression, it is of great interest to predict the timing of the pubertal growth spurt in the individual patient with adolescent idiopathic scoliosis.

Furthermore, in severe scoliosis, surgical fusion is still the gold standard and for the prevention of complications like the crankshaft phenomenon[3], the operation, if possible, has to be postponed until the pubertal growth spurt of the patient for the most part has passed.

The pubertal growth spurt is known to take place between 10 and 14 years in 95% of the girls, and between 12 and 16 years in 95% of the boys[4-6]. This range holds for a large population, but is too wide to make an accurate prediction in the individual patient.

Several methods have been studied to predict the timing and magnitude of the pubertal growth spurt in the individual child. Different maturity indicators can be used like skeletal age in different areas, the Risser sign, status of the triradiate cartilage, Tanner stage of sexual maturation, age of the thelarche and menarche, and several body length dimensions. Furthermore, the trend in total body height for an individual child can be used in a mathematical growth model to predict the timing and magnitude of the pubertal growth spurt[7]. These indicators of maturity are all signs that reflect growth or remaining growth of the patient and can be useful in predicting the timing of the pubertal growth spurt in the individual patient.

Researchers have tried to find different ways to predict curve progression in AIS as well, besides relating progression to the pubertal growth spurt. A promising method was shown by Cheung et al[2,8], who found a relationship between curve progression and altered electromyography ratios of the convex and concave sides of the curve. This will be discussed later.

This chapter provides a concise outline of several indicators of growth and curve progression in order to be able to provide a clear overview of which indicators can be useful in predicting the timing of the pubertal growth spurt and therefore the timing of possible scoliosis progression.

2. Skeletal age dimensions

Any skeletal region with consistent physeal markers can be determined for skeletal age. The most commonly used markers of skeletal age in patients with idiopathic scoliosis are the hand and wrist, the ossification of the iliac apophysis (Risser sign), the status of the triradiate cartilage, and the ossification of the epiphysis of the elbow.

Determination of skeletal age by hand and wrist X rays is usually done by the method of Greulich and Pyle or Tanner and Whitehouse.

The Greulich and Pyle method as originally described involves a complex comparison of all of the bones in the hand and wrist against reference "normal" radiographs of different ages. In most institutions a modified version of this technique is used, whereby the overall appearance of a given radiograph is compared with the reference radiographs and the nearest match is selected. Although this modified approach is considerably faster than the original it may be less accurate. The Tanner and Whitehouse method relies on the systematic evaluation of the maturity of all the bones in the hand and wrist. The Tanner Whitehouse classification can predict well if the patient is before or after the pubertal growth spurt. The Greulich and Pyle method of assessing skeletal age is easier to use but less precise and the atlas was compiled from radiographs made in the 1930's[9].

The Risser sign describes the ossification of the iliac apophysis (Figure 1). It continues to be an accepted prognostic sign in the evaluation of growth of patients with idiopathic scoliosis. More controversy is arising since Risser stage 1 occurs after the growth spurt in 85% of patients and the distribution is fairly wide. Its predictive value is therefore low[10,11]. However, some recent studies showed that taking the lateral spinal X-ray in consideration as well, the accuracy of the Risser sign can be improved and it can therefore be helpful for predicting the spinal growth potential[12].

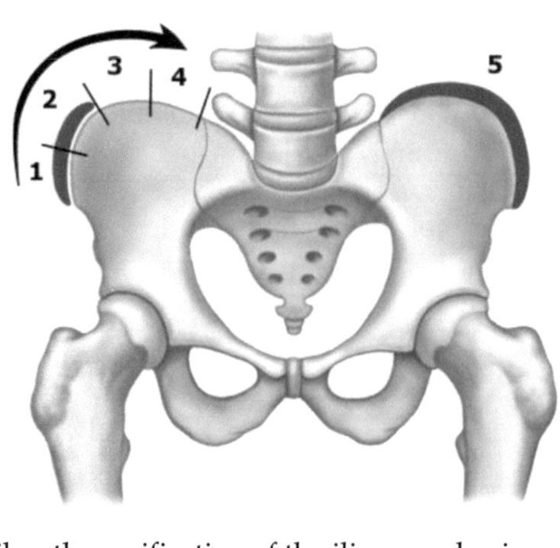

Fig. 1. Risser sign describes the ossification of the iliac apophysis.

Sanders et al.[13,14] found the status of the triradiate cartilage (Figure 2) to be more predictive for the timing of the peak growth velocity of total body height, though it is only predictive whether the patient is before or after the pubertal growth spurt. Once the patient has closed triradiate cartilages, he or she is very likely past the pubertal growth spurt. However, the predictive value of open triradiate cartilages is less clear.

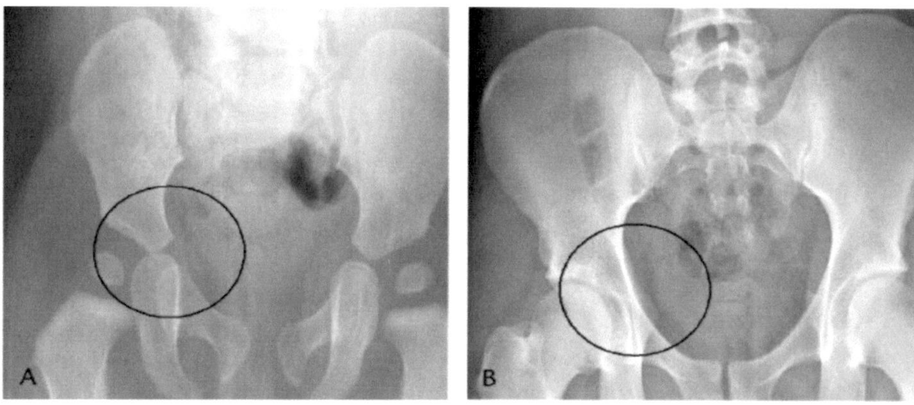

Fig. 2. status op the triradiate cartialge.

A different method for describing skeletal age is the Sauvegrain method (Figure 3), in which skeletal age is determined using a scoring system for four anatomical landmarks of the elbow. At the onset of puberty, the elbow is still largely cartilaginous. Two years later, fusion of the elbow growth centers is complete. This period is critical since it is marked by the pubertal growth spurt. This method was found to be more accurate and detailed than the Greulich and Pyle atlas[15]. Furthermore, it is easier to use and it allows the evaluation of skeletal age in six-month intervals, in contrast to one-year intervals in the most commonly used methods of Greulich and Pyle, and Tanner and Whitehouse.

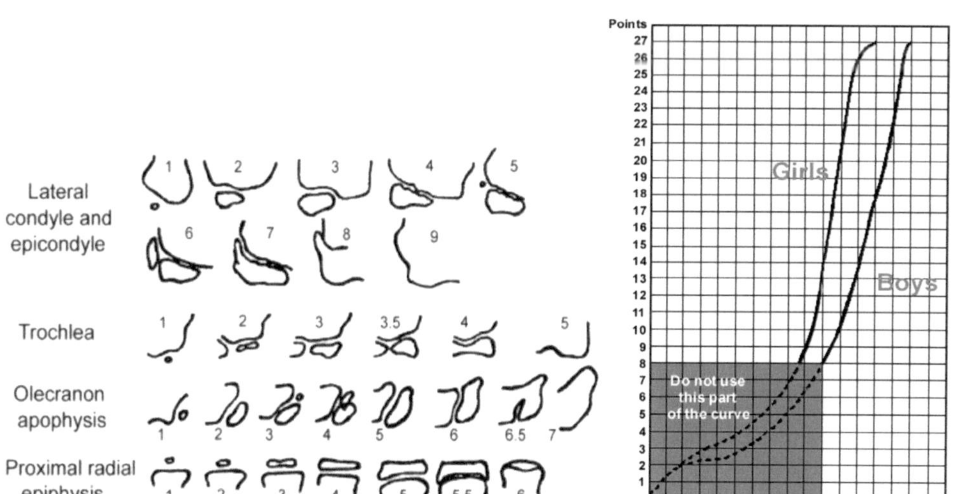

Fig. 3. The Sauvegrain method describes the skeletal age using four anatomical landmarks of the elbow.

3. Secondary sexual characteristics

Another hallmark of maturation is the development of secondary sexual characteristics, often classified by Tanner (Figure 4). Thelarche, the first stage of secondary breast development, marks the beginning of puberty and usually takes place 1 year before the pubertal growth spurt[16-19]. Girls typically experience their pubertal growth spurt between stages 2 and 3 of breast development and pubic hair development. The pubertal or Tanner stages are good measurements of maturity. Timing of menarche, the first menstrual period, can be used in girls, but most often takes place 1 year after the growth spurt and is therefore always retrospective.

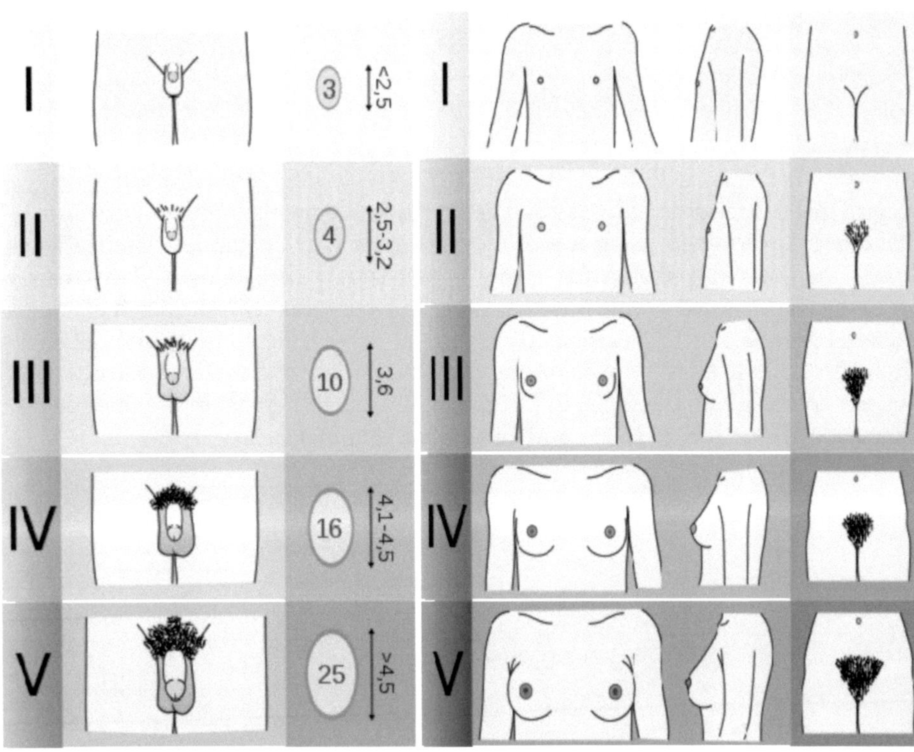

Fig. 4. Tanner stages of sexual maturation.

4. Body length dimensions

It is generally accepted that different body length dimensions each have their own typical growth pattern influenced by age- and gender-related factors. Research has been done by Welon and Bielicki[19], Cameron et al.[21], Dimeglio[22], and Rao et al.[23] to the sequences of peak growth velocities of different length measurements of children from 1-18 years. They all confirm the distal-to-proximal growth maturity gradient as described by Tanner[24]. Body parts that are more distal will have their pubertal growth spurt earlier in adolescence.

However, Busscher et al.[25] showed that this growth gradient theory is not always applicable to the individual child. On average it holds for large groups, but individual variations make it less useful for predictions of the pubertal growth spurt in the individual child.

Furthermore, in order to calculate growth velocities of a body length dimension, access is needed to longitudinal growth data of the patient. Usually patients who visit the outpatient clinic for the first time do not have growth data over the last years and it takes years to gather the data.

However, a different study from Busscher et al.[26] showed that the shoe size can be helpful in predicting the timing of the pubertal growth spurt in children. Since patients and their parents can recall the course of their shoe size for the last year or two, the clinician already has some longitudinal data at the first visit. In particular the fact that the shoe size does not increase any further when the pubertal growth spurt takes place in both boys and girls can be helpful, even in the individual child.

A complete different way of predicting the timing of the pubertal growth spurt was recently shown by using a mathematical growth model[7]. A new model was presented in which a small part of the available growth velocity curve of an individual child was linked to a known generic growth velocity curve. The generic curve was shifted and stretched or shrinked, both along the age-axis (X-axis) and the height velocity axis (Y-axis). In this way, a new complete growth velocity curve for that individual child was obtained and the individual timing of the pubertal growth spurt could be determined. The results were highly promising even when using just few available growth data of an individual patient.

5. Electromyography of the paraspinal muscles

As mentioned earlier, Cheung et al[2,8] found a relationship between curve progression and altered electromyography ratios of the convex and concave sides of the curve. An electromyography was made of the paraspinal muscles in order to determine the ratios of muscle activity on the convex and concave side of the main scoliotic curve.

For the electromyographic measurements, 12 EMG electrodes were placed symmetrically along the superficial erector spinae muscles at three levels, 30 mm from the midline, and parallel to the spinous processes. The electrode levels correspond to both end vertebrae of the curve (most tilted ones), and the apex vertebra.

The paraspinal activity (EMG) ratio was defined as the EMG activity of the erector spinae muscles between a convex electrode pair divided by the EMG activity between a contralateral concave electrode pair.

Enhanced EMG ratios were observed at three levels of the scoliotic curve (lower end vertebra, apex, and upper end vertebra) at the start of progressive periods. At the start of a non-progressive period, such an enhanced EMG ratio was only observed at the level of the apex vertebra[2].

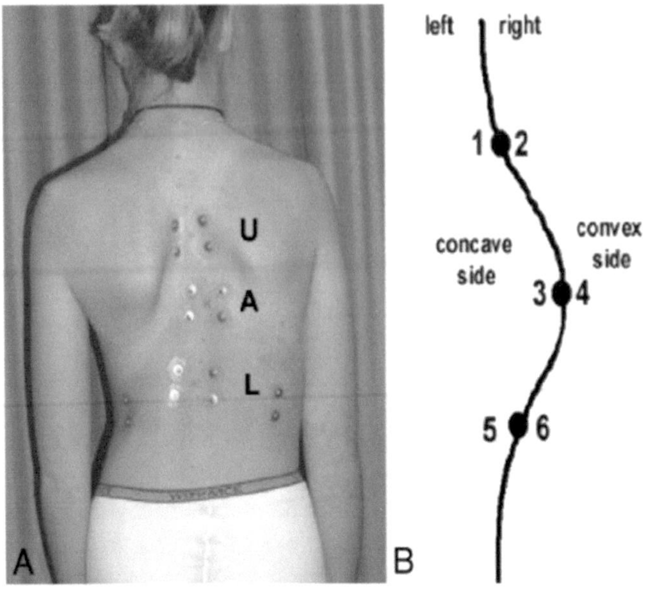

Fig. 5. Measurement of electromyography ratios of the paraspinal muscles of the convex and concave side of the curve.

6. Conclusion

This chapter provided an outline of several indicators of growth and curve progression in patients with adolescent idiopathic scoliosis. Some are useful, others are less useful. A problem in finding useful indicators for predicting the timing of the pubertal growth spurt is that several indicators are only useful for large groups of children. On average they can help, but individual variations are large and therefore predictions for the individual child are difficult.

Useful indicators should be easy to use, fast and should not place a large burden on the patient or the clinician. For example, EMG measurement of the paraspinal muscles is a highly promising method but it is fairly time consuming.

A combination of several indicators of growth and curve progression can help the orthopaedic surgeon in planning the treatment of adolescent idiopathic scoliosis in the individual child.

A combination of the Sauvegrain method for skeletal age, the Tanner stages of sexual maturation, the individual course in shoe size, and the use of a new mathematical growth model is most likely to be helpful in predicting the timing of the pubertal growth spurt and the timing of curve progression in the individual patient with adolescent idiopathic scoliosis.

7. References

[1] Wever DJ, Tonseth KA, Veldhuizen AG. Curve progression and spinal growth in brace treated idiopathic scoliosis. Stud.Health Technol.Inform. 2002;91:387-92.

[2] Cheung J, Veldhuizen AG, Halbertsma JP et al. The relation between electromyography and growth velocity of the spine in the evaluation of curve progression in idiopathic scoliosis. Spine (Phila Pa 1976.) 2004;29:1011-6.

[3] Sanders JO, Little DG, Richards BS. Prediction of the crankshaft phenomenon by peak height velocity. Spine 1997;22:1352-6.

[4] Gerver WJ, de Bruin R. Paediatric morphometrics: a reference manual. Second extended edition ed.UPM Maastricht, 2001.

[5] Gerver WJ, de Bruin R. Growth velocity: a presentation of reference values in Dutch children. Horm.Res. 2003;60:181-4.

[6] Tanner JM, Davies PS. Clinical longitudinal standards for height and height velocity for North American children. J.Pediatr. 1985;107:317-29.

[7] Busscher I, Kingma I, de Bruin R, et al. Prediction of the peak growth velocity in the individual child, validation of a new growth model. Eur Spine J 2011; 10.1007/s00586-011-1845-z

[8] Cheung J, Halbertsma JP, Veldhuizen AG, Sluiter WJ, Maurits NM, Cool JC et al.: A preliminary study on electromyographic analysis of the paraspinal musculature in idiopathic scoliosis. Eur Spine J 2005, 14: 130-137.

[9] Bull RK, Edwards PD, Kemp PM, Fry S, Hughes IA: Bone age assessment: a large scale comparison of the Greulich and Pyle, and Tanner and Whitehouse (TW2) methods. Arch Dis Child 1999, 81: 172-173.

[10] Little DG, Sussman MD: The Risser sign: a critical analysis. J Pediatr Orthop 1994, 14: 569-575.

[11] Shuren N, Kasser JR, Emans JB, Rand F: Reevaluation of the use of the Risser sign in idiopathic scoliosis. Spine 1992, 17: 359-361.

[12] Kotwicki T: Improved accuracy on Risser sign grading with lateral spinal radiography. Eur Spine J 2008, 17 (12): 1676-85.

[13] Sanders JO, Browne RH, Cooney TE, Finegold DN, McConnell SJ, Margraf SA: Correlates of the peak height velocity in girls with idiopathic scoliosis. Spine 2006, 31: 2289-2295.

[14] Sanders JO, Browne RH, McConnell SJ, Margraf SA, Cooney TE, Finegold DN: Maturity assessment and curve progression in girls with idiopathic scoliosis. J Bone Joint Surg Am 2007, 89: 64-73.

[15] Dimeglio A, Charles YP, Daures JP, de Rosa V, Kabore B: Accuracy of the Sauvegrain method in determining skeletal age during puberty. J Bone Joint Surg Am 2005, 87: 1689-1696.

[16] Loncar-Dusek M, Pecina M, Prebeg Z: A longitudinal study of growth velocity and development of secondary gender characteristics versus onset of idiopathic scoliosis. Clin Orthop Relat Res 1991, 278-282.

[17] Little DG, Song KM, Katz D, Herring JA: Relationship of peak height velocity to other maturity indicators in idiopathic scoliosis in girls. J Bone Joint Surg Am 2000, 82: 685-693.

[18] Karlberg J, Kwan CW, Gelander L, Albertsson-Wikland K: Pubertal growth assessment. Horm Res 2003, 60: 27-35.

[19] Tanner JM: Foetus into Man. Physical Growth from Conception to Maturity. OBP London; 1978.

[20] Welon Z, Bielicki T: The timing of adolescent growth spurts of 8 body dimensions in boys and girls of the Wroclaw growth study. Stud Phys Anthrop 1979, 5: 75-79.
[21] Cameron N, Tanner JM, Whitehouse RH: A longitudinal analysis of the growth of limb segments in adolescence. Ann Hum Biol 1982, 9: 211-220.
[22] Dimeglio A: Growth in pediatric orthopaedics. J Pediatr Orthop 2001, 21: 549-555.
[23] Rao S, Joshi S, Kanade A: Growth in some physical dimensions in relation to adolescent growth spurt among rural Indian children. Ann Hum Biol 2000, 27: 127-138.
[24] Tanner JM: Growth at Adolescence, 2nd Edition edn. Oxford: Blackwell Scientific Publications; 1962.
[25] Busscher I, Gerver WJM, Kingma I, et al. The growth of different body length dimensions is not predictive for the peak growth velocity of sitting height in the individual child. Eur Spine J 2010; 20(5): 791-797
[26] Busscher I, Kingma I, Wapstra FH, et al. the value of shoe size for prediction of the timing of the pubertal growth spurt. Scoliois 2011; 6(1):1

11

The Impact of Spinal Deformity on Gait in Subjects with Idiopathic Scoliosis

Agnieszka Stępień
Józef Piłsudski University of Physical Education in Warsaw, Poland

1. Introduction

Walking is one of the most coordinated activities of a human being. It is a natural way of changing position among others, the avoiding or overcoming of obstacles, going upstairs and downstairs or changing directions. Efficiency of walking depends on mobility of the joints, activity of the muscles, coordination and rhythm of the movements as well as the ability to smoothly move the center of gravity. An ordinary gait pattern in healthy persons can be described by means of modern systems of movement analysis in space.

Any impairment in muscular, skeletal or nervous system can be the reason for which changes occur in an ordinary gait pattern. Different kinds of pathology in walking can be compensated by the movement of various body parts. They may involve greater forces and changes to the range of motion (ROM). Identification of a dysfunction follows recognition of any subtle substitute mechanisms and prediction of possible trauma. Scoliosis is one of the spine deformations affecting quality of movements and walking.

Scoliosis defined by the *Society on Scoliosis Orthopaedic and Rehabilitation Treatment* (SOSORT) is a lateral deviation of the normal vertical line of the spine which is greater than ten degrees when measured by x ray method. Scoliosis consists of a lateral curvature of the spine with rotation of the vertebrae within the curve. The changes in the frontal and transverse planes are associated with the lack of physiological alignment in the sagittal plane. Such a three - dimensional deformity results in changes to body mechanics and induces motion asymmetry.

The cause of idiopathic scoliosis and its development still remain unknown. Scientists tend to analyze scoliosis in three dimensions: frontal, sagittal and horizontal planes. There are many studies focusing on the structure of the spine and activity in subjects with scoliosis. They have been carried out according to the recommendations of WHO contained in the International Classification of Functioning, Disability and Health (WHO, 2001). Their results confirm the presence of structural disorders such as limitations of the range of motion, muscle dysfunctions, deep sensation and balance disorders. Some studies discuss the biomechanics of the spine in persons with scoliosis. Others point out activity abnormalities in a sitting or standing position leading to postural or movement asymmetry.

Some studies demonstrate the impact of spine deformity on gait in subjects with scoliosis. Their authors describe various walking disorders in subjects with different types of scoliosis measured by appropriate systems and instruments.

2. Stance ability and walking in subjects with scoliosis

It is reported that the patients with idiopathic scoliosis demonstrate balance problems in stance phase (Giakas, 1996) and have a poor postural stability and present higher sway area than the control group subjects (Chen, 1998).

Kramers -de Quervain et al.(2004) observed significant asymmetry in the trunk's rotational behavior in the transverse plane during double limb stance in girls with a left-lumbar and a right - thoracic curve. Syczewska et al. (2006) described abnormal position of the pelvis and an increased range of motion of the pelvis in the sagittal plane in girls with double curve idiopathic scoliosis. Lateral tilting in the frontal plane and improper position of the pelvis in the transverse plane were also observed during gait in the majority of the patients under assessment. Another abnormality revealed in this research was asymmetrical EMG of the greatest gluteal muscles and extensor muscles of the trunk along the lumbar and thoracic part of the spine. Mallau et al. (2007) noticed a decrease in the walking speed while performing different tasks and the disturbed stabilization of the head in patients with idiopathic scoliosis. Mahaudens et al. (2009) pointed out a significant decrease in muscle efficiency, reduction in shoulder, pelvis and hip motion and prolonged muscle activation in female subjects with left thoracolumbar or lumbar primary curves. Pasha et al. (2010) emphasized changes in three - dimensional pelvic movements during gait in female patients with adolescent idiopathic scoliosis and stated that different alignment of the pelvis dictated the biomechanics during movements.

Stępień et al. (2007) demonstrated that scoliosis induces asymmetry in feet load in subjects with scoliosis. It was assumed in that study that the effect of body weight while standing and walking was represented by the ground reaction forces and that spinal deformity had an impact on right and left foot load in separate gait periods. The authors observed various gait patterns depending on the type of scoliosis.

61 subjects, aged 10-18 (14,4), with idiopathic scoliosis were qualified to participate in the gait analysis. One of the conditions required to take part in the study was a diagnosis of right thoracic and/or left lumbar curve.

Three groups were formed for individual scoliosis type: L - 16 subjects with single left lumbar curve or double curve scoliosis with dominant left lumbar curve (difference between lumbar and thoracic curve from 5 degrees up), E - 17 subjects with equal double curve scoliosis with the same extent of right thoracic and left lumbar curve (difference between curves up to 5 degrees) and T - 28 subjects with single right thoracic curve or double curve scoliosis with dominant right thoracic curve (difference between thoracic and lumbar curve from 5 degrees up).

The Computer Dynography (CDG) system was used to assess feet load during walking. 8 sensors fixed in special shoes registered vertical reaction forces while walking (Figure 1). The values of the forces registered by the sensors were assigned to each gait phase of stance: Initial Contact (IC), Loading Response (LR), Mid Stance (MSt), Terminal Stance (TSt) and Pre Swing (PSw).

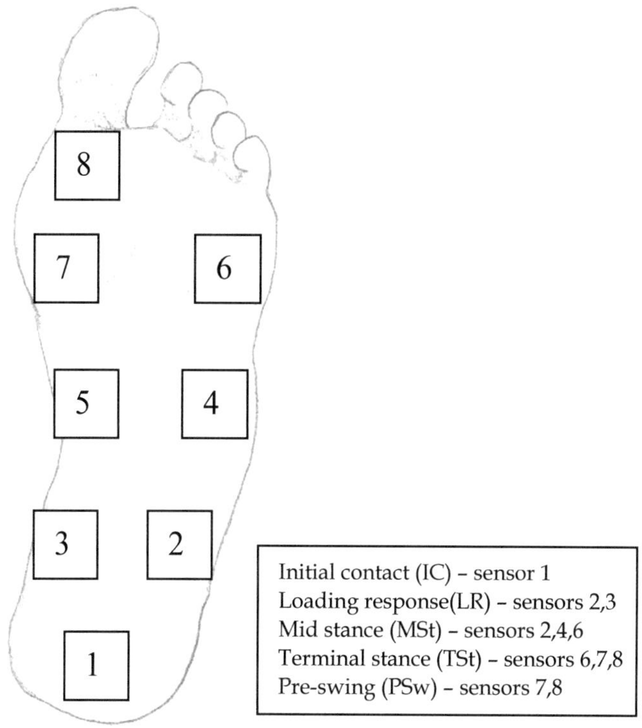

Fig. 1. Registration of vertical ground reaction forces - sensors localization depending on the division of stance phase.

The final results presented a specific and repeated pattern for the right and left foot load in each group. Some differences between the groups were recorded.

Increase in ground reaction forces for the lateral part of the right foot in thoracic scoliosis group (T) in MSt was observed in 75% subjects. In case of the lumbar scoliosis group (L) increasing ground reaction forces were found for the lateral part of the left foot in 63% subjects. No differences between feet load in E group were recorded.

Significant differences between the values of vertical reaction forces for the right and left foot were found in TSt and PSw. The ground reaction forces in TSt and PSw were bigger for the left foot than for the right one. Dominant left foot load compared with the right one was registered in over 90% subjects with double curve scoliosis. More significant differences between the left and right foot load were detected in these adolescents (T, E groups) than in the subjects with dominant left lumbar curve (L). Left foot load was significantly bigger in T group than in the subjects with dominant left lumbar curve. It suggests that the thoracic curve provokes the increasing differences in feet load in TSt and PSw phases during walking.

2.1 Reasons for change of gait pattern in subjects with scoliosis

What is the cause of walking asymmetry in people with idiopathic scoliosis? There are a few hypotheses for each gait phase that explain this phenomenon. The capability to remain in upright standing position is fundamental to develop the ability to walk. The stability in quiet standing is determined by keeping the vertical axis of the body, proper muscle activity, joints mobility, balance, feet structure and others. These factors are essential also for gait pattern.

2.1.1 Alignment of the body

Proper alignment of the head, trunk and pelvis is a necessary factor to improve effectiveness of sitting, standing and walking (Adler et al., 2008) in the light of the concepts in the field of physiotherapy of international renown such as PNF (represented by International Proprioceptive Neuromuscular Facilitation Association - IPNFA) or The Bobath Concept (represented by International Bobath Instructors Training Association - IBITA) are.

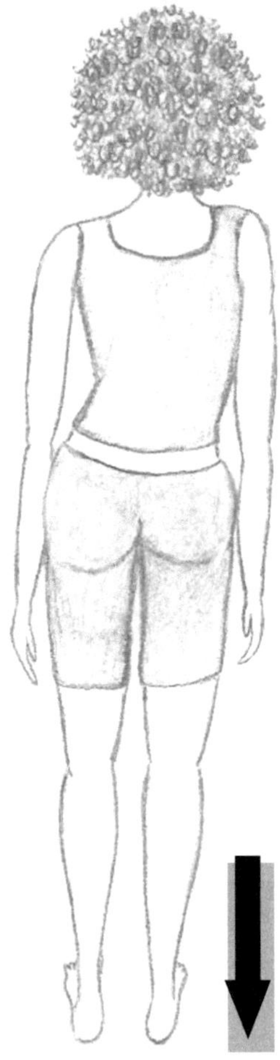

Fig. 2. The lateral shift of the body overloads the lower limbs unilaterally.

Continuous effort to bring the center of mass forward is one of the biomechanisms which is specific for walking. The alignment of the body decides on the localization of the center of mass (COM) and the quality of ground reaction force. Any deviation from the physiological curves of the spine, lateral, forward and backward shift from the upright posture results in changes to feet load in standing position and decides on the stability in stance phase. Forward or backward link of the body carries the center of plantar pressure to the anterior or posterior part of both feet, respectively. A lateral shift of the COM in relation to the pelvis and the base of support increases weight bearing to the unilateral lower leg (Figure 2).

Scoliosis is defined as three - dimensional change in spinal alignment. Some studies took into consideration three - dimensional changes of the body in people with scoliosis.

Mac - Thiong et al. (2003) found out changes in physiological curves of the spine and the pelvic incidence in the sagittal plane. Stępień (2008) observed increased anterior pelvic inclination in adolescent girls with idiopathic scoliosis compared to girls without scoliosis. The lower thoracic kyphosis and higher lumbar lordosis observed in subjects with scoliosis can hinder the activity of the muscles responsible for the stability, upset the postural control of the body and change the feet load in stance (Figure 3).

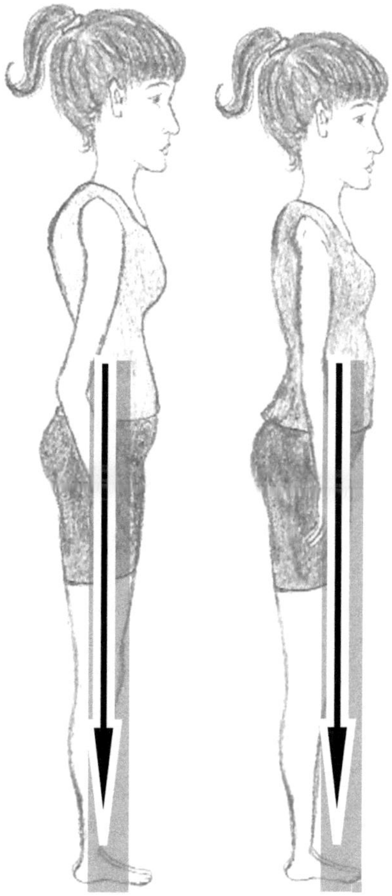

Fig. 3. Influence of the spine alignment in the sagittal plane on feet load in stance. Lower thoracic kyphosis and higher lumbar lordosis move the center of mass forwards changing the feet load.

Zabjek et al. (2008) demonstrated that persons with different types of the spinal curvatures (right thoracic, left thoracolumbar and right thoracic - left lumbar curve) were characterized by disparate posture in the space, represented by different orientation of the pelvis, shoulders and shoulder blades. It was also noticed that persons with scoliosis had larger amplitude of anterior - posterior displacement of T1 - S1 spinous processes in reference to the base of support in comparison with the subjects with no pathology (Zabjek et. al., 2005). Some investigators gave their attention to improper pelvic alignment (Gum et al., 2007).

These significant differences in the sagittal, frontal and transverse plane can have an effect on the quality of feet load in the standing position and stance phase in gait .

A few authors demonstrated in their studies that spine deformations provoke displacement of the center of mass (COM), change the placement of the center of pressure (COP) and disturb balance. A decrease in standing stability was observed by Nault et al. (2002) as an increase in displacement of COM, COP and a greater neuromuscular demand. Dellau et al., (2007) also found out higher variability in COP in adolescent girls with scoliosis in comparison with the control group. Szulc et al. (2008) observed a specific pattern of the plantar pressure in scoliotic persons in the standing position. Dalleau et. al. (2011) revealed high values of COP range and COP speed in adolescent girls with idiopathic scoliosis. Stępień et al. (2007) found out the correlation between the displacement of the vertical plumb of the body and the lateral - medial feet load in girls with dominant lumbar or dominant thoracic curve.

2.1.2 Muscle activity

Muscle activity is another determinant influencing the stability in quiet standing and gait pattern. The primary function of muscles is to stabilize the body. Postural control depends on cooperation of many muscles and muscular chains. Important role in body stability is played by the following muscles: multifidus muscles, m. transversus, m. obliquus external, m. obliquus internal, m. gluteus medius and minimus, muscles of the pelvic floor and the diaphragram (Haase, 2006).

M. transversus is regarded as the main muscle responsible for the stability of lower trunk, which is active just before every movement of the upper and lower limbs (Hodges & Richardson, 1996; 1997). Any dysfunction of these muscles results in the worsening of postural control which may influence walking. Muscle stability is difficult especially in single limb support as body weight transfers over the supporting limb.

Some authors focused their attention on muscle activity in people with scoliosis. Lin et al. (2010) described abnormal position of scapulas and different muscle contraction activity on both sides of the thoracic curve in the standing position during arm elevation in female patients with scoliosis. They identified higher contraction activity of lower trapezius muscle on the convex side and lower contraction activity of lower trapezius and serratus anterior muscles on the concave side in comparison with the control group.

Well coordinated movements of shoulder blades and arms are essential for economic gait. Alternating arm swing supports the lower legs in their motions during the stance or swing phase and it is coordinated with the trunk muscles changing activity. Anterior elevation of the scapula supports the unilateral lower limb to keep the weight of the body in stance phase. On the other hand posterior depression of the scapula supports stance phase on the contralateral lower limb. Alternating movements of the scapulas reinforce rotational control of the trunk and stability in single and double limb stance (Proprioceptive Neuromuscular Facilitation - Adler et al., 2008).

Any muscle dysfunction around shoulder blades can be the cause of walking disturbance. New physiological and biomechanical theories state that human body acts through stimulation of muscle chains activity and any impairment of muscle function can provoke changes in the whole body and trigger new movement patterns in daily activity. This knowledge is the base in physiotherapeutic concepts like PNF (Adler et al. 2008; IPNFA) and close to the theories of muscle chain activity (Myers, 2009).

Haumont et al. (2011) found significant differences in posture control under perturbation conditions between female patients with scoliosis and the control group. Differences were observed especially as earlier onset and prolonged activation of the left multifidus on the lumbar convex side and the right gastrocnemius on the lumbar concave side. The results of these studies are useful for gait analysis, because both the multifidus and the gastrocnemius muscle play a significant role in walking.

2.1.3 Optimal mobility

Optimal mobility in hip joints is one of the conditions necessary for efficient and coordinated walking. Any limitation on passive or active range of motion (ROM) with regard to extension, abduction or rotation disturbs symmetry of walking. The above-mentioned limitations will influence MSt, TSt and PreSw phases in particular and provoke a chain of compensations. Some authors showed in their studies that there were hip joints dysfunctions in persons with scoliosis. The results of their studies imply that most patients with idiopathic scoliosis have asymmetric range of passive hip rotation arising due to transposition of the sector of motion in both hip joints (Kotwicki et al., 2008). The dysfunction of the hip joints in the transverse and sagittal plane in patients with idiopathic scoliosis also occurs during walking (Syczewska et al, 2006). Asymmetrical position and range of motion in the hip joints in many patients with scoliosis is a consequence of incorrect spatial orientation of the pelvis.

2.1.4 Feet structure

Feet are the base for human body. Any deviation from the proper structure of a foot/ feet has a negative impact on the correct position of the whole body. The feet and the body influence each other. Improper alignment of the body results in the change of feet load, consequently, incorrect feet structure changes the orientation of the trunk and pelvis. Orientation of the pelvis in the transverse plane is one of the essential determinants affecting the feet position. Rotation of the pelvis to the right moves the load to the lateral part of the right foot and lowers the medial arc of the left foot. That explains the type of feet asymmetry in subjects with scoliosis characterized by the right pelvic rotation noticeable mainly in patients with the main right thoracic curve (Figure 4). Structural feet asymmetry in patients with scoliosis may influence the feet load during walking.

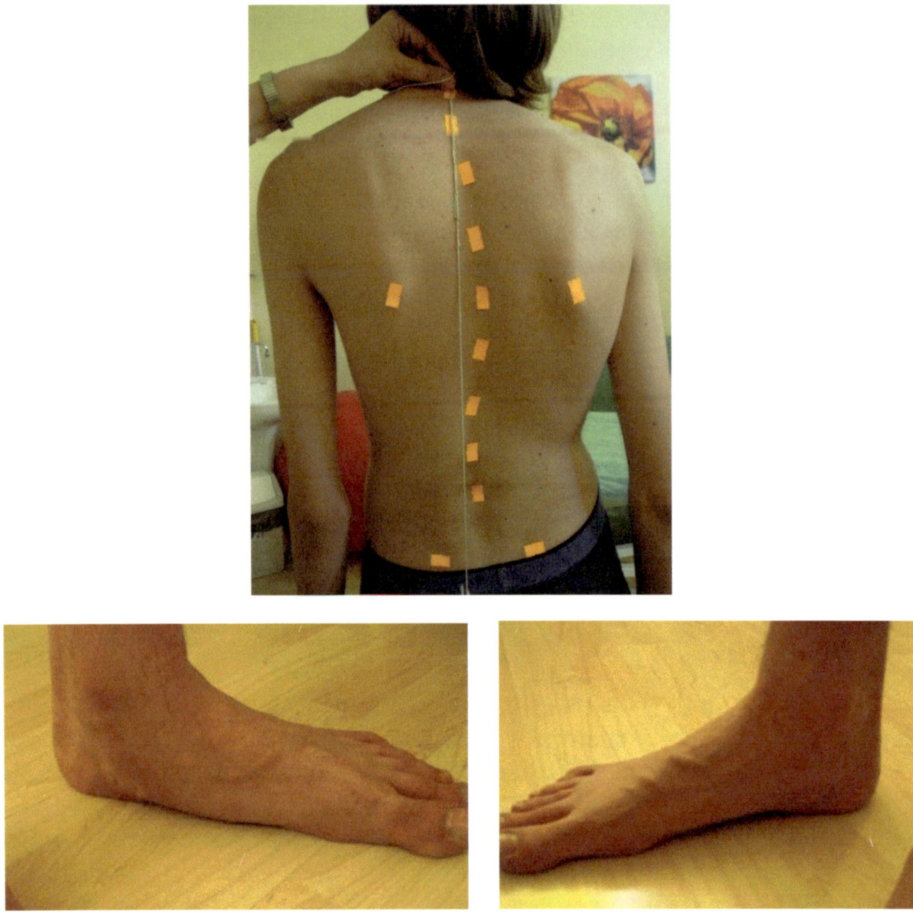

Fig. 4. Example of asymmetrical feet structure in the boy with scoliosis.

2.1.5 Disturbed counter rotation

Disturbed counter rotation of the upper trunk in relation to lower trunk and pelvis can be one of the factors resulting in gait asymmetry in TSt and PSw (Stępień et al., 2007) in subjects with scoliosis. Double limb stance with the right lower limb moved forward and the left one behind the body requires rotation of pelvis and vertebrae in the lower part of lumbar spine to the left, which is in harmony with thoracic vertebrae movement to the right. Stepping forward with the left lower limb is combined with the rotation of the pelvis and lumbar vertebrae to the right and the rotation of thoracic vertebrae in the opposite direction. It means that stepping forward with the right lower limb is in harmony with rotation of the left lumbar curve and rotation of the right thoracic curve in subjects with double curve scoliosis. On the other hand swing phase of the left lower limb requires activity in these persons against deformity of the lumbar curve in the frontal and horizontal plane and rotation of thoracic curve in the opposite direction. This situation can lead to occurrence of asymmetry in alternating movements of the trunk, pelvis and limbs in walking. All movements in those "with" scoliosis are easier for skeletal and muscular system, so any step forward with the right lower limb is associated with higher values of left foot load. It is likely that ground reaction forces in stance for the right foot in subjects with double curve scoliosis in TSt and PreSw are reduced due to the movement being in discord with the rules of the mechanics present in scoliosis.

Disturbed counter rotation was taken into consideration as the basic hypothesis in the following study project (Stępień, 2008). The aim of that study was to determine the influence of a spine deformation type on the trunk and pelvis range of motion in horizontal plane in adolescent girls with idiopathic scoliosis (Stępień, 2011). The additional aim was to describe the trunk and pelvis angular motions in the sagittal plane that occur during rotation.

59 girls with adolescent idiopathic scoliosis and 30 asymptomatic girls at the age of 10-18 participated in the study. Right thoracic curve or/and left lumbar curve in spine radiography were the criteria for further measurements in the girls with scoliosis. Four groups were formed of the girls with different types of deformity: L - single left lumbar curve or double curve scoliosis with dominant left lumbar curve (14 girls), E - equal double curve scoliosis (16 girls), T1 - double curve scoliosis with dominant right thoracic curve (22 girls), T2 – single right thoracic curve (7 girls).

Measurements were made in quiet standing and in the standing position with the left or right lower limb at the front (position imitating double limb stance). The pelvis was fixed when the trunk was rotating and the shoulder girdle with upper trunk was stabilized during the pelvic motions. A specially designed prototype axial rotation tester with a computer system was used to assess ROM of the trunk and pelvis rotation and the angular coupled motions in the sagittal plane. An angle of rotation and associated motions were registered by the unit placed on the thorax and thoracic vertebrae (Th5 - Th7) or on the pelvis and lumbar vertebrae (L4 - S1). Special sensors placed under the first metatarsal bones signaled movements of the feet while rotation of the pelvis came about. Each participant's task was to perform pelvic rotation without taking metacarpal bones away. 6 movements of the trunk and 6 movements of the pelvis (3 right, 3 left) were taken in account into the analyses. The results were presented in numerical and graphic form (Figure 5).

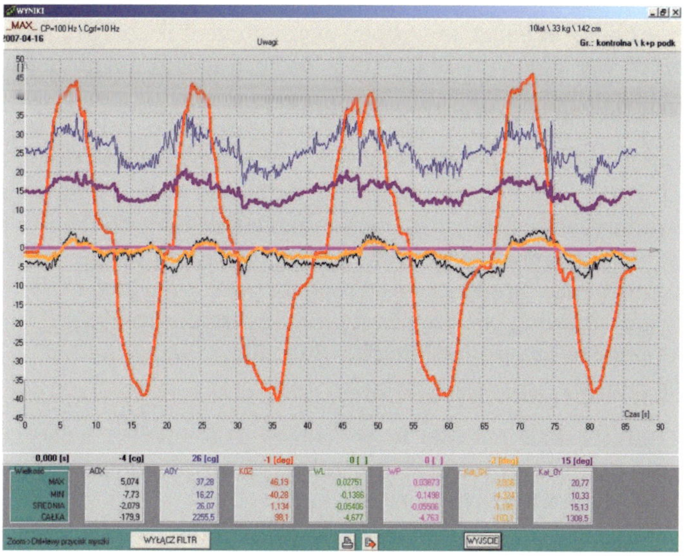

Fig. 5. Exemplary results in a graphic form - a range of trunk rotation in the transverse plane and coupled angular motions in the sagittal and frontal plane.

The results indicated many significant differences, particulary, between the girls with double curve scoliosis with dominant right thoracic curve (T1), the girls with single or double curve scoliosis with dominant left lumbar curve (L) and those from the control group.

A significant limitation of the trunk and pelvis rotation in the horizontal plane was observed in the girls with double curve scoliosis with dominant right thoracic curve. It was found that dominant left lumbar curve resulted in an increase of pelvic rotation compared to the control group and provoked asymmetries between ROM of the left and right rotation of the pelvis.

The limited rotation of the trunk and pelvis in the girls with double curve scoliosis was compensated in anterior - posterior movements in the sagittal plane.

Many significant differences between the values of the left and right rotation in each group and differences between the groups indirectly pointed out disturbed motions in the transverse plane as a potential reason of characteristic gait pattern in people with different spine deformations. The limited rotation in subjects with double curve scoliosis can affect the observed changes in feet load during walking in TSt and PSw. In both studies (Stępień et al., 2007; Stępień 2008) the adolescent subjects with scoliosis were grouped according to the same guidelines and the results of both projects showed the influence of dominant thoracic curve on increasing asymmetry.

2.1.6 Balance

One of determinants causing walking disorders in subjects with idiopathic scoliosis, taken into consideration by scientists, are balance disorders. It was stated that balance disorders in adolescent patients with idiopathic scoliosis could be the result of the detected morphoanatomical changes in the vestibular system (Shi et al., 2011).

Balance means the ability of equal or optimal distribution of the weight amount in different positions to keep proper alignment of the body. Balance activities require integration of the visual, auditory, kinesthetic, tactile, and vestibular senses to effect the proprioceptive processes that help to reduce injuries and improve performance. Balance is a global reaction of the body, when the head is positioned over the sacrum and pelvis, shoulders tend to stay horizontally and the mass of the trunk is transferred to the vertical axis of the body. That is possible thanks to three dimensional reaction of the whole body in the frontal, sagittal and tranverse plane. Any dysfunction or local biomechanical failure of the spine results in disturbance of balance and compensations. Proper balance is the base for human daily living activities in sitting or standing position. Every forward, backward, lateral trunk leaning and movements of upper and lower limbs involve three dimensional reaction of the body. Also walking requires complex reaction of the body.

Some authors study balance reaction in patients with idiopathic scoliosis in stance and walking but the first step in analysing the balance should involve three dimensional assessment of the body in sitting position.

The alignment of the spine in sitting is associated with the pelvic position. Improper alignment of the pelvis in the sagittal plane has influence on the position of the cervical, thoracic spine, sternum and ribs (Kiebzak et al., 2010). The lateral displacement in the frontal

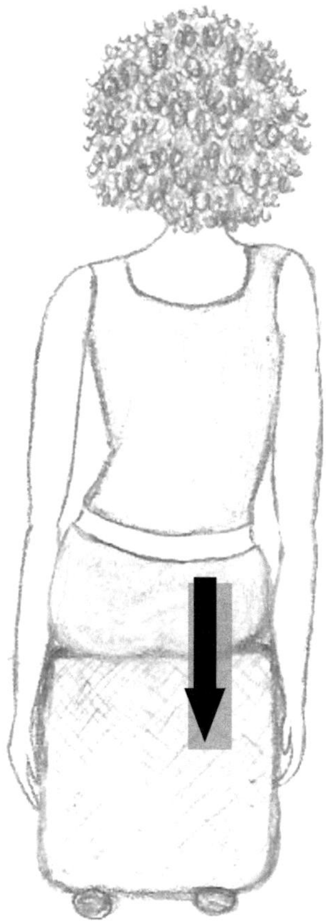

Fig. 6. Improper sitting position. The lateral shift of the trunk to the right increases load onto the right ischiadic tuber.

plane causes a different load of the right and left ischiadic tuber (Figure 6). It creates different position in the right and left hip joints (Stępień, 2010a,b). Tubers load depends on the type of scoliosis. The patients with left lumbar curve have a tendency to transfer load toward the left ischiadic tuber while the persons with thoracic curve usually shift the weight in the direction of the right one. Asymmetry in sitting may increase while daily activities . Improvement of the trunk and pelvis control in the sitting position is the first step to regain better trunk control in stance and walking.

The preliminary results of the studies being currently carried by the author et al. involving girls with double curve (thoracic right and lumbar left curve) in sitting revealed balance disorders and possibility of compensation in this group. Each girl under the study had to demonstrate her usual sitting position and then shift her trunk laterally to the left and then to the right. The trunk's rotational behaviour in the transverse plane was analysed at the time of the lateral shift of the trunk.

The results showed that local lumbar limitation of the active lateral shift of the spine to the right in the sitting position was compensated in the transverse plane in the thoracic part of the spine. Compensation was noticeable as an increased rib hump (Figure 7 a,b,c).

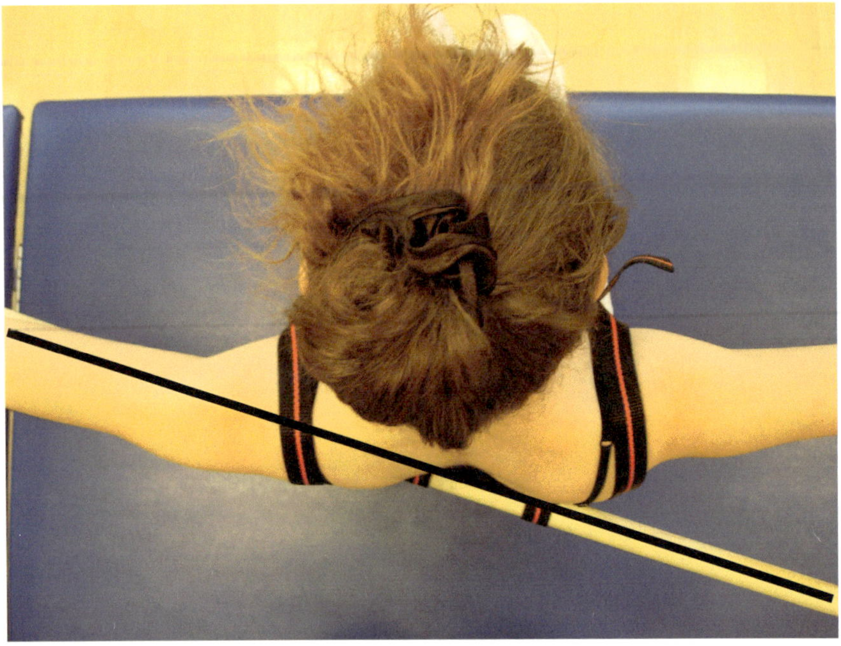

Fig. 7a. Sitting position. Top view.

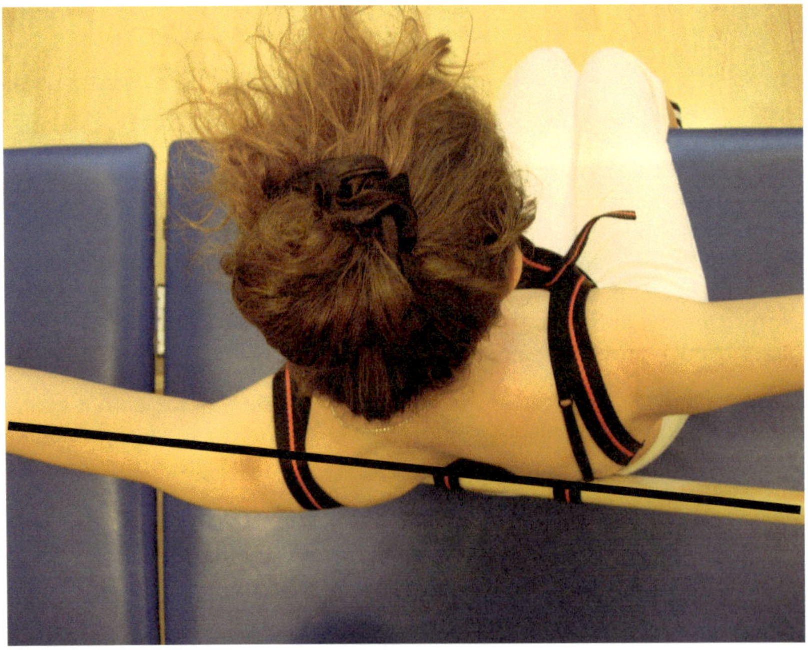

Fig. 7b. Lateral shift to the left in sitting. Top view.

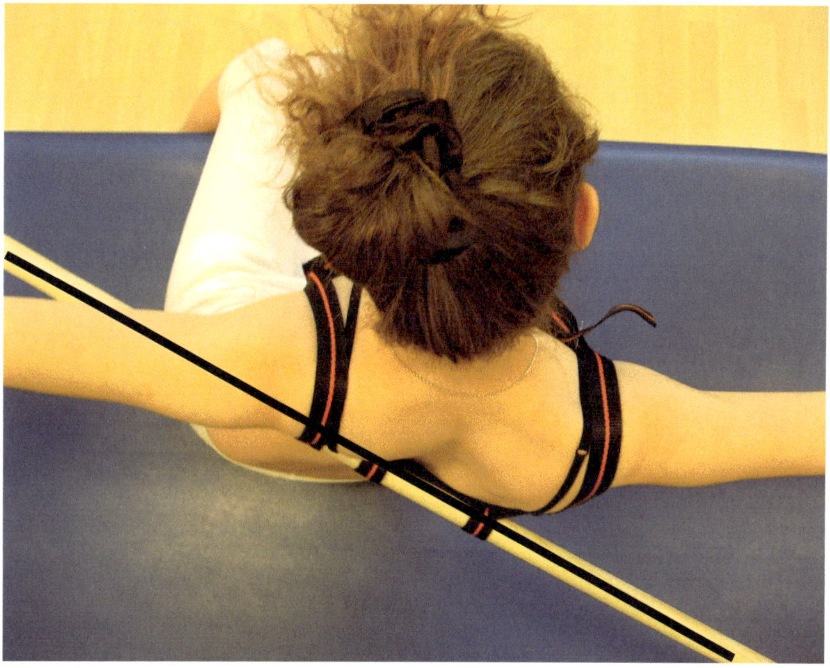

Fig. 7c. Lateral shift to the right. Top view.

The results suggested that the active shift of the trunk over the right lower limb during single limb support could provoke compensations noticeable in the thoracic spine rotation and anterior elevation of the right scapula.

These coupled motions of the spine can be the following factor which creates favorable conditions of development of walking disorders and acceleration of scoliosis progression.

A few authors have undertaken the studies to describe coupled motions in scoliosis. Stępień (2008) noticed coupled motions in the sagittal plane occurring during rotation of the spine. The relation between the movements in the frontal and transverse plane was described by Adam et al.(2008). These authors stated that lateral curve preceded vertebral rotation. Pasha et al. (2010) noticed that movement of the pelvis in one plane caused the change of position in the other two planes.

All these findings mentioned above can be accepted as hypothetical disorders resulting in gait asymmetry.

2.2 Gait pattern in subjects with scoliosis

There are two basic periods in every gait stride: a stance and swing phase. The proportion of the two phases is about 60% to 40% of the time between consecutive heel strikes of the same lower limb (Perry, 1992). The stance is more demanding phase due to the need of shock absorption at the time weight acceptance and recovery of the stability during single limb support. The stability during single and double limb support phases depends on many factors such as the alignment of the spine and lower limbs, muscle strength, joint mobility, coordination or balance of the body.

The stance phase includes: Initial Contact (IC), Loading Response (LR), Mid Stance (MSt), Terminal Stance (TSt), Pre Swing (PSw). The swing phase is divided into: Initial Swing (ISw), Mid Swing (MSw) and Terminal Swing (TSw). On account of the importance of stance phase including weight acceptance and involvement of many structures keeping dynamic stability of the body, the stance phase will be mainly discussed below.

2.2.1 Stance phase

Initial Contact (IC)

It is a very short and difficult phase which lets the balance be retained after lower limb swing. The peak of arms displacement during walking occurs at IC (shoulder extension) and TSt (shoulder flexion), so any difficulties in IC and early LR can be compensated in the range of arm motions what is noticeable in persons with scoliosis, dependent on the speed of walking.

Initial Contact requires proper muscle activity around the lower trunk. Multifidus is bilaterally active at the time of every contact of the heel with the floor, so any functional impairment of multifidus, observed in stance under balance perturbation conditions (Haumont et al.,2011) can result in walking disorders. Initial Contact is characterized by asymmetric activity of extensors muscle along the lumbar part of the spine (Syczewska et al., 2006) and increased knee flexion what was observed in girls with double curve scoliosis.

Loading Response (LR)

Weight acceptance and acceleration in LR require a very compound mechanism of the body control. A rapid lateral drop of the pelvis of the contralateral side observed in this phase in healthy people forces higher muscle activity (mainly hip extensors, abductors and knee extensors) to decelerate this movement. A disturbed function of hip abductors and extensors can be the next cause of gait asymmetry in LR and MSt what was pointed out in the studies (Syczewska et. al, 2006).

Prolonged muscle contraction of the qudratum lumborum, erector spinae, gluteus medius found by Mahaudens et al.(2009) in AIS female patients suggests modification in gait in LR, MSt and TSt compared with the persons without scoliosis although, no kinematic or EMG left-right asymmetry was observed in this study.

At the moment of pelvic drop the pelvis begins its rotation forward. The differences in pelvis position in the transverse plane in persons with specific scoliotic deformation (Pasha et al., 2010) at the beginning of forward rotation on the right and left side can be the cause of the asymmetric gait pattern in LR and PreSw.

Also the preliminary results of the study conducted in our University pointed out the differences between 13 girls with double curve scoliosis (thoracic right and lumbar left) and 11 girls from the control group of the same age, height and weight. The goal of the study was to measure acceleration of the pelvis along the vertical, anterior - posterior and transverse axis of the body in individual gait phases in both groups. A measurement unit was placed on the pelvis and measurement was taken during walking with normal speed on a flat ground. Significant differences between the groups were mainly noticed along the anterior- posterior axis of the body in LR, MSt and PSw phases. The girls with scoliosis were characterized by lower values of acceleration when compared to the control group (Żyłka, 2010). Further studies are necessary to discover the reasons for the lower values of pelvic acceleration in girls with scoliosis.

Proper activity of the quadriceps and well - coordinated cooperation of the trunk muscles associated with the change of direction of arm movements are necessary for dynamic stability in LR. Until now no studies have demonstrated abnormalities in these structures.

Mid Stance (MSt)

The centre of gravity normally moves over to the foot being on the ground during walking in MSt, while the other limb moves forward. Feet load in MSt is influenced by body alignment.

In the study Stępień et al. (2007) observed evident relation between the body vertical axis shift and feet load in stance phase. The lateral displacement of the plumb line in adolescent with dominant right thoracic curve (T) and dominant lumbar left curve (L) was linked to the direction of dominant curve of scoliosis – the plumb line displacement to the left was observed in L group, whereas in case of T group – to the right. The shift of upright posture line of the body in subjects of the groups under study was correlated with the greater load on lateral edge of the foot at the same side, i.e. more often the lateral edge of the left foot in subjects from L group and the lateral edge of the right foot in subjects from T group were loaded additionally. It means that any lateral deviation of the plumb line from proper upright posture of the body is an important determinant influencing the feet load value in MSt and any action taken to correct the upright posture in persons with scoliosis can contribute to the improvement of their walking.

Bringing the center of gravity over the supported foot is possible thanks to proper muscle activity of such muscles as gluteus medius, gluteus maximus, tensor fasciae latae. The precise evaluation of physical condition of the person with scoliosis in single limb support often demonstrates weakness of hip joint abductors, mainly on the concave side of the lumbar curve. The left lumbar curve is usually associated with excessive pelvic tilt to the left during single support on the right limb (Figure 8). Any muscle dysfunction of these muscles increases the pelvic drop of the contralateral side of the body and changes the gait pattern.

Terminal Stance (TSt)

TSt is completed by the other foot support on the ground to regain stability. Forward transfer of body weight requires proper balance reaction, muscle coordination and undisturbed movements of the spine and lower limbs. The lumbar and thoracic components of the erector spinae in healthy people begin their coordinated action in TSt and continue through PSw. M. multifidus is active whenever any heel strike. Increasing muscle activity around the ankle joint and foot is necessary in this phase. This increased muscle activity observed in terminal double limb stance, demonstrated in higher values of the ground reaction forces, also depends on the ability to change the direction of trunk rotation and upper limbs movements.

It has been established that there is a significant asymmetry between the right and left foot load in TSt and PSw in adolescents with scoliosis, and the observed differences were conditioned by the type of scoliosis (Stępień et al., 2007) (Figure 6).

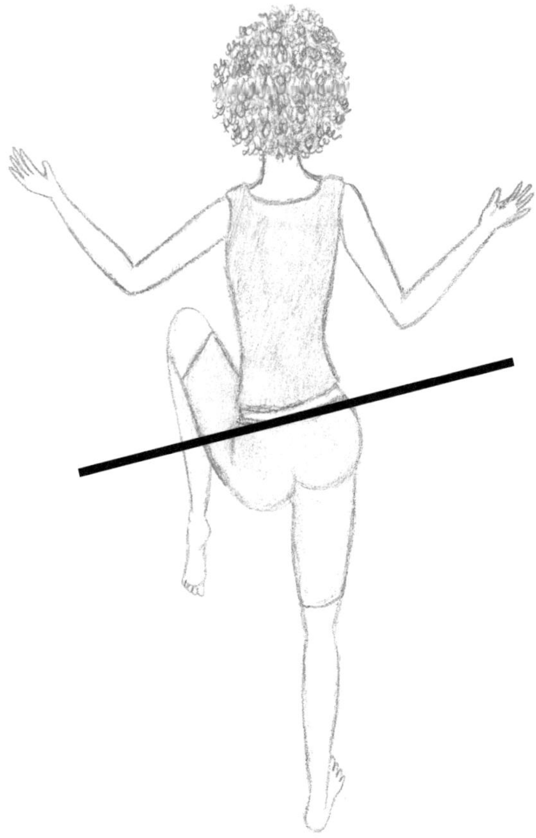

Fig. 8. Example of abnormal lateral pelvic tilt in a patient with scoliosis.

Other authors also indicate that structural spine impairments influence gait abnormalities in double limb stance in the subjects with scoliosis. Kramers- de Quervain et al. (2004) revealed asymmetry in the trunk rotation in the transverse plane during double limb stance in girls with left lumbar and right thoracic curve. Pasha et al. (2010) noted significant changes in pelvic motions during walking in female patients with idiopathic scoliosis compared with persons without spine deformation. It was observed that differences were especially noticeable in subjects with the thoracic right and lumbar left curve. One of achieved results were differences in pelvic motions in the transverse plane. In the majority of the evaluated patients the dominant direction of pelvic rotation was the same as the major curve (right). The authors concluded that the change to one parameter in one of the planes resulted in changes in the other two planes. This conclusion is unanimous with observations made by Stępień (2008), presented above.

Studies carried out by Syczewska et al. (2006) and Kotwicki et al. (2008) showed the differences between the range of rotation in the right and left hip joint in the majority of the assessed patients with idiopathic scoliosis. This mechanism stands for the compensation of

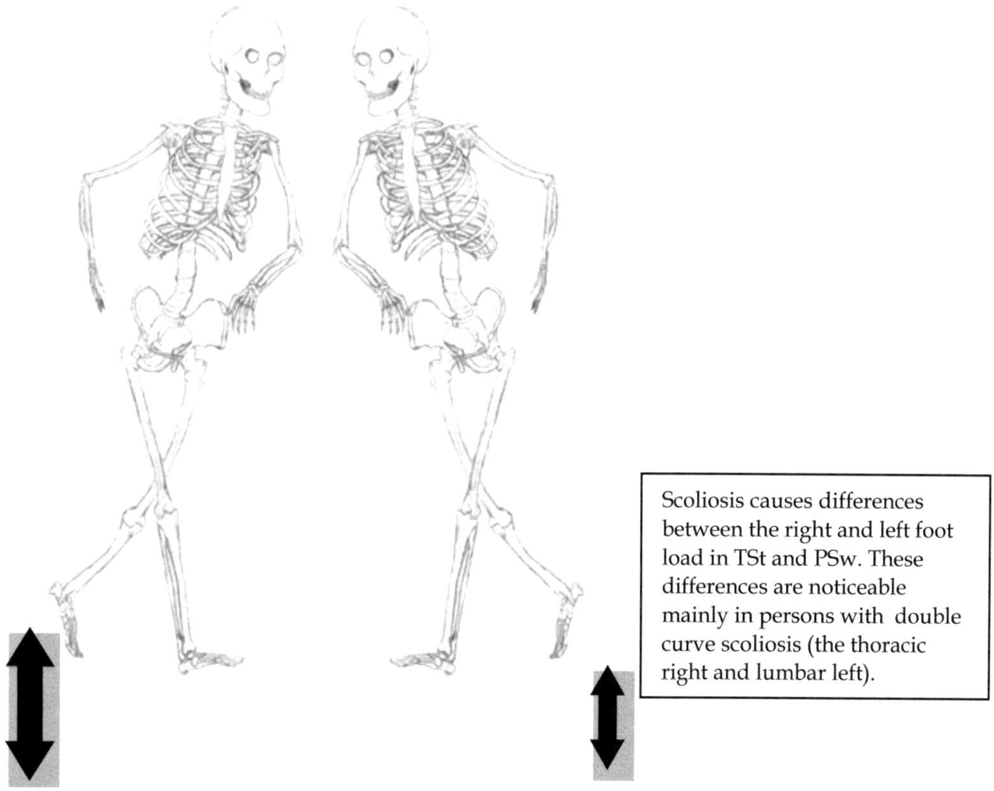

Fig. 6. Differences between the values of the vertical ground reaction forces for the left and right foot in the patient with double curve idiopathic scoliosis.

scoliosis rather than the cause of deformity but it may influence walking and cause differences in feet load in TSt and PreSw.

Pre Swing (PSw)

The load of the foot rapidly decreases in this phase as a result of weight acceptance by the other lower limb. Optimal range of motion in the hip joint is still one of the conditions required for normal gait.

2.2.2 Swing phase

Unfortunately it is not well known what occurs in swing phases in persons with scoliosis. Many authors analyze stance phase considering it to be the most important issue for walking. In normal gait the peak action for abdominal muscles (external oblique muscles) occurs during late Mid Swing and early Terminal Swing. Structural deformations of the spine and rib cage in persons with scoliosis can be the factor disturbing the proper functioning of the muscle chain including external oblique muscles nevertheless it has not been assessed until now.

Improper position of the feet was established in one study of adolescents with idiopathic scoliosis. Syczewska et al. (2006) observed that the feet were dorsiflexed in the ankle joints in the swing phase and there was an internal rotation of the feet with relation to the shanks.

3. Conclusion

The studies presented in this chapter show that gait pattern in subjects with scoliosis depends on the parameters of the spine deformity such as the number of curves in scoliosis, extent and direction of the dominant curve. It is likely that the observed asymmetries during walking are a sign of compensatory mechanisms and they can be a factor leading to pathology and trauma. There are many types of scoliosis under different classifications, so it is necessary to describe the pattern of walking in people with each type of scoliosis. The next step is to correlate the structural dysfunctions related to them. The structures and functions are interrelated. On the one hand, any structural disorder provokes asymmetry or limitation of the movement as well as a change to the quality of an activity. On the other hand a spontaneous position of the body and asymmetry of movements in everyday activities can cause structural dysfunction therefore walking can be one of the reasons for scoliosis progression. The most essential issues, i.e. the reasons of gait asymmetry and those of scoliosis- remain unanswered. Some potential hypotheses are still waiting for research and explanation.

Further studies are necessary to form physiotherapeutic programs to prevent increasing compensations and other secondary deformations such as ribs asymmetry (Zhu et al., 2011) or the temporomandibular joints dysfunctions (Smieciuch, 2011). Another goal is to concentrate on the improvement of gait pattern in persons with idiopathic scoliosis as long as the modern physiotherapy has appropriate means to facilitate gait in patients with different pathology (Adler et al., 2008) including scoliosis.

4. Acknowledgment

The chapter is the result of the efforts of many people. I am especially grateful to Professor Andrzej Seyfried who was my teacher and my thesis supervisor.

Some studies of the author presented in this chapter were carried out thanks to the financial support granted by the Minister of Science and Higher Education, Poland (2006).

5. References

Adam CJ, Askin GN, Pearcy MJ: " Gravity-induced torque and intervertebral rotation in idiopathic scoliosis". Spine (Phila Pa 1976). 2008 Jan 15;33(2): E30-7.

Adler SS, Beckers D, Buck M: "PNF in Practice". Springer Medizin Verlag Heidelberg 2008.

Chen PQ, Wang JL, Tsuang YH, Liao TL, Huang PI, Hang YS: "The postural stability control and gait pattern of idiopathic scoliosis adolescents". Clin Biomech (Bristol, Avon). 1998;13(1):52-58.

Dalleau G, Allard MS, Beaulieu M, Rivard CH, Allard P: " Free moment contribution to quiet standing in able-bodied and scoliotic girls". Eur Spine J. 2007; 16(10) Oct; 1593-9.

Dalleau G, Damavandi M, Leroyer P, Verkindt C, Rivard CH, Allard P: " Horizontal body and trunk center of mass offset and standing balance in scoliotic girls". Eur Spine J.2011 Jan;20(1):123-8.

Giakas G, Baltzopoulos V, Dangirfield PH, Dorgan JC, Dalmira S: "Comparison of gait patterns between healthy and scoliotic patients using time and frequency domain analysis of ground reaction forces". Spine 1996;21(19): 2235-2242.

Gum JL, Asher MA, Burton DC, Lai SM, Lambart LM: " Transverse plane pelvic rotation in adolescent idiopathic scoliosis: primary or compensatory? " Eur Spine J. 2007 Oct; 16(10): 1579-86.

Haase G: Der Stellenwert der posturalen Kontrolle in der Neurorehabilitation. 2006 Vortrag im Rahmen des Kongresses: Bobath aktuell, Hamburg.

Haumont T, Gauchard GC, Lascombes P, Perrin PP: " Postural instability in early stage idiopathic scoliosis in adolescent girls" Spine (Phile Pa 1976) 2011, Jun 36(13): E 847-54.

Hodges PW, Richardson CA,1996: "Inefficient muscular stabilization of the lumbar spine associated with low back pain. A motor control evaluation of transversus abdominis". Spine; 21(22): 2640-2650.

Hodges PW, Richardson CA, 1997: "Contraction of the abdominal muscles associated with movement of the lower limb". Physical Therapy; 77:132-144.

Kiebzak W, Kowalski MI, Kassolik k, Opuchlik A, Zarzycki D, Kiljanski M, Śliwiński Z: „ Wpływ ustawienia miednicy na dolegliwości bólowe w okolicy serca". Orhopedic Quarterly 2010; 77(1): 56-67.

Kramers - de Quervain IA, Muller R, Stacoff A, Grob D, Stussi E: " Gait analysis in patients with idiopathic scoliosis" Eur Spine J. 2004 aud; 13(5): 449-56.

Kotwicki T, Walczak A, Szulc A:" Trunk rotation and hip joint range of rotation in adolescent girls with idiopathic scoliosis: does the "dinner plate" turn asymmetrically?". Scoliosis 2008,3:1.

Lin JJ, Chen WH, Chen PQ, Tsauo JY : " Alteration in shoulder kinematics and associated muscle activity in people with idiopathic scoliosis" Spine (Phila Pa 1976) 2010, May 15 ; 35(11): 1151-57.

Mac -Thiong JM, Labelle H, Charlebois M, Huot MP, de Guise JA: " Sagittal plane analysis of the spine and pelvis in adolescent idiopathic scoliosis according to the coronal curve type". Spine (Phila Pa 1976). 2003 Jul 1;28(13):1404-9.

Mahaudens P, Banse X, Mousny M, Detrembleur C: " Gait in adolescent idiopathic scoliosis: kinematics and electromyografic analysis". Eur Spine J. 2009 Apr;18(4):512-21.

Mahaudens P, Detrembleur C, Mousny M, Banse X: " Gait in adolescent idiopathic scoliosis: energy cost analysis". Eur Spine J. 2009 Aug;18(8):1160-8.

Myers TW, 2009. "Anatomy Trains. Myofascial Meridians for Manual and Movement Therapist". Churchill Livingstone Elsevier, ISBN: 978-0-443-10283-7.

Nault ML, Allard P, Hinse S, Le Blanc R, Caron O, Labelle H, Sadeghi H: Relation between standing stability and body posture parameters in adolescent idiopathic scoliosis" Spine (Phila Pa1976). 2002 Sep 1;27(17):1911-7.

Perry J, 1992: "Gait analysis", SLACK Incorporated, ISBN: 1-55642-192-3, New York.

Shi L, Wang D, Chu WC, Burwell GR, Wong TT, Heng PA, Cheng JC: "Automatic MRI segmentation and morphoanatomy analysis of the vestibular system in adolescent idiopathic scoliosis". Neuroimage.2011 Jan;54 (1):180-8.

Śmieciuch KD: " Dysfunkcje stawów skroniowo-zuchwowych u osób ze skoliozą". Jozef Pilsudski University of Physical Education, Warsaw, Poland, 2011. Not published master degree study.

Stępień A, Seyfried A, Krawczyk M, Graff K: "The impact of spinal deformity on feet load during the gait in subjects with scoliosis". Advances in Rehabilitation. 2007; (2), 13-20.

Stępień A: "Zakresy rotacji tułowia i miednicy u dziewcząt ze skolioza idiopatyczną". Jozef Pilsudski University of Physical Education, Warsaw, Poland, 2008. PhD dissertation.

Stępień A : „Ocena pacjenta ze skoliozą idiopatyczna na poziomię struktur i aktywności dla potrzeb planowania procesu fizjoterapii. Kręgosłup". Praktyczna Fizjoterapia i Rehabilitacja. 2010; 2/10; 40-43.

Stępień A: „Ocena pacjenta ze skolioza idiopatyczna na poziomie struktur i aktywności dla potrzeb planowania procesu fizjoterapii. Miednica i kończyny dolne ". Praktyczna Fizjoterapia i Rehabilitacja. 2010; 3/10; 58-62.

Stępień A:" The range of rotation of the trunk and pelvis in adolescent girls with idiopathic scoliosis". Advances in Rehabilitation.2011, 25(3): 5-12.

Szulc P, Bartkowiak P, Lewandowski J, Markuszewski J: "The influence of idiopathic scoliosis on load distribution in the feet". Chir Narzadów Ruchu Ortop Pol. 2008 May-Jun;73(3): 187-91.

Syczewska M, Łukaszewska A, Górak B, Graff K: „Changes in gait pattern in patients with scoliosis". Medical Rehabilitation 2006, 10 (4): 12-21.

World Health Organization: "International Classification of Functioning, Disability and Health", Geneva, 2001.

Zabjek KF, Leroux MA, Coillard C, Rivard CH, Prince F: " Evaluation of segmental postural characteristics during quiet standing in control and Idiopathic Scoliosis patients". Clin Bomech (Bristol, Avon) 2005, Jun; 20 (5): 483 - 90.

Zabjek KF, Leroux MA, Coillard C, Prince F, Rivard CH: " Postural characteristic of adolescent with idiopathic scoliosis". J Pediatr Orthop. 2008 Mar; 28(2):218-24.

Zhu F, Chu WC, Sun G, Zhu ZZ, Wang WJ, Cheng JC, Qiu Y: " Rib length asymmetry in thoracic adolescent idiopathic scoliosis: is it primary or secondary?" . Eur Spine J. 2011 Feb;20(2):254-9.

Żyłka J: „Ocena przyspieszen na poziomie miednicy podczas chodu u dziewcząt ze skoliozą idiopatyczną". Josef Pilsudski University of Physical Education, Warsaw, Poland, 2010. Not published master degree study.

www.ibita.org – International Bobath Instructors Training Association (IBITA)

www.ipnfa.org – International Proprioceptive Neuromuscular Association (IPNFA)

www.sosort.mobi/ - Society on Scoliosis Orthopaedic and Rehabilitation Treatment (SOSORT)

12

Characteristics of Body Posture in Children and Youth with Hearing Disorders

Elżbieta Olszewska and Dorota Trzcińska
The Unit of Corrective Therapy
The Department of Theory and Methodics of Physical Education
Józef Piłsudski University of Physical Education in Warsaw
Poland

1. Introduction

Beginning at birth, and until the moment of death, changes in the shape of one's spine are conditioned by the processes of posturogenesis. Posturogenesis (postural development) is a process of the form a body posture during the development. It is very intensive process, especially during the children life (Wolański 2005, Angelakopoulos et al., 2008) . The specificity of the construction of the spine, which has anterior-posterior spinal curvatures, is connected with its function, as well as with the fact that humans adopted an upright position (Iwanowski, 1982; Kiwerski, 2009; Lewandowski, 2006;).

Body posture constitutes a motor habit that is typical for an individual (Kutzner-Kozińska et al. 2001). For that reason, it is difficult to specify only one pattern of body posture, especially if it is change through ontogeny (Wolański 2005, Lewandowski 2006). Researchers are still looking for a pattern of correct body posture, and the first typologies were introduced at the end of the 19th century (Babakhani 2011, behind Staffel 1889). At present, the size of physiological spinal curvatures, as well as abnormalities along the cephalocaudal axis, can be assessed by means of visual inspection. This includes a point-based method and an orthopaedic check-up, as well as with measuring apparatuses such as Moire's method, an S-posture meter, and a electrogoniometer Penny & Giles with modification of Boocock. S-posture meter is a polish devices to measures physiological curves (ryc.1). [Boocock, et al., 1994; Iwanowski, 1982; Kasperczyk, 2004; Kasperczyk & Waleszek, 2009; Śliwa, 1993; Wilczyński, 1999).

The most important element of assessing the course of posturogenesis is diagnosing children and adolescents, with special attention given to detecting postural defects.

Postural defects are not conditioned by climatic or geographical factors. They affect children and youth from various countries and social environments to the same degree (Goldberg et al., 1995; Karachalios et al., 1999). Scoliosis is one of the most dangerous abnormalities in body posture. According to the Scoliosis Research Society (www.srs.org), scoliosis is considered a systemic disease. Many authors in their studies have shown that a scoliotic curves , which is of the spine is accompanied by an asymmetric construction of the brain stem, sensory and balance disorders, as well as blood and collagen function disorders

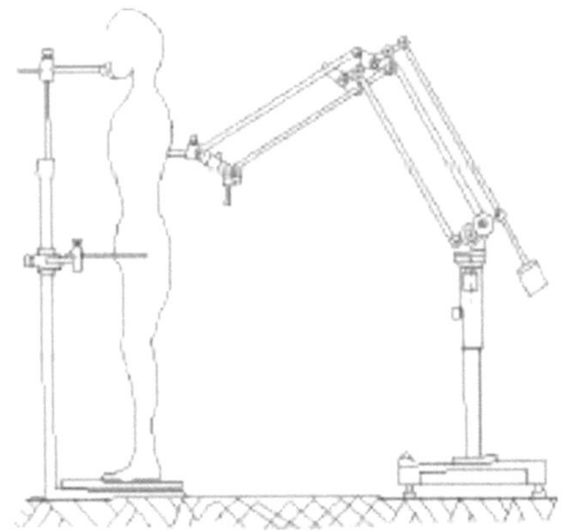

Fig. 1. S-posture meter - the polish devise to measures body posture.

(Cailliet 1975, Romano et al., 2008). Most cases of scoliosis have an idiopathic character, which makes it difficult to define both the progression of the spinal curve as well as the chances for posture correction. There is a conviction that the only efficient methods of treating progressive, sideways curvature of the spine are by wearing corsets or by conducting surgery. In the case of children with scoliosis, kinisiotherapy can only contribute to the increase of the physical fitness and functioning of youth and children (Maruyama et al., 2008; Negrini et al., 2008; Romano et al., 2008; Weiss & Goodall, 2008).

Treating scoliosis is incredibly difficult, and physiotherapeutic treatment can be inconclusive as well as sometimes inefficient. Thus, the early diagnosis of children and youth, with special attention given to abnormalities along the cephalocaudal axis of the spine, allows for preventive action to be taken in the period when abnormalities are not permanent. It can be assumed that, beginning in early childhood, influencing the development of the habits of good posture can have a positive influence on the physical and motor development of the young organism. It is accepted that body posture is an indication of physical and mental state as well as an indication of neuromuscular balance and coordination (Dega, 1996; Kutzner-Kozińska, et al., 2001; Nowotny et al., 2008; Szczygieł et al., 1999;).

Epidemiological studies have shown that bad posture also occurs, or is even more common, in disabled children and youth. Many authors suggest that visual and hearing impairment, mental disabilities, neurological disorders, or any other abnormalities, both congenital and acquired, can cause changes in the processes of posturogenesis (Kasperczyk, 1988; Szczygieł et al., 1999; Śliwa et al., 1999; Zwierzchowska & Gawlik, 2006).

Hearing impairment is one of the sensory defects that cause abnormalities in the physical, motor, and psychosocial development of children and youth. There are many criteria pertaining to the degree of hearing loss.

The International Bureau for Audiophonology established a line at 90 decibels of average value that delineates the difference between serious hearing impairment and deafness. Complete and partial deafness were distinguished:

- mild hearing impairment - 20-40 decibels;

- moderate hearing impairment - 40-70 decibels;
- severe hearing impairment - 70-90 decibels;
- profound hearing impairment - above 90 decibels (Szczepankowski, 1999).

Another criteria, commonly applied in the relevant literature, are the division according to human speech reception. Flower's classification, combined with Van Uden's categorization, distinguishes the following:

- mild hearing impairment - inaudible whisper (0-20dB);
- moderate hearing impairment - troubles with hearing colloquial language;
- not very severe hearing impairment - moderately laud speech in most cases inaudible (40-60 dB);
- severe hearing impairment - loud speech inaudible (60-80 dB);
- extremely severe hearing impairment - scream inaudible (above 80 dB);
- complete deafness - very loud scream inaudible (hearing loss) (Skarżyńska et al., 1997).

Hearing impairment is a factor that negatively influences the processes connected with shaping physiological spinal curvature. Maintaining correct body posture in an upright position requires cooperation between the middle ear, sight, proprioception, and the central nervous system (Błaszczyk, 2004; Dudek & Szczygieł, 1999; Woods et al., 1995). The central nervous system receives limited information from peripheral centres due to hearing impairment, and this leads to the disturbance of dynamic processes connected with maintaining balance (Sipko, 1999; Sipko & Skolimowski, 1997, 1998). The loss or impairment of hearing can damage an individual's motor functions and cause disturbances in balance, plasticity, and speed of movements. The pace of physical and motor development in deaf children is slower. Many authors explain that this results not only from hearing impairment but from social and living conditions as well (Maszczak, 1977; Shephard & Berg, 1986; Umsławska & Staniszewska, 2006; Zwierzchowska et al,. 2008).

Abnormalities in the physical and motor development of children and youth are reflected in body posture, which is contingent upon morphological, functional, and environmental conditions (Kutzner-Kozińska et al., 2001).

Relevant literature reports the presence of numerous abnormalities in the body posture of children and youth with developmental defects. That is why the authors decided to conduct research on body posture of children and youth with hearing impairment.

The purpose of the present paper is to assess the body posture of children and youth with hearing impairment, with an emphasis on the frequency of the occurrence of abnormalities. Subjects were students at the Institute for the Deaf in Warsaw. Defining the percentage of abnormalities in the body posture of the examined group allows for corrective work to be planned.

2. Material and testing methods

Tests were conducted at the Institute for the Deaf in Warsaw in 2005. Children and youth who participated in the study were hearing impaired and were aged between 7 to 18 years. Altogether, 88 persons were examined. All subjects had severe or profound hearing impairment. This information was procured from the child's health card in the institute.

Moreover, the subjects took part in speech corrective classes; most of them had difficulties communicating verbally, whereas all of them had a command of sign language.

Table 1 presents the number of subjects.

girls	N	%	boys	N	%
	41	100.0		47	100.0
prepubertal period	11	26.8	prepubertal period	11	23.4
the puberty period	23	56.1	the puberty period	30	63.8
the postpubertal period	7	17.1	the postpubertal period	6	12.8

Table 1. The number of deaf subjects in the studied group with view to gender and developmental periods.

The number of students in individual age classes was diverse, causing the results to be presented in three developmental brackets: before puberty, at puberty, and after puberty. The classical division, acknowledged by both anthropologists and psychologists, was accepted (Wolański 2006; Birch & Malim, 2007). The age of puberty was determined in girls between 10.51 and 10.50 years; in boys, between 11.51 and 15.50 years.

The majority of children and youth in the Institute for the Deaf in Warsaw live in the Mazowieckie Voivodship and come from both the urban (65%) and rural (35%) environments. Some subjects (63%) stay at the boarding house during the week, the rest stay at home and come to classes at the Institute for the Deaf in Warsaw.

The socioeconomic status is diverse due to the specificity of the examined group. Research participants came from both the city and the country. The education level of the parents of the children and youth can be determined as low, taking into account the fact that 36% of the subjects live in Warsaw. Among the parents, 54% of the fathers and 51% of the mothers received a vocational education. The lowest educational status was observed in 27% of the parents. Only one mother had higher education. The material status of the families was described on the basis of an assessment by the parents. They usually defined the material status of the family as average (42.5%). This meant that a family could afford to cover the basic living needs. Roughly one-third (36.8%) of the parents determined their living conditions to be good, i.e., after fulfilling their basic living needs, the family could afford to send their children on summer holiday.

Moire's photogrammetric technique was applied to assess body posture (Nowotny et al., 1992). This technique uses the refraction of the source of light on a given object. All accepted parameters that assess body posture were presented as a function of body height.

The following parameters were used to assess the body posture of the deaf children:

- the angles of individual segments of the spine in relation to perpendicular (α, β, and γ) (Fig. 2a);
- the angle of chest kyphosis (KP);
- the angle of loin lordosis (LL);
- the asymmetries of shoulder and scapula placement (Fig. 2b);
- the angle of the pelvis turn;
- the angle, localization, and direction of scoliosis.

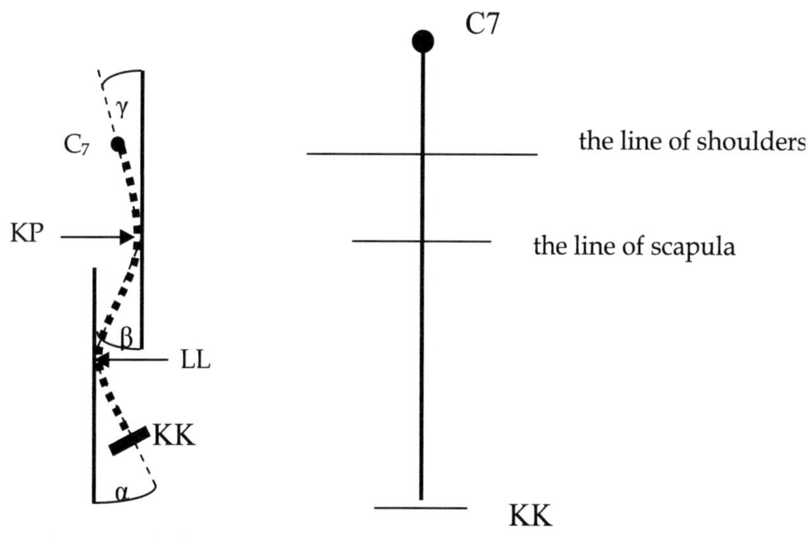

a. The sagittal plan b. The coronal plane

Fig. 2. The angles of individual segments of the spine in relation to perpendicular. (C7 - seventh cervical vertebra, KK - the beginning of sacrum).

The age of children was accurate to 0.01 years and calculated on the basis of the difference between the date of birth and the date of the test. The gathered results were statistically analysed, and the following parameters were calculated:

- the average formed values of the angles of individual parts of the spine in relation to perpendicular (the value of the angles α, β, γ of each subject were brought to the arithmetic mean and the standard deviation of the examination of the children from Gdansk, with emphasis put on their age and sex);
- the percentage distribution of the selected features of body posture;
- the correlation factor between the angles of individual parts of the spine in relation to perpendicular and the angle of the torso in relation to the cephalocaudal axis;
- the percentage distribution of the frequency of defective posture occurrence.

3. Results

3.1 The body posture of the subjects in the sagittal plane

The physiological curvatures of the spine have an indisputable influence on one's existence, yet it is difficult to clearly determine their size on the sagittal plane They support an individual, and help to maintain an individual's balance and steadiness in various situations (Adams et al., 2002; Hof, 2003).

The angles, as well as the length of chest kyphosis and loin lordosis, depend on numerous factors: the stage of biological development, the body height, the pelvis position, and the pectoral girdle, among other things. It needs to be mentioned that physiological curvatures do not constitute a sector, which causes another problem when defining their proper size. However, the fact that defects can occur in the body posture of children and youth brings about the need to define at least the general criteria that would allow body posture to be assessed. In the present paper such criteria was also applied; they served as a basis for assessing the body posture in children and youth with hearing impairment.

The characteristics of the body posture in the sagittal plane of deaf children was predicated on the analysis of the angles of individual spinal segments in relation to perpendicular as well as the size of the angles of chest kyphosis and loin lordosis (Fig. 2). The torso angle in relation to the cephalocaudal axis was determined as well. Maintaining silhouette in the body axis allows the mechanical balance to be maintained. The inclination of the torso to the front or to the back can disturb the upright position as well as contribute to the occurrence of abnormalities in physiological spinal curves. The description of this parameter, especially in deaf children, can have a crucial significance from the perspective of introducing corrective and compensating exercises, which contribute to maintaining the optimal physical fitness of children with hearing impairment.

The analysis of the position of the silhouette in the body axis showed the inclination of the torso to the front in over 50% of the subjects, a little more often in the boys than the girls. Taking into consideration periods of development, it has been noticed that the inclination of the torso to the front was more common in the subjects who had reached puberty 68.4% (over 14.5 years in the girls and over 15.5 years in the boys). Such a silhouette also characterises 53.8% of the children before puberty. The inclination of the torso to the back from the main axis pertained to only 8% of the subjects (Table 2).

The position of the torso in the vertical axis.	girls		boys	
	N	%	N	%
the position of the spine in the vertical axis.	16	39.0	17	36.2
the inclination of the spine to the back	4	9.8	3	6.4
the inclination of the spine to the front	21	51.2	27	57.4

Table 2. The position of the torso in the vertical axis.

A correlation rate was calculated in order to characterise a connection between the inclination of the torso in relation to the cephalocaudal axis and the angle parameters of the physiological spinal curves (the angles α, β, γ and the angles KP and LL). Table 3 presents the values of the correlation rate.

A negative correlation was observed in case of the angle β (the inclination of the section conjoining the apex of chest kyphosis with the apex of loin lordosis). It can be assumed that the torso of the subjects moves closer to perpendicular with the increase of the β angle. The correlations showed a positive direction of change in cases of the inclination of the torso and the angles α and γ. The axis of the spine diverges from the cephalocaudal axis with the increase of the angle of the outermost segments of the spine (especially the one conjoining C7, the seventh cervical vertebra, with the apex of chest kyphosis). Its significant inclination may have an influence on the maintenance of the mechanical balance as well as the deterioration of the body posture of the subjects (Table 3).

	α angle	β angle	γ angle	KP angle	LL angle
The angle of inclination of the torso	- 0.11	0.81*	-0.42*	-0.39*	-0.42*

* - p≤0,05; KP angle – the angle of kyphosis, LL angle – the angle of lordosis

Table 3. The correlation rate.

The inclination of individual segments of the spine in relation to perpendicular (Fig. 2) determines the size of the physiological spinal curve and might be applied to assess the frequency of defective posture occurrence in the sagittal plane.

Due to the differentiation of the number of the examined children in individual age classes, the value of the angles α, β, and γ of each subject were brought to the arithmetic mean and the standard deviation of the examination of the children from Gdansk (Zeyland-Malawka, 2003).

The analysis of data showed that in a group of deaf boys, the values of the discussed angles are on average a little higher in comparison with hearing boys (fig. 3). The differences amount to 0.26 SD, 0.57 SD, and 0.22 SD, respectively. In the size of the β angle, the differences are significant statistically. Higher values of the discussed angles may signify that there is an enlarged physiological spinal curve in a subject.

Taking into consideration developmental periods, it was observed that the size of angles α, β, and γ in the boys with hearing impairment, aged between 11.5-15.15 years, are closest to the average values of hearing children.

The γ angle that influences the size of chest kyphosis had similar values in all the mentioned groups. A difference of 1.97 SD was observed in the sizes of the α angle between the boys aged 7-11 and those aged 16-18 years. The deaf boys aged between 16 and 18 are characterised by smaller values of the α angle in comparison with the boys aged between 7 and 11, as well as their healthy peers (Fig. 3). This result may suggest that there is a tendency to the reduction of the loin lordosis in the boys between the ages of 16 and 18 years with hearing impairment. Nevertheless, the small number of the examined boys in this age group does not allow conclusions to be generalised.

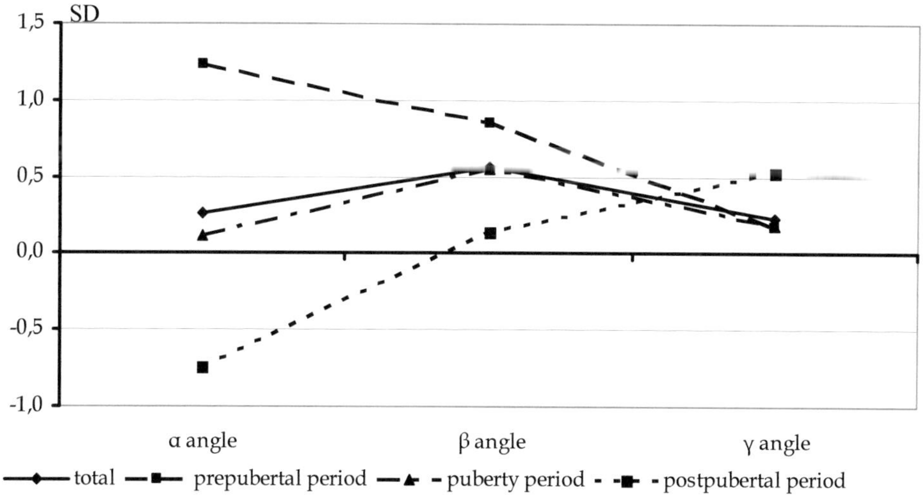

Fig. 3. The normalized values of the angles α, β, and γ of the tested boys.

The sizes of the angles of chest kyphosis and loin lordosis were also applied to assess the frequency of abnormalities of the spine on the sagittal plane. The abnormal size of the physiological spinal curvatures only occurs in around 40% of the tested hearing-impaired boys; the most common defects comprise concave back or roundly-concave back. The frequency of the excessive physiological spinal curves decreased with the age of the subjects. Body posture defects on the sagittal plane occurred in about 20% of the subjects, in the boys aged between 16 and 18. At this stage of development only excessively enlarged chest kyphosis was observed (Fig. 4).

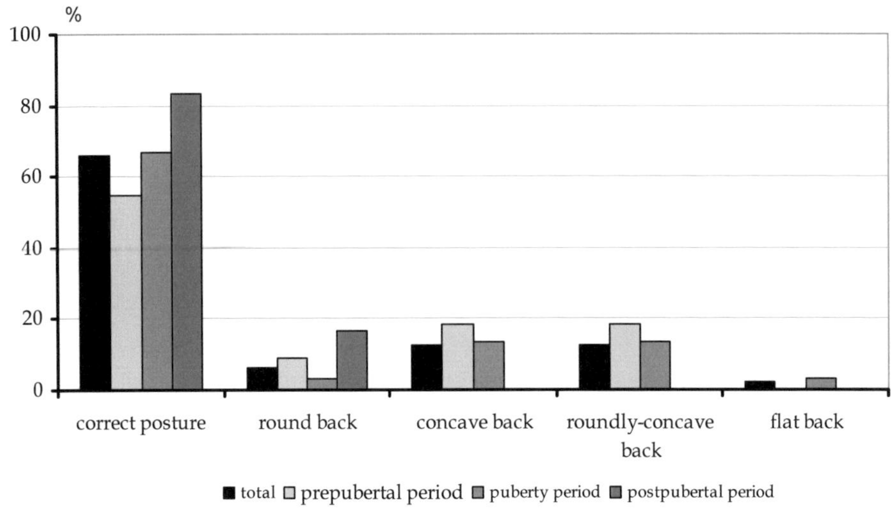

Fig. 4. The frequency of defective posture occurrence on the sagittal plane in a male group.

In the group of hearing-impaired girls, the assessment of the angles of individual spinal segments in relation to perpendicular, showed that they have bigger values of the angles α, β, and γ compared to the hearing girls. Changes in the size of these angles are presented in Figure 5. Despite the fact that the values of the discussed angles are varied in the given age groups, no statistically significant differences were observed.

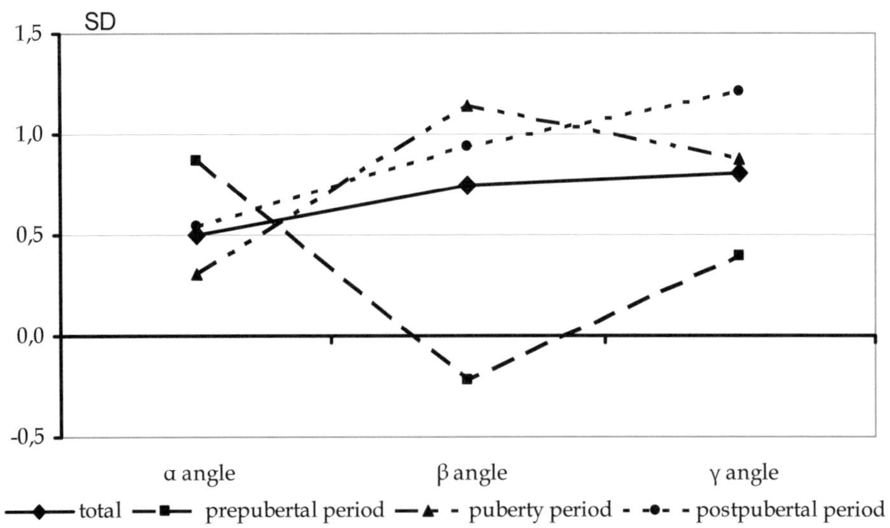

Fig. 5. The normalized values of the angles α, β, and γ of the tested girls.

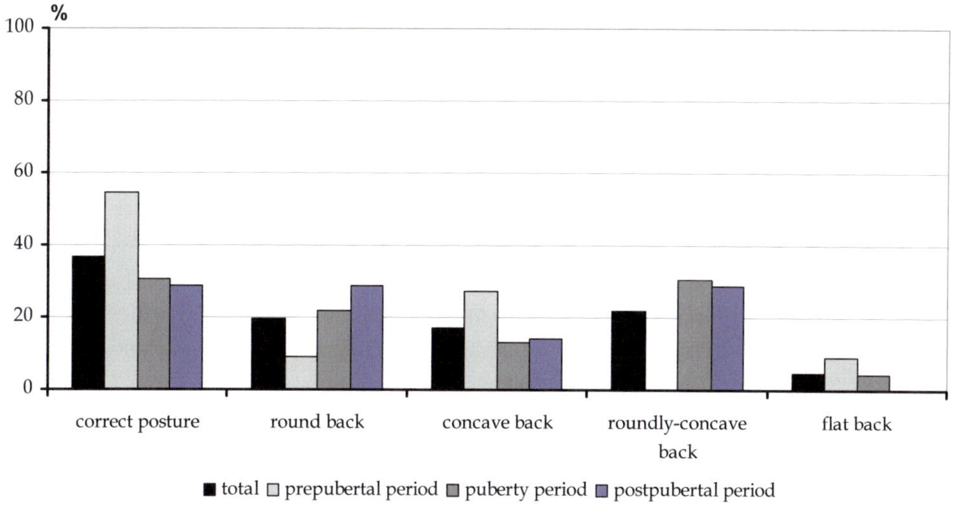

Fig. 6. The frequency of defective posture occurrence in the sagittal plane in the female group.

A disturbance of physiological spinal curve in the hearing-impaired girls was observed in the case of 62% of the subjects. The most common defects were round back, concave back, and round-concave back. Taking into consideration developmental periods it was observed that abnormalities in the size of the curvature of the spine were most common in the girls aged between 12 and 18 years. The frequency of defective posture occurrence increased with age. Round and round-concave back was observed in about 60% of the girls aged between 14.5 and 18.5 years (Fig. 6).

Additionally, a comparative analysis was conducted of the features of the body posture on the sagittal plane of the subjects with hearing impairments, with emphasis put on the sex of the students. No significant changes in the size of the angles β and γ were observed; whereas the differences in the angles α and loin lordosis were on the border of statistical significance, which can indicate a more frequent occurrence of body posture defects in hearing-impaired girls rather than boys. A small number of subjects in individual developmental periods could lead to the lack of significant differences in the discussed parameters, but the percentage values indicated that the enlargement of curvature was more common in the group of girls rather than boys at every developmental stage.

3.2 The body posture on the coronal plane

The assessment of the body posture on the coronal plane allows the asymmetric position of the individual segments to be identified, which then determines the course of the cephalocaudal axis. Disorders of the spine and other posture segments on the coronal plane can cause scoliosis. The sideways curve of the spine is considered a systemic abnormality because it can cause not only hearing disorders but disorders of other systems as well, for example, respiratory or cardiovascular ones. According to the definition by the Scoliosis Research Society, scoliosis is understood as a structural curvature of the spine where a rotation took place, and with the Cobb angle greater than 10 degrees. However, when analysing a child's body posture during a developmental period, it is worth considering the problem of the liability of body posture, which sometimes is typical of children with a limp and asthenic build. Disorders of the tension of the postural muscles can cause abnormalities in body posture to occur. These abnormalities, as well as a child's intensive development and growth, can contribute to scoliosis. For that reason, the present research comprises subjects with scoliotic posture. Such an abnormality was characterised by a slight curvature of the spine (4-9 degrees in a photogrammetric picture) and lack of rotation. The curvature bore no signs of consolidation, and in most cases could be actively corrected.

Body posture defects and scoliosis often occur together with some other disorders, such as visual or hearing impairment, as well as mental disorders. There is the need for an early diagnosis of children and youth with various developmental defects, as well as in terms of postural defects and scoliosis (Woods et al., 1995).

In the present paper, the body posture research in terms of scoliosis had a screening character. The applied method of assessment did not allow a thorough diagnosis of the sideways curve of the spine, which is possible when using an X-ray machine, for instance. That is why the subjects whose photogrammetric picture showed a significant sideways curve of the spine were referred for a more specialised diagnosis.

The present study provides an analysis not only of the course of the cephalocaudal axis but also of the symmetric position of shoulders, scapulas, and pelvis. Moreover, the turn of the pelvis in the transverse plane was assessed.

The results of the hearing-impaired boys showed that asymmetry of the shoulders occurred in about 53% of the subjects; whereas the asymmetry of the scapulas pertained to 43% of the boys. The abnormalities in most cases pertained to the left side. The turn of the pelvis characterised around 33% of the students with hearing organ dysfunction (Fig. 7).

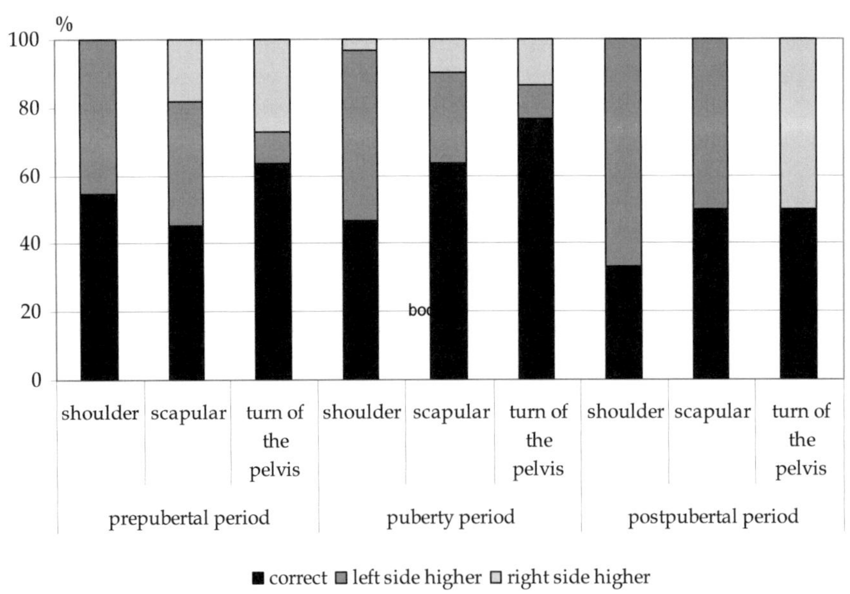

Fig. 7. The occurrence of shoulder and scapular asymmetry as well as the turn of the pelvis in the hearing-impaired boys, according to their developmental periods.

Taking into consideration the subjects' developmental periods, it was determined that the most frequent asymmetry of the discussed segments occurred in the boys aged between 15.5-17.5 years (Fig. 7).

When the course of the cephalocaudal axis was being analysed, it was accepted in the testing methodology, that children with the angle of curve over 10 degrees would qualify for the groups of scoliosis. The subjects with the angle between 5 and 10 degrees and the asymmetric position of shoulders, scapulas, or pelvis were qualified for the group with scoliotic posture.

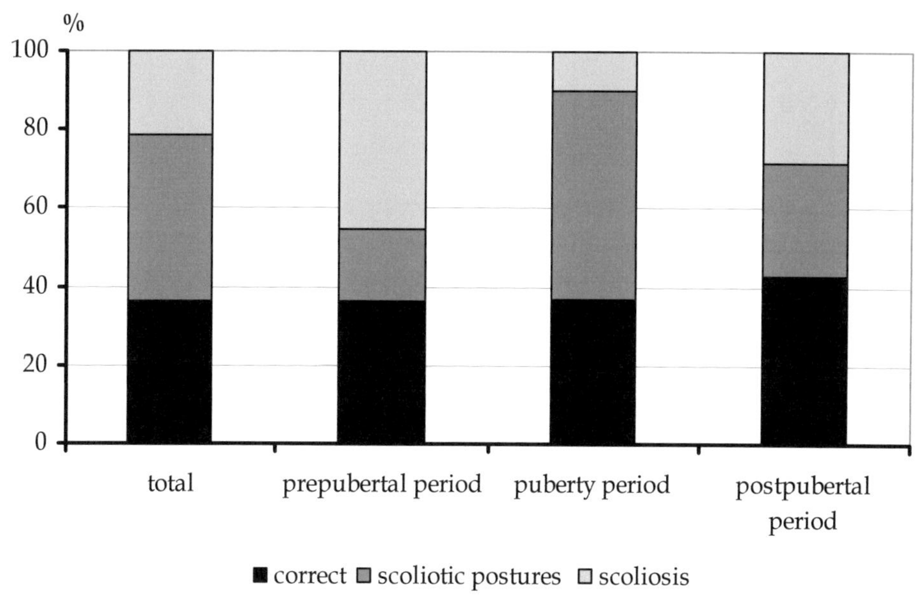

Fig. 8. The occurrence of the sideways curves of the spine in the group of boys.

Scoliotic postures and scoliosis occurred in around 63% of the subjects. The degree of the advancement of changes was in most cases small, these abnormalities could be determined as trace scoliosis. Altogether, it was diagnosed in around 27% of the hearing-impaired boys. A consolidated sideways curve of the spine, with asymmetric outline of the back, was diagnosed in 4.3% of the boys Taking into consideration their developmental periods, no consolidated scoliosis was detected in the group of the oldest boys. The highest percentage of the most advanced sideways curve of the spine was observed in a group of the youngest boys (Fig. 8).

The results of the tests in the group of girls showed that the asymmetry of shoulder position was typical for 51% of the subjects. The left shoulder was positioned higher than the right one much more frequently. An abnormal position of scapulas in the girls was less common than an abnormal position of shoulders. It pertained to around 22% of the subjects. The turn of the pelvis was observed in around 46% of the hearing-impaired girls. The pelvis was more often turned to the right, i.e., left anterior superior iliac spine was more moved to the front compared to the right one. Similar concurrences were observed when the discussed segments were being analysed, with emphasis put on the developmental period.

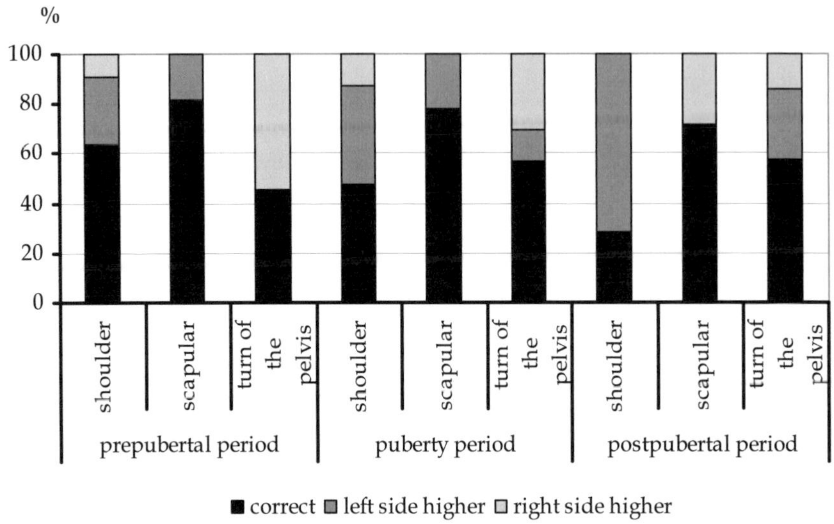

Fig. 9. The occurrence of shoulder and scapular asymmetry as well as the turn of the pelvis in the hearing-impaired girls, with a focus on developmental stages.

The percentage of shoulder and scapular asymmetry in the examined girls increased with their age. Also, the number of the subjects with a turn of the pelvis was on the increase (Fig. 9).

Abnormalities of the course of the cephalocaudal axis on the coronal plane were observed in around 64% of the examined hearing-impaired girls. Scoliotic posture was typical for around 30% of the deaf; whereas scoliosis occurred in around 37% of the subjects. This was, most frequently, scoliosis of a lower degree, with no asymmetry of the back outline. Consolidated scoliosis, with spine rotation (positive results in the Adam's Forward Bend Test) was observed in only 4% of the girls (Fig. 10).

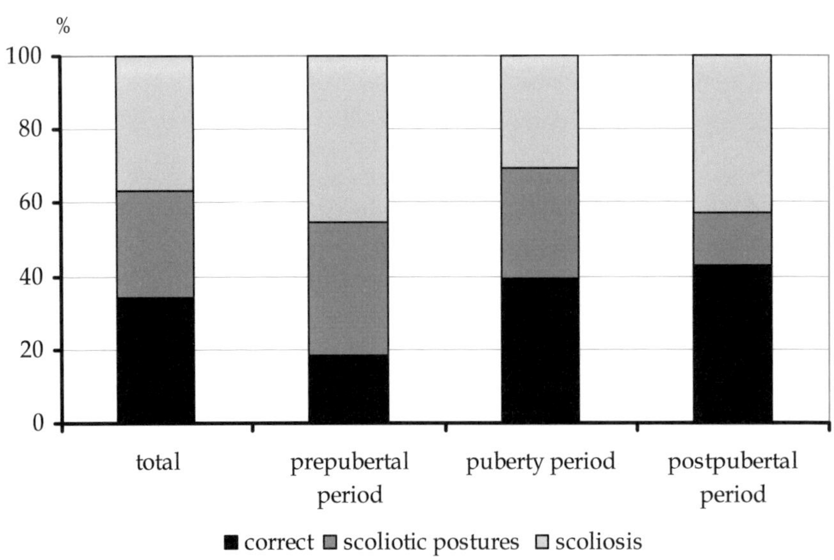

Fig. 10. The frequency of occurrence of the sideways curve of the spine in the group of girls.

The number of abnormal postures declined with age, but simultaneously, the percentage of more advanced scoliosis, with a tendency for asymmetric back outline, increased.

4. Discussion

Human body posture depends on many factors: morphological, functional, as well as environmental (Kasperczyk, 2004; Kutzner-Kozińska et al., 2001). There are numerous studies where the authors emphasise that various developmental disorders of children and youth influence, most often negatively, the process of posturogenesis. Among such abnormalities we may list: mental disorders, visual and hearing impairment, as well as short height. In Poland, the assessment of body posture with developmental dysfunctions was studied by Szczygieł, Śliwa, Kasperczyk, Grabara, Zwierzchowska, and Gawlik (Kasperczyk, 1988; Szczygieł et al., 1999; Śliwa et al., 1999, Zwierzchowska & Gawlik, 2006; Grabara, 2006). The analysis of posturographic parameters was primarily subjected to the assessment of sideways curves of the spine as well as the asymmetry of the position of individual segments of the body.

Wilińska and Kasperczyk (1990) claimed that abnormal body posture occurred in around 40% of hearing-impaired children. A much bigger percentage of defects in a group of deaf-mute and hard of hearing were observed by Szczygiel (Szczygieł et al., 1999). The frequency of disorders in the discussed tests was present in around 80% of the boys and girls. These abnormalities in majority pertained to the coronal plane and had a small degree of advancement (the angle of the sideways curve reached up to 10 degrees. Body posture disorders were also quite frequent in the examination of the children from Wroclaw aged between 7 and 15 years. In most cases, this was trace scoliosis. Consolidated sideways curve of the spine occurred in 35% of the hearing-impaired subjects (Śliwa et al., 1999). According to Zwierzchowska and Gawlik, 44% of children and youth with hearing impairment had sideways curve of the spine, girls more frequently than boys. Apart from the changes in the course of the cephalocaudal axis, the authors observed an asymmetric position of shoulders, scapulas, and pelvis (Zwierzchowska & Gawlik, 2006, 2007; Grabara, 2006). Moreover, the present study showed an abnormal position of such segments of the body as shoulders and scapulas, as well as a turn of the pelvis. The percentages of abnormalities among the subjects are bigger in comparison with hearing children (Olszewska & Trzcińska, 2005; Olszewska & Trzcińska, 2007). The discussed asymmetries accompany sideways curves of the spine. Scoliosis was observed in a considerable number of subjects with hearing impairment, with similar frequency among the boys and girls. It needs to be emphasised, though, that in the group of girls a percentage of the most advanced abnormalities along the course of the cephalocaudal axis occurred in the oldest group. There was no such correlation in the group of boys. In the discussed test, the percentage of scoliotic postures in the developmental stages did not change significantly. Hearing impairment can have a negative influence on the processes of posturogenesis, especially due to the connection between deafness and maintaining balance. According to the tests, the mechanism for maintaining balance is impaired in deaf and hard-of-hearing persons. The results of the Fleming's test conducted in a group of hearing and hearing-impaired showed that the time that balance can be maintained is considerably shorter in a group with hearing impairment. Many authors showed a correlation between the correct body posture and maintaining balance. Some tests show a smaller percentage of scoliosis among hearing-impaired children in comparison with hearing children. According to the authors, this results from the fact that hearing-impaired are "protected" from scoliosis by neurological disorders that accompany deafness. For that reason, a need exists to undertake actions to prevent postural defects as well as incorrect movement habits.

5. Conclusions

The results of the present research allow the following conclusions to be drawn:

1. Body posture defects among children and youth with hearing impairments are rather common. The frequency of occurrence of abnormalities increased with the subject's age, which should alarm people who look after children with hearing impairment.
2. There is a need to undertake actions that will shape correct movement habits, including those pertaining to body posture, as well as to correct the existing abnormalities in body posture in children and youth with hearing impairments. Creating programmes of preventive and corrective actions in postural defects should be the responsibility of the teachers working in facilities for hearing-impaired children and youth, as well as of doctors and education authorities.

6. References

Adams, M. (2004). Biomechanics of back pain. *Acupuncture in Medicine* vol. 22 No 4 pp.178-188, ISSN 1759-9873

Angelakopoulos, T. Georgios, Savelsbergh, Geert J. P., Bennett, Simon J., Davids, Keith W., Haralambos, Tsorbatzoudis, & George, Grouios (2008). Systematic review regarding posture development from infancy to adulthood. *Hellenic Journal of Physical Education and Sport Sciences (68)*, pp. 35-43.

Babakhani, F. (2011). The effect of backpack load on the posture of children and its relationship to trunk muscle activity during walking on a treadmill. Dissertation submitted to the faculty of the social and applied human sciences at Saarland University, Saarbrücken. Behind: Staffel, F. (1889). *Die menschlichen Haltungstypen und ihre Beziehungen zu den Rückgratverkrümmungen*. Wiesbaden: Bergmann.

Birch, A.& Malim, T.(1988). Developmental psychology. From infancy to adulthood, The Macmillan Press Ltd., ISBN 83-01-11938-1, Houndmills, Basingstoke, London

Błaszczyk, JW. (2004). Biomechanika kliniczna, PZWL, ISBN 83-2002917-1 Warszawa, Polska

Boocock, MG , JA Jackson, AK Burton, Tillotson KM, (1994), Continuous measurement of lumbar posture using flexible electrogoniometers. Ergonomics, 37. pp.175-185, ISSUE 1

Cailliet, R. (1975). Scoliosis, Philadelphia, F. A. Davis Co, 1975

Dega, W. (1996). Ortopedia i rehabilitacja, PZWL, ISBN 83-200-2823-3, Warszawa, Poland

Dudek, J. & Szczygieł, A. (1999). Poprawianie zaburzeń statyki ciała u dzieci niesłyszących w wieku 11 - 15 lat, *Postępy Rehabilitacji*, vol. 13 No 4, pp. 137 - 145, ISSN 0860-6161

Hof A.L. (2003). Muscle mechanics and neuromuscular control. *J. Biomechanics*, vol. 36, No 7, pp.1031-1038, ISSN: 0021-9290

Goldberg, CJ. Dowling, FE. Fogarty, EE. & Moore, DP. (1995). School scoliosis screening and The Unite State Preventive Services Task Force. An examination of long - term results. *Spine*, vol. 20, No 12, pp. 1368 - 1374, ISSN 1529-9430

Grabara, M. (2006). Dysfunkcje narządu słuchu a asymetria postawy ciała. *Fizjoterapia Polska* vol. 6, No 4 pp. 121-125, ISSN 1642-0136

Iwanowski, W. (1982).Kształtowanie się fizjologicznych krzywizn kręgosłupa. AWF, PB 3545/83, Wrocław, Poland

Karachalios, T. Sofianos, J. Roidis, N. Sapkas, G. Korres, D. & Nokolopoulos, K. (1999). Ten years follow-up evaluation of a school screening program for scoliosis. Is the forward-bending test an accurate diagnostic creation for screening of scoliosis. *Spine*, vol.24 , No22, pp. 2318-2324, ISSN 1529-9430

Kasperczyk, T. (1988) Postawa ciała a wybrane cechy morfologiczne i funkcjonalne u dzieci w wieku 8 - 15 lat. AWF, ISSN 0860-0643 Kraków, Poland

Kasperczyk, T. (2004). Wady postawy ciała - diagnostyka i leczenie. Kasper, ISBN 83-90977-0-7, Kraków, Poland

Kasperczyk, T. & Waleszek, R. (2009). Przydatnośc metod punktowania w ocenie wad postawy ciała. In: Wady postawy ciała u dzieci i młodzieży. J.Nowotny (Ed.), pp. 57-63 ,WSA, ISBN 978-83-60430-32-3 Biesko - Biała, Poland

Kiperski, J. (2009). Diagnostyka i terapia wad postawy ciała. In: Wady postawy ciała u dzieci i młodzieży. J.Nowotny (Ed.), pp.25-30 ,WSA, ISBN 978-83-60430-32-3 Biesko - Biała, Polska

Kutzner - Kozińska, M. Olszewska, E. Popiel, M. & Trzcińska, D. (2001). Proces korygowania wad postawy. AWF, ISBN 83-87210-42-0, Warszawa, Poland

Lewandowski, J. (2006). Kształtowanie się krzywizn fizjologicznych i zakresów ruchomości odcinkowej kręgosłupa człowieka w wieku 3 - 25 lat w obrazie elektrogoniometrycznym. AWF, ISBN 83-88923-63-3, Poznań, Poland

Maruyama, T. Takeshita, K. Kitagawa, T. (2008). Side - shift exercise and hitch exercise. *Stud Health Technol In form*. Vol.135, pp.246-251, ISSN 0926-9630

Maszczak T.1977: The somatic and Motor Level of Deaf Children in Poland. PZGl, Warszawa, Poland

Negrini, S. Zaina, F. Romano, M. Negrini, A. & Parzini, S. (2008). Specific exercises reduce brace prescription in adolescent idiopathic scoliosis: a prospective controlled cohort study with worst-case analysis. *J Rehabil Med.* Vol. 40, No 6 pp. 451-455, ISSN 1650-1977

Nowotny, J. Zawieska, D. & Saulicz, E. (1992). Fotografia z wykorzystaniem rastra optycznego i komputera jako sposób oceny postawy ciała. *Postępy Rehabilitacji* vol. 6, No 1, pp. 17 - 26, ISSN 0860-6161

Nowotny, J. Nowotny - Czupryna, O.& Czupryna, K. (2008). Reedukacja posturalna w systemie stacyjnym. WSA, ISBN 83-60430-76-4, Bielko - Biała, Poland

Olszewska, E. & Trzcińska, D. (2005) Postawa ciała dzieci i młodzieży w różnych okresach rozwojowych. In: Korektywa i kompensacja zaburzeń w rozwoju fizycznym dzieci i młodzieży. K. Górniak (Ed.), pp66-75, Vol.2, ISBN 83-920273-7-X, Biała Podlaska, Poland

Olszewska, E. & Trzcińska, D. (2007). O potrzebie korekcji wad postawy ciała u młodzieży gimnazjalnej. *Wychowanie Fizyczne i Zdrowotne* No 3, pp. 18 - 22, ISSN 0860-8075

Przewęda, R. (1962) Przegląd ważniejszych metod oceny postawy ciała. Roczniki Naukowe AWF vol. 2, Warszawa, Poland

Romano,M. Ziliani, V. Atanasio, S. Zaina, F. & Negrini S. (2008).Do imbalance situations stimulate a spinal straightening reflex in patient with adolescent idiopathic scoliosis? Stud *Health Technol Inform*. vol 40, pp. 307-309, ISSN 0926-9630

Shephard Roy J. & Berg F.S., 1986, Characteristic of the target population. Educational audiology for the hard of heating child. Grune & Stratton, inc. New York, Boston, London).

Sipko, T. (1999). Regulacja równowagi ciała w pozycji stojącej osób z upośledzeniem wzroku lub słuchu. *Medycyna Sportowa*, vol. 16, No 4, pp.35-39, ISSN 1232-406 X

Sipko, T. & Skolimowski, T. (1997). Wpływ chwilowej i trwałej utraty kontroli wzrokowej położenia ciała w przestrzeni na proces regulacji równowagi ciała w pozycji stojącej. *Fizjoterapia* vol.5, No 2, pp. 25-30, ISSN 1642-0136

Sipko, T. & Skilimowski, T. (1998). Równowaga ciała w pozycji stojącej osób niesłyszących. *Fizjoterapia* vol.6, No 1-2, pp. 40-43, ISSN 1642-0136

Skarżyński, H. Mueller-Malasińska, M. & Wojnarowska, W. (1997). Klasyfikacja zaburzeń słuchu. Audiofonologia vol. 10, PKA, ISSN 1425-3089, UMCS Lublin, Poland

Szczepankowki, B. (1999) Niesłyszący - głusi - głuchoniemi. Wyrównywanie szans. WSiP, ISBN 8302073962, Warszawa, Poland

Szczygieł, A. Dudek, J. Janusz, M. Kilar, Z. Ridan, T. & Snakowski, T. (1999). Postawa ciała dzieci i młodzieży niepełnosprawnej w zależności od rodzaju dysfunkcji i stopnia aktywności ruchowej. In: Sport w rehabilitacji niepełnosprawnych, J. Ślężyński (Ed.), pp.141-150, Polskie Stowarzyszenie Osób Niepełnosprawnych, ISBN 83-87252-10-7, Kraków, Poland

Śliwa, W. (1993). Posturometr - S urządzenie diagnozująco - pomiarowe. In: Powstawanie wad postawy ciała, ich ocena i postępowanie korekcyjne. W. Śliwa (Ed.). pp. 5-16, Posmed Wrocław, Poland

Śliwa, W. Chlebika, E. & Kowal, M. (1999). Postawa ciała dzieci głuchych w wieku 7 - 15 lat. In: Sport w rehabilitacji niepełnosprawnych. Ślężyński J. (Ed.), pp. 151 - 154, Polskie Stowarzyszenie Osób Niepełnosprawnych, Kraków, Poland, , ISBN 83-87252-10-7

Umławska, W. Staniszewska, A. (2006). Physical growth of children and youth with hearing impairment. *Med Wieku Rozwoj.*, No10, No 3, pp. 913-922, ISSN 1428-345X

Weiss, HR. & Goodall, D. (2008). Thetreatment of adole scentidio pathicscoliosis (AIS) according to present evidence. A systematic review. *Eur J Phys Rehabil. Med.* Vol.44, No2, pp. 177-193, ISSN 1017-6721

Wilczyński, J. (1999). Nowoczesne metody badania postawy ciała. In: Rozwój fizyczny i motoryczny oraz postawa ciała dzieci i młodzieży niepełnosprawne Ślężyński J. (Ed.), pp.161-171, AWF, Katowice, Poland

Wilińska K, & Kasperczyk T. (1990). Czucie równowagi dynamicznej a postawa ciała dzieci i młodzieży z dysfunkcją narządu wzroku i słuchu. In: Postawa ciała, jej wady i sposoby korekcji. J. Ślężyński (Ed.) AWF, Katowice, Poland

Woods, Laura A.; Haller, Randy J.; Hansen, Paul D.; Fukumoto, Dave E.; Herman, & Richard M. (2008). Decreased Incidence of Scoliosis in Hearing-Impaired Children | Implications for a Neurologic Basis for Idiopathic Scoliosis. *Spine*, vol. 20, No7, pp. 776-780, ISSN 1529-9430

Wolański, N. (2005) Rozwój biologiczny człowieka. Podstawy auksologii, gerontologii i promocji zdrowia. PWN, ISBN 830114422X, Warszawa, Poland

Zeyland - Malawka, E. (2003). Wyniki pomiarów krzywizn kręgosłupa jako układ odniesienia w badaniu postawy ciała. *Fizjoterapia* vol. 11, No 3, pp. 5 - 12, ISSN 1642-0136

Zwierzchowska, A. & Gawlik, K. (2006). Korektywa dzieci i młodzieży z dysfunkcją wzroku i słuchu. AWF Katowice, ISBN 83-87478-88-1, Katowice, Poland

Zwierzchowska, A. & Gawlik, K. (2007). Deaf children and adolescents and defective posture. *New Medicine*, vol. 2, pp.37-39, ISSN 1427-0994

Zwierzchowska, A. Gawlik, K. & Grabara, (2008). Deafness and motor abilities level. *Biology of Sport* vol. 5, No 3, pp. 263-274, ISSN 0860-021X

Section 3

Treatment of Idiopathic Scoliosis

13

Scoliosis Idiopathic? The Etiologic Factors in Scoliosis Will Affect Preventive and Conservative Therapeutic Strategies

Piet J.M. van Loon
Dept. of Orthopedics, Medical Spectrum Twente, Enschede, The Netherlands

1. Introduction

Scoliosis is a three dimensional deformation of the complete spine and trunk, only present in humans, with its start and progress occurring during childhood. It still puzzles the medical world.

All medical (=human) conditions that lack a clear set of etiological factors will suffer ongoing discussions if the existing or new therapeutic measurements will be the right ones. Of course a massive change in form of the spine like in scoliosis or hyperkyphosis must be related to multiple causative factors inside and outside the afflicted body. In the last six decades very little attention is given to the variability in sequence in presentation of these factors in time and the severity of their action in otherwise healthy children. Also the fact that, besides in clear neurological diseases, deforming forces are exogenous or under influence (by muscles) of external circumstances stayed widely underestimated. With the wish to erase the pronoun "idiopathic", used in scoliosis for sixty years, there should be awareness of these shortcomings in knowledge among orthopedic and related scientists.

There is ongoing discussion and research in the modern scientific world of Orthopedics on causes and thus on strategies of therapy in idiopathic spinal deformities (Wang et al., 2011). The discussion on pathogenesis is evolving quickly towards more physiologic neuromuscular events. Looking into genetic aspects is also popular, but the fact that the unique genome of an animal effects all cells and tissues makes that genes cannot be directly related to a gross asymmetric deformation of half a body in otherwise healthy children. This focus on chromosomal blueprints and concomitant biochemical substrates can prevent the discovery of practical solutions in spinal deformities.

There was quit common knowledge in the nineteenth century, that most spinal deformities were caused by children's labor in industry and on farms and accelerated by tuberculosis or rachitis (Hohmann et al, 1957). For phycisians looking to girls and young tailors it was obvious that prolonged sitting is a strong deforming factor, but all this basic observations disappeared out of the academic point of view in the search for etiologic factors. Because of known differences in qualities of tissues for girls (lower mean weight, lesser mean muscle strength, increased mean ligament and capsular laxity, earlier spurt of growth) in concordance with a different neurohormonale system compared to boys, a preference for the occurrence of scoliosis in girls is clear and only in that way as causative "genetic" factor foreseen by clinicians (Jansen, 1912).

Especially on the conservative pathways, like bracing, orthopedics are apparently on a crossroad (Negrini et al., 2010; de Mauroy et al., 2010). Is the fact most physicians still try to brace under discussion, or are there reasons to look specifically to the way or technique we do it? Does the three point correction with pushing forces on the apical ribs, like in contemporary bracing techniques, correspond with the pathogenesis of deformities and patient specific type of curves? Dealing with a multitude of factors and theories and the lack of a plausible (and correctable) factor in etiology is troublesome and not helpful in all day practice and transparency towards patients. Scoliosis and kyphotic deformities are no radiological events for children and parents, but are in general still "products" of complex clinical processes (fig. 1.). Most value and attention is given by patients and doctors to what can be seen and measured in standing X-rays.

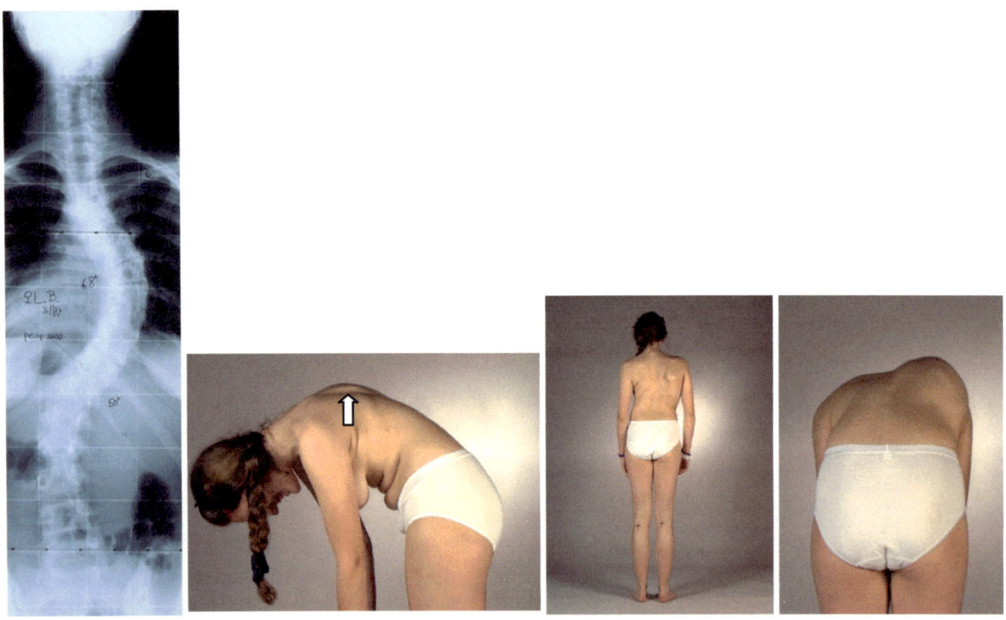

Fig. 1. Normally used radiological and clinical studies in scoliosis. The AP whole-spine radiograph (gold standard since Cobb) shows a serious right sided thoracic curve of 68° in a girl of almost fourteen year with an early menarche at 11.6 year. No other afflictions. Very late referral and a short period of TLSO before surgery in 2000. The typical clinical manifestations (on the day before surgery) show a right sided thoracic gibbus by bending (left and right), waist asymmetry and very pronounced right scapula in stance (middle). Not mentioned in textbooks is the shown inability to bend further from the hips, because of thight hamstrings. The aggravation of mainly the thoracolumbar kyphotic curve is responsible for the visible creases at the higher abdominal wall (left). A small part of the thoracic spine itself still looks hypokyphotic (according to Dickson's axiom) in bending on the level of the apex of the gibbus (arrow).

Even upgrading the imaging of the deformation from two dimensional radiographic to three dimensional proportions, like in modern CT scanning or EOS is not enough to understand the full clinical and morphologic presentation.

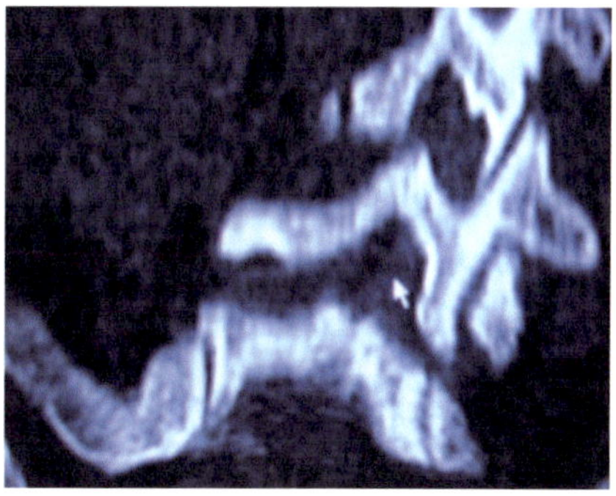

Fig. 2. AP slice of a spiral CT scan in scoliosis. In this 18 year old girl with a painful left lumbar curve the surplus value of CT scanning above plain X-ray shows details of the rotated pars interarticularis L4, sequelae of prolonged compressive forces as arthritic changes and subluxation in the facet joints in the concavity under the left sided thoracolumbar curve. It is important to state that the final configuration of any piece of bone is achieved by all (mainly muscular) forces on it during childhood (Wolff's Law), so that the morphology (also the radiologic) we see in adulthood is the resultant of all compressive and tensile forces during growth (Hohmann et al., 1957).

MRI brought even a lot more: imaging of the soft tissues and its relationships with bone. MRI can show the intriguing cohabitation and reciprocal influence of neural and skeletal tissues in all deformities in a more advanced way. But the fourth dimension, time, and the sequence of morphogenetic events in time and the level of penetration of their causative factors, so important in understanding any affliction during growth, is not visible, but can be deducted. Even MRI shows only the resultant of previous processes.

The processes of growth are not only to increase volumes and masses, but it also copes with energy and asks for storage of energy by incorporating elastic properties in any part of a body, from cell to the complete loco motor system. Movement isn't possible without these properties in energy- processing. Only one organ is capable of multidimensional control of these processes: the central nervous system (CNS). As part of obvious natural manifestations of human growth, in the absence of diseases, spinal deformations will have their biology based explanation in a deviation or adaptation of the natural arrangement of forces, masses and energy during growth. There is no modern biomedical scientific field around the neuromuscular skeletal system, in which the natural tendency of any organism towards optimalisation in form and function, broadly accepted in evolutionary biology, are starting points. But it is just what every growing organism, so even the human species, strives for. It is the observed variation that is called "natural". Inherited variation as can be seen in color of hair and eyes or elasticity of the skin is only indirectly related to the wide variation in the visible end stages of the phenotype. Environmental / external factors should be the most influential factors in individual deviations of growth and phenotype as they are in all evolutionary changes in form and function. The human species creates its own environmental factors by its constant and rapidly changing lifestyle (sedentation,

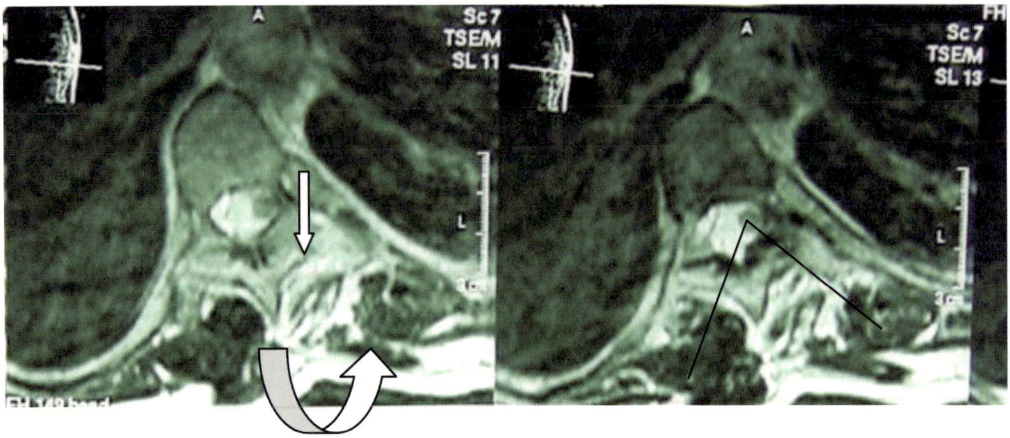

Fig. 3. MRI (transverse slides) in scoliosis. According to the findings of Milan Roth with pneumomyelographic studies, on MRI in the lower thoracic spine in an otherwise healthy female patient of 38 year with a never treated scoliosis, the very asymmetric position of the central cord is seen in the concavity of the curve. Also the slender caliber of the cord is not normal, as is the contact zone of the cord to the bony boundaries of the spinal canal. The picture of a bony canal that spiralizes around the precious cord (Roth), that stays by itself in the middle of the total body has in MRI its modern way of assessing concomitant features of the neural tissue in scoliosis. Of paramount importance to understand the message of Roth's work and taken consequences in TLI is the flattening of the vertebral groove at the left, concave, side (arrow) and the luxated erecting musculature (curved arrow) out of it, compared to the right side. The rope is dislodged from its groove in the trolley. The right muscle shows already some fatty disuse degeneration. The estimated distance from the centre of the cord to the centre of the muscles still show an equilateral triangle (right).As a fact the musculature (dynamic stays) balance the cord (the regulator) via the flexible spine (mast).

urbanization, industrialization and mechanization) in which unnatural tools and circumstances are repulsing the natural ones. Its structural body has to follow in fenotypical alterations, not in genotypical changes. In the lifestyle of the human species prolonged sitting on chairs is a novel circumstance for the majority of people since less than a century. The availability of chairs and the explosive habit of prolonged sitting in childhood started its demographic "normalization" or "incorporation" only in the second half in the nineteenth century (schooling, school laws) and shows its foreseen effects in our spines (fig.4).

2. Goal

Our goal is to support the development of etiology related therapeutics in spinal deformities with help of forgotten or apparently neglected science and some own observations.

In this chapter, we follow a way back to our predecessors whose results are still undisputed. Then we try to look for more original thoughts and existing science on scoliosis and growth nowadays. We go first back to the (guiding) article of Robert Dickson were the presence of lordosis in the thoracic spine got its place as causative factor and a factor to be addressed in therapeutic strategies in scoliosis. It seems a firm starting point (after a standstill in science

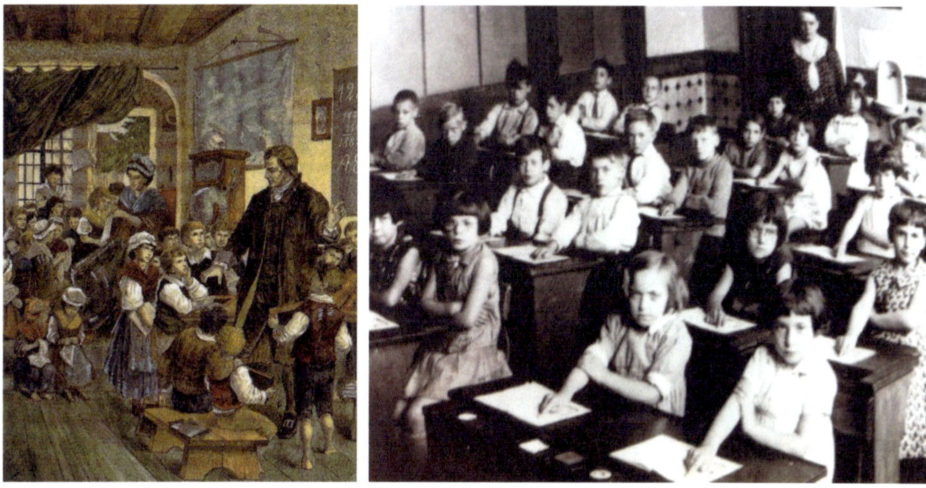

Fig. 4. Two pictures on schooling and the role of sitting with a century in between. On the left an idealized portrait of Georg Fröbel, a pioneer in guiding proper development of physical and cognitive capacities even in the youngest children by organized playing (Kindergarten). On the right just a class in an elementary school around 1950 showing the furniture once advised by the Swiss orthopedic W. Schulthess around 1850. It is obvious care is taken by teachers to look after a good posture for everybody. First in the Montessori and Dalton school systems and later on generalized by introducing loose chairs again, this discipline on posture was loosened and faded completely.

on scoliosis during and between the World Wars) were the most used biomechanical models and techniques of modern bracing and surgical procedures got their scientific background (Dickson, 1988). Had all what was investigated or used in the centuries before lost its value? Was looking to deformities of the human spine as understandable disfeatures of natural growth, as Andry already did in looking to trees (fig.5), a false start (Andry,1741) ? There came awareness in the nineteenth century, that in mechanical structures, certainly living ones with autonomic loco motor functions, all events or processes will have to respect the Natural Laws (Gordon, 1991). Besides those initiated by Isaac Newton on dynamics, the modern (extended) laws of Robert Hooke (on energy and springs)dealing with conservation of energy, momentum and angular momentum leading to regulation of equilibrium (mainly by torque or rotational forces) are part of this. This homoeostatic process in balancing masses and energy should nowadays be taken into account in understanding deformations in a given body during its developing period.

Till the research of Milan Roth came unexpected in the medical world, knowledge on how the, also growing, nervous system (in all "higher" forms of life) regulates the interrelated processes of skeletal growth was (and is?) a blind spot in Medicine(van Loon P,2008b). Homoeostasis (important in growth) combines static (anatomical and functional posture) and dynamic muscle-actions (movement), and the spring like functions (energy preservation) of joints and discs in stance and voluntary locomotion. The osseous spine is only part of the complete neuro-loco motor system but is the most important and has an understandable construction in the view of mechanical engineers if they recognize the original functions. Only in living creatures there are natural developing processes in which form follows function.

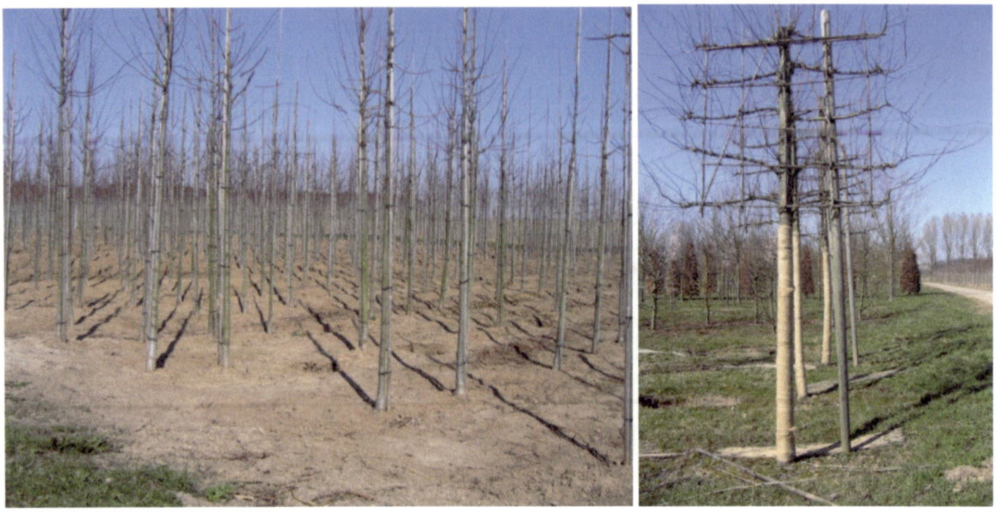

Fig. 5. Young trees connected with straight poles. As Andry took a young deformed tree as an allegory for the orthopedic way of looking towards human growth, it must be emphasized that the only reason for placing poles attached to trees by gardeners is to protect them for deforming forces like winds. By guiding branches of a young tree tied to sticks almost any form can be obtained. In old anatomic textbooks the morphology of bones is attributed to the ever moulding action of the intrauterine pressures and the postnatal action of muscles in movement. The logo of Orthopedics is more about protection, forces, growth and time, not so much on a technique of correction of deformities.

The spine has unchanged capabilities in evolution between all vertebrate species, according to Gracovetsky, as primary engine in locomotion (Gracovetsky& Farfan, 1986). The main change in function of the spine between quadrupeds and bipedals is that the coupling mechanism at the thoracolumbar joint (cauda equina) changed. From coupling a pair of pendulums with ground contact steered by counter wise directed torsional movements at this joint towards the coupling of one pendulum with ground contact and a free moving reversed pendulum. Balancing the weight of (an impressive) skull connected on top of the same spring- like spine in between plays an important role. Homo erectus is the only animal with a conus-cauda at the thoracolumbar joint, and this had much to do with this evolution, which makes counterwise torques possible (Roth, 1985). Still by the use of torsional forces, men are amblers, not gallopers (Gracovetsky& Farfan, 1986). But men achieved a powerful and efficient locomotion in thousands of years. Thanks to the right evolution of their spines.

3. Method

We searched in older available studies and descriptions of deformities from the Renaissance on and followed the gradually developing knowledge in ethiopathogenesis by leading European institutions. By that we can now highlight some forgotten or misinterpret pieces of evidence brought by researchers who brought biologic, evolutionary and biomechanical science in a proper sense together in the nineteenth century. As mentioned a missing link in underlying knowledge how a living animal or human actually grows persisted till our time. By the use of own observations in clinical practice (orthopedics) some connections between clinic and underlying biology can be postulated along this older knowledge, which lost much of its value and penetration in modern Medicine. The ongoing science on ethiopathogenesis of scoliosis was apparently interrupted by the global social disturbances in the period 1914-1945. Traumatology attracted all focus and manpower in Orthopedics.

We under scribe evolutionary knowledge in which the human spine has the same origin, development (phylogenetic and ontogenetic) and functions in locomotion as any other vertebrate and will have to face the same (forming and deforming) forces to grow, to keep balance in stance and while moving. Walking of men is indeed bipedal, but balancing only on hind legs is shared with all birds, quadrupeds like kangaroo's and to a certain degree some other primates. On this point the search for proper knowledge which organ organizes all this features in individual development and how scoliosis as a deviation should be under control of the nervous system too, the work of Roth became disclosed. Further exposure of the work of Roth, who in a way attached the old knowledge in many biomedical fields into a comprehensive explanation how growth is organized and regulated by the oldest organ (phylogenetic and ontogenetic) of animal life: the central nervous system with its precious brainstem-cord-roots complex in vertebrates in his concept of the "Nervous Skeleton" and its very intriguing way of growth, is undertaken (Roth, 1985; van Loon, 2008b).

4."Lost" historic knowledge on spinal deformities and natural scientific evidence on morphogenesis in pre-Pubmed literature

Only a few highlights in orthopedic history will be referred to in this chapter.

In **1792** the surgeon of the city of Amsterdam David Van Gesscher published his book on "Observations on Deformations of the Spine" (in Dutch and assigned to the German surgeon at the court of King George III of England). His clinical studies on form and function and postmortem observations in kyphosis and scoliosis are written down and seem a start for a concise system in understanding scoliosis. He postulated two important concepts in the non consumptious (the old name for Tuberculosis was Consumption) deformated spine: the optimalisation of the balancing forces towards a healthy posture in the human bipedal ways of standing and walking needs a certain optimal sagittal curvature. He even postulated a mathematical formula for the description. This optimal curvature is necessary to keep the weight of the head and the shoulders balanced in an energy saving way above the hips in stance and during walking. He postulated already that a long up-going lumbar lordosis to Th10 in the sagittal contour was the mainstay of a good posture. In postmortem studies he found the weakening and ventral deformations in discs, apophyses and wedging vertebrae mainly at the thoracolumbar area as was found in our days too in serious kyphosis and scoliosis. The second concept was on the role of prolonged sitting and the relation with the found changes around the discs at the thoracolumbar spine. He observed that (mainly) girls, especially those with "a weak constitution" who spent their days by knitting or with embroidery in a flexed position on chairs or stools can develop scoliosis more easily around their compressed and easily deformable thoracolumbar elements(van Gesscher,1792). Looking afterwards this "weak constitution" was caused in some cases by rachitis (English disease), but even in those days, many girls were not allowed to play outside and was the nutrition quit badly. Van Gesscher invented an extending corrective corset. This was used for more than 100 years in The Netherlands and abroad before the use of Plaster of Paris (invented by A. Mathijsen) became popular (cheap, easy, changeable). This corset shows a lordotic configuration in its complete length.

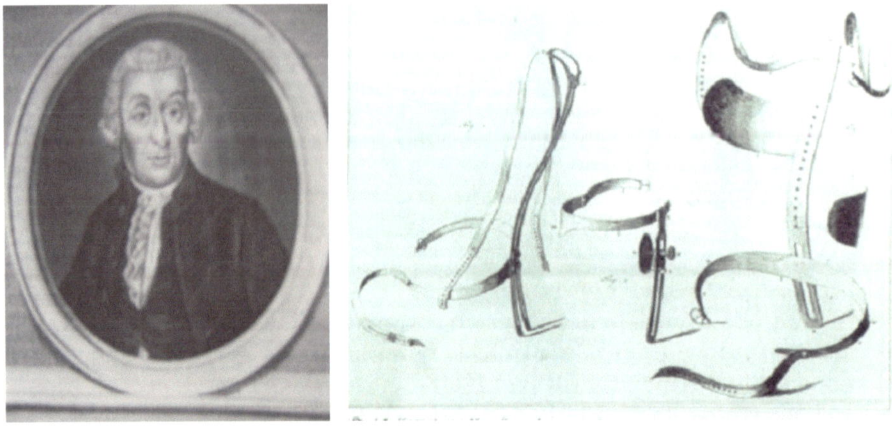

Fig. 6. Portrait of the surgeon of Amsterdam, David van Gesscher (1735-1810) and a picture of his successful brace for scoliosis out of his book from 1792.

In France Nicolas Andry already hypothesized in the same era the possibilities of guidance and correction young growing human spines and skeletons by using the moulding capability of muscular forces towards more optimized posture and function. As in tree-growing by gardeners his guidance by extending corsets was a proven method to withstand deformating external forces (like wind in young trees). With exercises and symmetrical extension at the thoracolumbar joint in corsets (for "weak" girls) he managed a good deal of deformities as scoliosis (Andry, 1741). This was followed by Vernel and later on popularized in many European orthopedic institutions. Extension of the spine and avoidance of sitting in flexed position (bad posture) became a mainstay in Orthopedics (and educational environments) until the mid twentieth century (Hohmann et al., 1957). When cosmetic aspects became popular for this guidance with corsets of posture in girls and young women, the scientific background of its original purpose faded quickly.

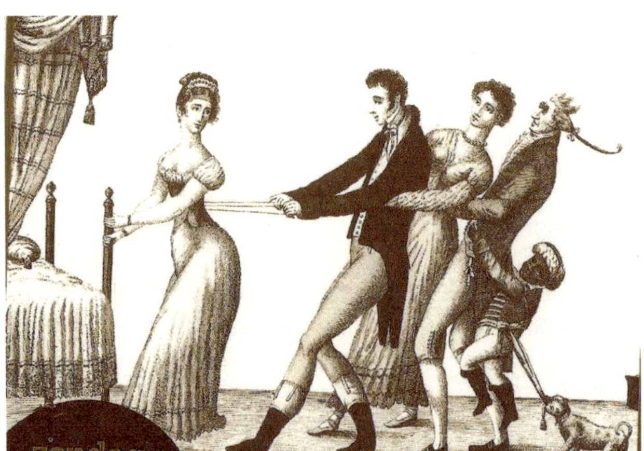

Fig. 6. Caricature from the early nineteenth century.At the time it became popular to put any young woman in higher classes in a constricting but extending corset, the original purpose or indication in children with deforming spines and a "weak constitution" according to Andry and Vernel was on its way to be forgotten. In countries like Germany and Sweden special gymnastics and postural excersises replaced these corsets in girls and young women.

In 1907 one of the first hospital surgeons in Germany treating scoliosis, L. Wüllstein described his animal experiments in young dogs to show how forced flexion can produce all now well known characteristics of kyphotic deformities in the midportion of the canine spine. Thorough macroscopic and microscopic investigations were done at sacrifice of these young dogs after a different amount of weeks. They functioned with the spine brought in forced flexion (Fig.7) All pathologic features ,afterwards describing the changes in Scheuermann's disease, were present in only a few weeks (from Hohmann et al.,1957)

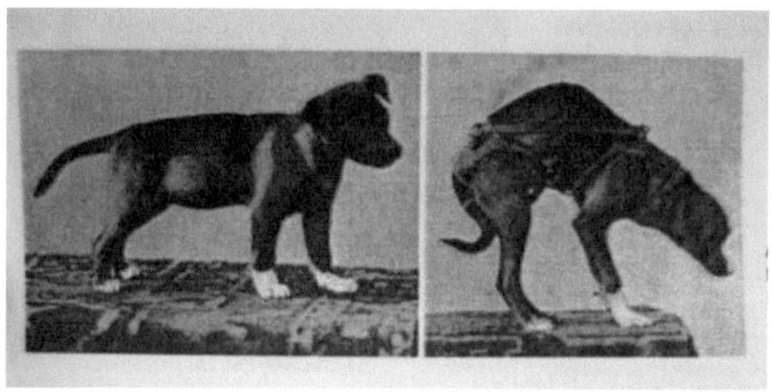

Fig. 7. Photograph from the described animal experiment to create serious spinal deformations in dogs by Wüllstein.

In 1912 one of the co-founders of the SICOT, the Dutch orthopedic surgeon Murk Jansen, published his book "The Physiologic Scoliosis and its causes "(in Dutch). Besides a thorough but also critical review of all available published knowledge on scoliosis and kyphosis by scientists like Lorenz, Schulthess, Nicolodani, Schanz, Volkmann and Hueter, own research was done. Out of postmortem studies (partly in Liverpool with Robert Jones) it was suggested strongly, that the anatomic and physiologic asymmetry in the left and right crurae diafragmaticae act as a creator of asymmetrical rotational forces at the thoracolumbar area in ventilation. This was seen as an explanation of the quit dominant presence of right sided thoracic and left sided lumbar curves in scoliosis. Moreover, he did in vivo tests with children to show the sometimes very early presentation of a thoracolumbar kyphosis with angular configuration if siblings are put too much and too soon in sitting positions. The stiffening of this area in kyphosis he observed and explained as contractures around the (later called) "neutral" vertebra creates a fulcrum (a functional bar of some vertebrae) to cantilever the now opposing rotational forces by the diaphragm in lateral curvatures. He did in vivo experiments with young children suspended under vertical head traction to show the right sided torsional movements of the ribcage in respiration. In animal experiments in hares (even so suspended, now on their ears), he performed intrathoracic pressure measurements and showed consequent lower intrathoracic pressure in the right pleural cavity.

In conclusion of all this, Jansen plead strongly for preventive measurements by restriction of passive sitting (flexed posture) in siblings and young children before their muscular strength to extend the spine was properly established (by playing, crawling and sleeping in prone positions!) and the thoracolumbar lordosis has established itself firmly. All, to prevent the development of this early kyphotic deformity (Jansen, 1912). Alertness of parents and teachers, optimalisation of static and dynamic posture building by influencing lifestyle factors (school furniture designed by Schulthess and others) and exercises (gymnastics, reinforcement of the muscles extending the spine) were advised in those days. Some of this holistic approach and relation with gymnastics still survives or struggles for survival in parts of Europe (Weiss, 2008; Zahner et al., 2006; Bas et al., 2011).

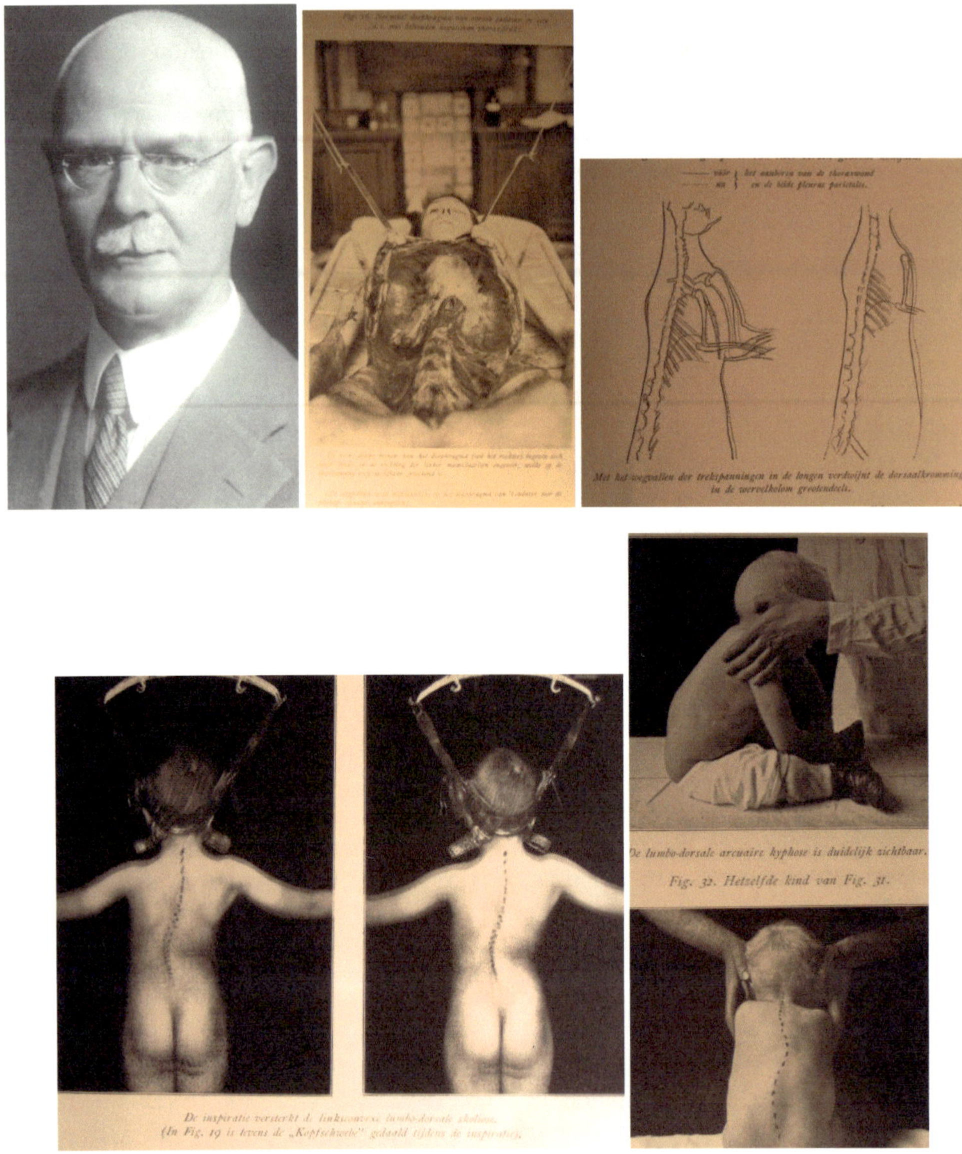

Fig. 8. Portrait of Murk Jansen (and the most illustrative figures in his monograph on scoliosis(1912).Clockwise: portrait of Murk Jansen (1867-1935); Ventrally opened cadaver with suspension of the asymmetric configuration of the left and right crux diaphragmatica; Drawing of the idea of his animal study in hares to confirm that almost the same asymmetry in the diaphragm in these mainly bipedal animals gives asymmetric but side-consequent higher intrathoracic pressures; A boy with a scoliosis, suspended on his head. The rotational movement in inspiration is visibly increasing the left lumbar curve; an in vivo demonstration of early kyphosis of the thoracolumbar spine in a young child in sitting position. Even at this age this is already a sign of structural changes in height and form of vertebrae and discs. The slight right sided coronal curve above this kyphosis is also depicted.

Unhappily the prevailing way of correcting structural and serious scoliosis in Jansen's time has changed in Europe to prolonged bedridden periods on corrective plaster shelves. Cobb mentioned it even as the "Murk Jansen plaster shelf". Sayre's method of corrective plastering in suspension, leaving mobility for walking was apparently overruled in Europe by Calot's corrections in prone position under anesthesia and plaster shelves (Gelbke, 1883). The corrective action was still a quit symmetrical thoracolumbar lordotic hyperextension. Only the gravity forces during stance were ruled out. In his review Jansen actually connected the various scientific knowledge brought by dozens of scientist and argued on the value of the discussion between Volkmann and Hueter. Their "principle" was never written down in one sentence by both of them, there was even an argue on the exact role of the resilience of the deformable structures in the spine, e.g. the discs, the apophyses, ligaments and the cartilage in the facet joints. But the "principle" reflects in retrospection to the Conservation Laws mentioned on which the deformation of growing cartilage in other joints is also theoretically based. Orthopedics knew, as generalists, around 1900 the way "the system" works, but were unaware of the exact role of the central nervous system as constructor and controller of its own housing. A black box.

Because of the World Wars and other political disturbances a longstanding gap in evolution of knowledge on spinal deformities is visible in produced literature. The sources in German language got dusted in libraries. When Cobb in the United States presented the value of radiographic measurements of curves he did warn seriously not to forget the clinical and physiological/ functional aspects of scoliosis, but such a fate seems to have happened for quit some time (Cobb, 1958).

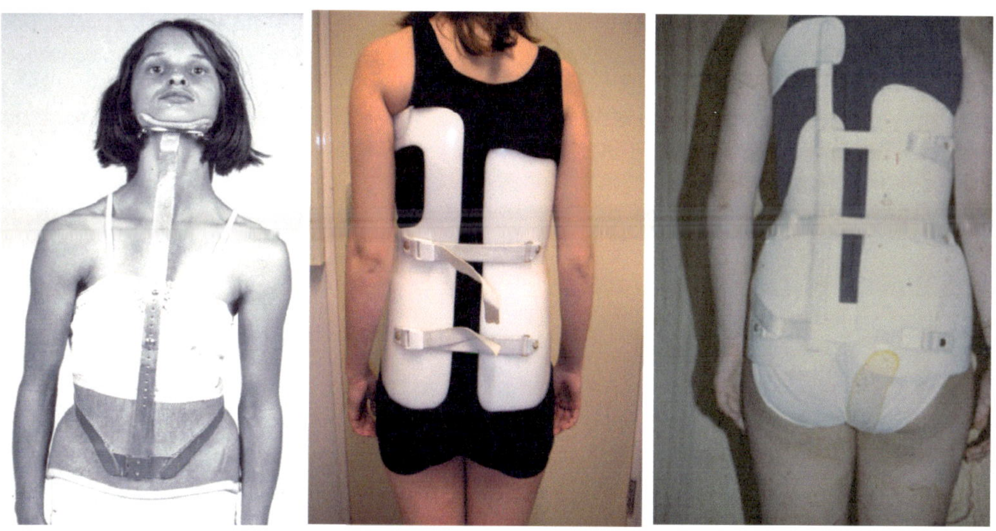

Fig. 9. Pictures of popularized braces. On the left an early Milwaukee brace based on a leather lumbar corset and the chin-head superstructure stretching the upper spine. In the middle a Boston brace with apparently orthotist dependent modifications. At the right a modified Boston brace with a so called Edelmann superstructure.

So the international research into causes of spinal deformities went away for a long time from the black box, the biological process of growth still was. This is also what hapens with the known effects of lifestyle in terms of quantity and quality of movements and forces during all childhood (if you don't sit) and the role basic posture plays.

Maybe disconnected from this knowledge, from the USA two types of braces using distraction (Milwaukee brace) or thoracic flexion and lateral pressure on the apical zones (modular Boston brace) were globally popularized, and dozens of alternatives with their way of action following grossly the three point correction with pressure on apices of the different curves are also still in use.

5. Dyscongruency of neurovertebral growth relations in spinal deformity disclosed by Milan Roth

Undetected till 2001 by the mainstream of orthopedic scientists Milan Roth of Brno developed between 1960 and 1985 his concepts on neurovertebral and neuro-osseous growth relations and the tension driven system of reciprocal influence between the two tissues. If this system is hindered by endogenous or exogenous influences, incongruence of growth can occur, leading to spinal deformities and alterations in morphology and function of the nervous system too. It was based on thorough knowledge of biological literature on growth in vertebrates, basic orthopedic knowledge and own research. Roth was a neuroradiologist and as professor in this field, he created a small research department with focus on spinal deformities and their background.

Roth returned for the orthopedic knowledge on scoliosis and the existing science on growth back to the gathered European science around 1900. Where concerning the way our loco motor system grows and functions and how pathways to run into trouble, the scientists involved were reaching each other quit well. Roth provided thoroughly revisited and new biological knowledge (in Czech, German and English) on how growth appears to happen on more conceptual scale for the parts doctors cannot see: the influence of time and all internal and external forces on an embryo or born vertebrate and how this is arranged. His main and most striking achievement is the discovery of the way the two different types of growth in Nature work together. The volume and mass increasing mitotic growth of all cells in all tissues during the whole process of growth, next to the extending type of growth of the neural tissues, whilst its amount of cells (billions) is already reached in the early stages of embryological life.

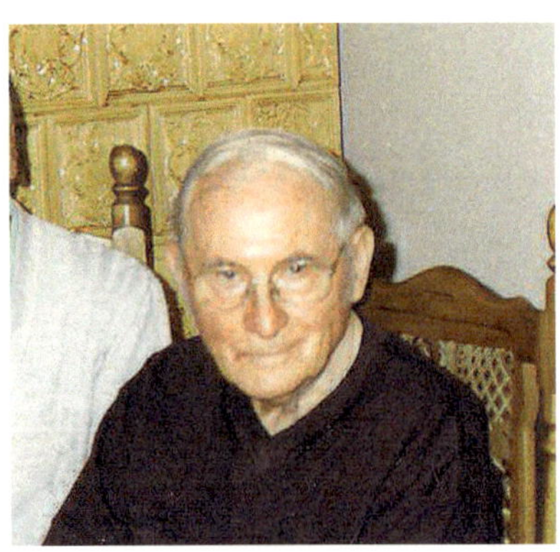

Fig. 10. Portrait of Prof. Milan Roth (1923-2006), neuroradiologist and scientist at the (now) Masaryk University of Brno, Cech Republique.

In this he supported the clinical observations on growing children made during the centuries before by orthopedics and gymnasts. Roth accepted the evolutionary theories completely and used them often by comparing the conditions of spine and cord in other animals. As is stated in anatomic science and embryology, the final form of bones is moulded by muscular action and the movement in joints. Roth proposed that all sorts of pulsating effects in the fluids around the embryo (heartbeat mother, respiration forces, intestinal mechanics and the motor activity of the mother are the first "moulders"of the early embryo. While the first differentiation in cells to occur is the formation of the neural stem cells organized in the notochord, the capacity of these cells will be the controlling and regulating tissue from that point on.

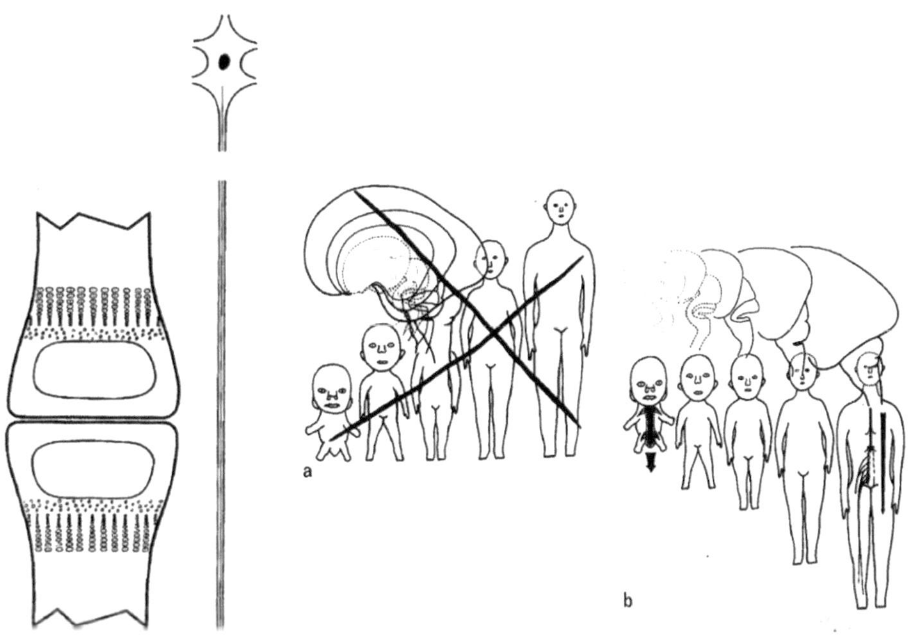

Fig. 11. Two drawings made by Roth on his most important researched issues and used in several publications on the way he learned to look to growth in vertebrates according to the discovered insights he brought into biomedical science. On the left a schematic drawing in which the osseous growth by celldivision, mitosis ,is depicted together with a simplified way to show, that a neural cell grows in the meantime by extension via continious attachement to mitotic growing tissue cells under their "guidance". An important dimension in growth is time. As Andry tried to catch time in his logo, Roth did this by drawing interruptions in the axons of the neural cell or in the periferal nerves.

In a huge amount of publications on observations in pneumomyelographic studies in scoliosis, animal experiments, mechanical modeling and post mortem in vitro tests he depicted the crucial role that the type of growth (namely by stretching) of the whole nervous system, "the nervous skeleton", has in the normal and abnormal formation of the spine. In teratogenic studies in animals, inhibitors of neural cell function and growth injected intrauterine, inevitably gave skeletal deformations. And the spines always spiralized into scoliosis.

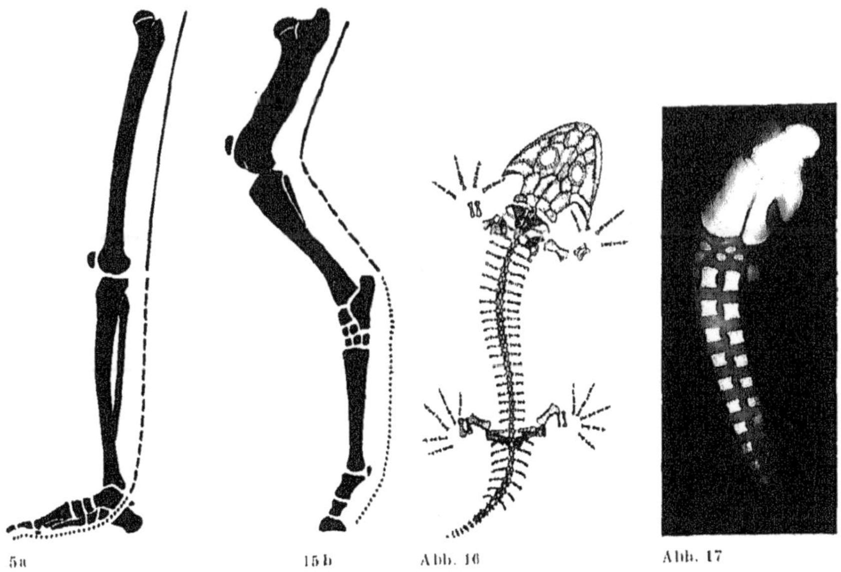

Fig. 12. Set of figures out of Roth's original articles in German. In a comparison between a hind leg of a man and a horse he illustrates the secondary length and width of bones to the primary lengthening of the nerves by stretching, on its turn induced by hormonal regulated increase in volume of the other tissues. In the two other pictures, a drawing of an extinct amphibian and an X-ray of a baby-whale with the similar skeletal build up of the cranial extremity, his vision on phylogenetic and ontogenetic morphogenesis around the nervous tissue is depicted.

A "short cord" can indeed cause scoliosis. Roth deducted the way Wolff's Law and the Volkmann Hueter principle works. Growth has to create flat (Platyspondylie) or wedged vertebral bodies in hindered stretch growth of the cord, in absence of too much torsional changes leading to kyphotic deformities. By this, he put Scheuermann's disease under the same etiological factors that are responsible for scoliosis (Roth1968,1969,1981,1985;van Loon,2008b). And he concepted the existence of a mechanical force like tension to be assessed from the outside to represent these interconnected subsystems. If there is increased tension in the cord, there must be increased tension in muscles to, if the energy is not used to deform the soft connecting parts (Volkmann Hueter principle) or the bones (Wolff's Law) of the spine.

Recently, the Hong Kong group lead by Chang and Chu published supportive reproducing studies with MRI in idiopathic scoliosis (Chu et al, 2008). Own, not published observations on clinical investigation and whole spine MRI in children who develop a hyperkyphosis are astonishing affirmative to Roth's research and mechanical models (van Loon 2008c).

In personal observations the presence of neuromuscular tightness or tension, well-known in hyperkyphosis (as Scheuermann's disease) is also present in the rapidly progressive scoliosis and bad postures (like flat spines). These are the clinical representants of the spine deforming and neuroprotective forces. Several tests can be done to assess this neuromuscular

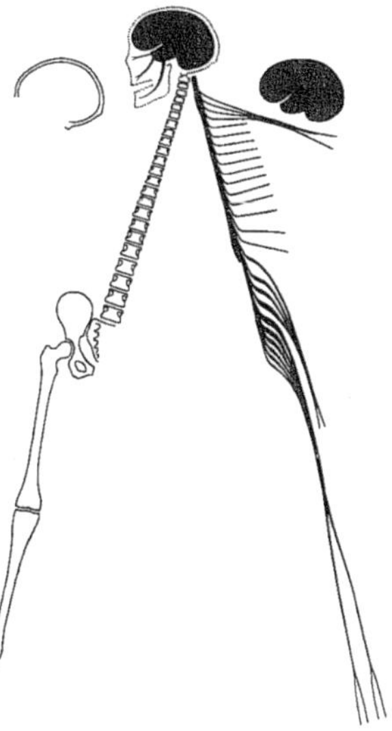

Fig. 13. Caricatured picture by Roth in the introduction of his book: Neurovertebral and neuro-osseous growth relations (1985). In this picture he satirized the greatest problem, in his eyes, existing in the biomedical and medical scientific fields with their diversity of developments and research: "The unfavorable existence of the interdisciplinary barrier". In case of his topic, the spine and its contents, with this caricature he complained over the complete barrier between orthopedics and neurology and neurosurgery to look to each others tissues in its developments and research into etiology. It looked if the two systems develop and function completely separated. He restored holistic knowledge.

tension (van Loon, 2008c). Like blood pressure in the cardiovascular system, this tension seems under influence of increasing (spurts, bad postures) and decreasing (sleep, stretching exercises, TLI bracing) factors.

The spring like storage of energy in these conditions can theoretically be a deforming force by itself. In a way Roth put these tensile forces in some of his mechanical models. Roth's only drawback (he was a radio neurologist) was a lack of clinical experience with healthy children with scoliosis or hyperkyphosis and thus a fruitful collaboration with orthopedics in a broader way. The ever existing and observed presence of neuromuscular tightness in children with deformities (well described for Scheuermann's disease) can be used in these proposed tests to evaluate increasing tension in the musculoskeletal system during growth of healthy children. They will give a further clue to the question of the chance of progression. Roth called it the growth in length inhibiting muscular forces if the mitotic increase of volume exceeds the speed of growth of the central neural tissues (brainstem, cord and cauda equina). It is the background between gross external body types as asthenia, athletic or pycnic. But also between children that are "lean" or "stiff" in their locomotion. Much of this can be understand by his plea to understand that any abnormal circumstance in the neural tissue has its effects in the musculoskeletal system. Is the cord tense, the muscles, especially those responsible for extension and balance, will be too?

These signs of neuromuscular tightness rapidly increases during growth spurts and can be addressed by physical therapy or gymnastics as neurodynamic tools. It fits in the radio

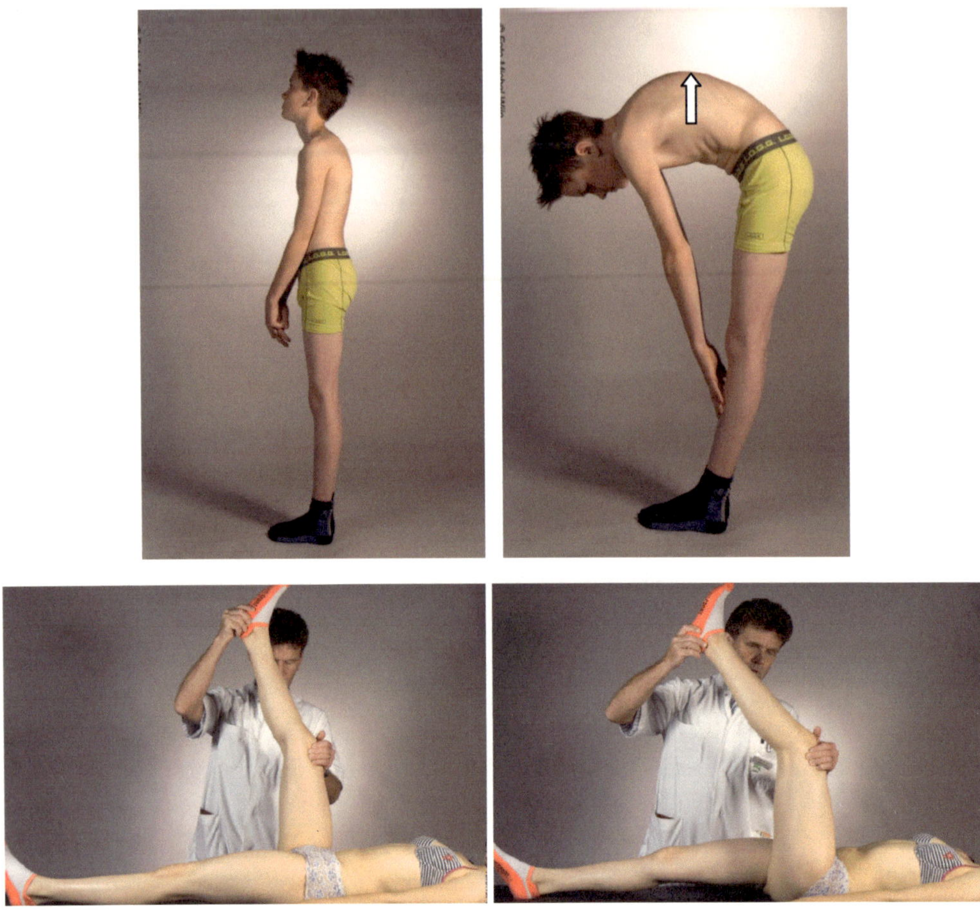

Fig. 14. Clinical test of neuromuscular tension. Above a boy of 12 presented with bad posture and muscular pains. From lateral an increased and long kyphosis can be seen. In bending because of "short hamstrings" and triceps surae a start of angulation in the kyphosis (arrow), leaning backwards in the ankles and a long finger ground distance can be seen. With his ankles in 90° he will loose balance. Below: healthy children with scoliosis as here in this girl show asymmetric straight leg raising or Femorotibiale angles. During growth spurts this is even more obvious.

diagnostic findings of a stretched, obvious tense central cord by Roth in his pneumencephalographic studies and the MRI findings recently published by Chu (Chu, 2008). In this publication observations are described on the relationship with Arnold Chiari malformations and scoliosis, by Roth already clearly stated (Roth, 1986). A nervous system that is stretched will have also have different clinical manifestations during life, all with secondary compensations and adaptations around it.

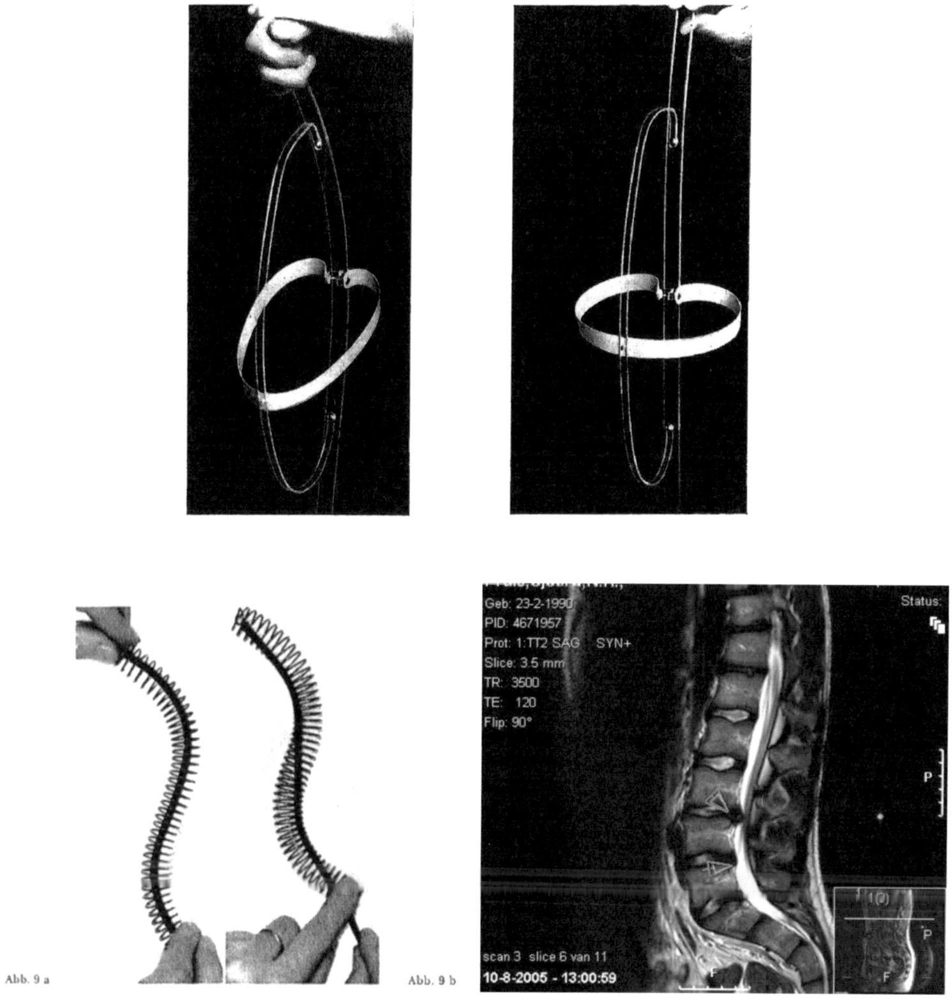

Fig. 15. For educational reasons and to show how tension between to systems can have consequences for both, Roth made different mechanical models. Above an eloquent model in which the relationship of creating the human lordosis, its concomitant vertebral grooves and the tensile forces to create and to hold this are condensed to mimic what happens in growth. The time factor and the increase in size cannot be shown. Below the most simple and illustrative model: a spring with a small rope inside. If the rope is shortened the curved spring shortens to but mainly by compressing the spirals in the concavities. To correlate with modern imaging at the right from own practice a sagittal T2 MRI from Th10 down. It is of a 15(!) year old boy who was seen for a bad sitting posture and low back pain. Straight leg raising was only 40° bilateral. Note the early changes as seen in Scheuermann at the TL joint and compressed discs at the posterior side lumbosacral. The complete posterior contact of the cauda in the canal and the stretched aspects looks similar to the spring model of Roth and were described already in his pneumomyelographies in Scoliosis and Scheuermann.

6. New facts on natural events around and deformations at the thoracolumbar joint and practical consequences in the evolution to proper treatment of scoliosis

The acceptance of the importance of all the events that take place, or evolves itself in the sagittal curvature in humans during growth gathered before 1914 helped us in the urge to go further than others to disclose the work of Roth. The acceptance of Roth's concepts because of their plausibility and their obvious representants in the all-day clinical practice with children and adolescents with postural and other spinal problems stimulated new ways of assessing and treating deformities like scoliosis in these children.

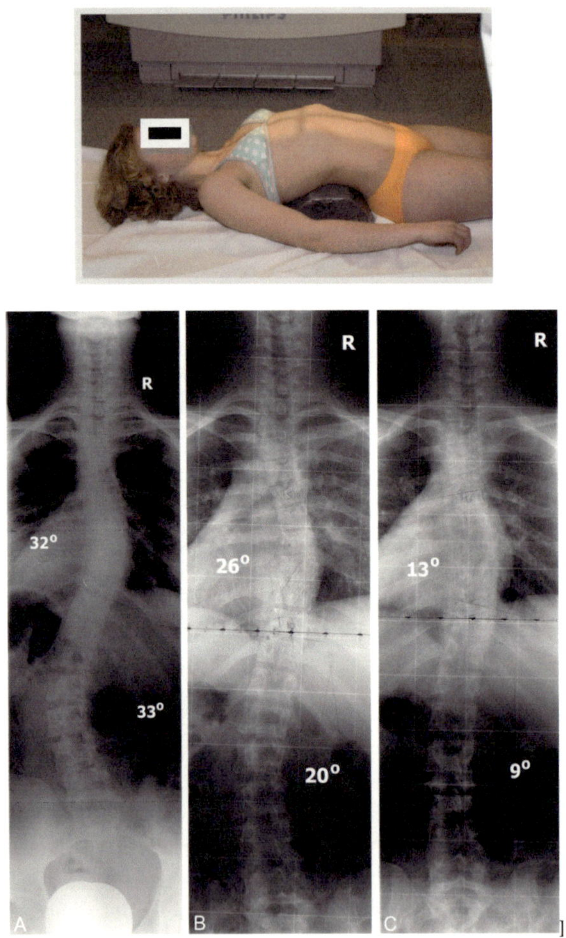

Fig. 16. Figures from the experimental study in Spine to proof the potential of correction by TLI principles in double major scoliosis. In 40 children with double major scoliosis (one curve at least 25°) the Cobb angles in standing position (left X-ray) were compared with those in supine position on a lordotic fulcrum under the thoracolumbar joint (picture left and right X-ray). In all cases both curves reduced very significantly. In a subgroup a third x-ray was made (middle X-ray) in just supine position, because of the well-known reduction of coronal curves if gravity is ruled out (van Loon et al., 2008)

In the found relation with the early events at the thoracolumbar joint (kyphosis in morphology, contracture in kinematics) and the possibility to come to etiology related therapeutic measurements the Thoracolumbar Lordotic Intervention (TLI) was developed. At first a brace technique with a new, unexpected way of successful correction in all deformities got into practice. In 2008 we presented in Spine a radiological study, demonstrating that forceful restoration of lordosis with a fulcrum under the thoracolumbar spine in supine children with double major scoliosis can correct instantaneous both curves significantly (van Loon, 2008a).

Its way of action of a TLI brace can be explained as to redirect the trunk extending long muscles in their original trail. The human spine is the only one that has such a trail in the form of the "vertebral groove", the concavities at each side of the spinal process in the vertebral lamina (Roth, 1969b). Also, for the first time, a consequent kyphotic curve in stead of the expected lordosis (in scoliosis) was found and described between the two coronal curves at the thoracolumbar spine in standing lateral radiographs. This finding is reproduced very recently by the study group of Sjanghai (Ni et al, 2010). With the, on these findings based corrective technique TLI (Thoracolumbar Lordotic Intervention) in braces, we brought promising results in a pilot study (van Loon et al, 2011).

TLI brings the older extending techniques back to stage and does not put the thoracic spine into flexion as is still advised based on Dickson's axiom. With the presence of any slight rotation in the spine or trunk, due to the asymmetric rotating forces of the diaphragm during respiration, a shortening and spiralisation will occur. This is according to Jansen and only proven by Dickson and his followers for the thoracic spine, because they overlooked apparently the events at the thoracolumbar spine. One of the main explanations can be that in developing kyphosis the proper deepening of the vertebral groove besides the spinal processus become shallow, and only slight, but persistent torsional forces (Jansen) the erector trunci will slip gradually out of this pulley-groove (see also fig.3).. The theory and experiments that dorsal shear forces are likely to be present in lordotic parts of a spine still holds.In our opinion they did not incorporate such a kyphosis in the thoracolumbar junction and this does not lean on older evidence in human spinal behavior and skeletal growth(Kouwenhoven et al,2006; Kouwenhoven & Castelein,2008). They describe the dorsal shear forces in fact in a "residual"- lordosis above a kyphotic change at the thoracolumbar joint. It does not say why it helps the M. erector trunci during growth spurts to force the spine and the complete trunk into an adaptive solution if the origin of the rotational forces that create even in non scoliotic a slight torsional aspect of the vertebrae. The location of the apices of sagittal curvatures is of paramount importance to assess if a human spine has developed along the ever present optimalisation processes

In common sense there was/is knowledge of this "beautiful posture" coming with optimalisation of the sagittal contour. Maybe because of developed aversion of the military and disciplinary aspects in "good posture", as not to speak of political abuse of this during the era's totalitarian regimes ruled peoples lives, discussions in academic Medicine on good and bad anatomical and physiological postures disappeared. For dealing with girls the fear not to be too much involved in "cosmesis"can be seen as a conflicting point of view to bring solutions. A more medieval acceptance of the presence of a good or a bad spinal posture slipped in, although tremendous efforts are done to cope in a very modern, increasingly "high tech" way, with our spinal problems.

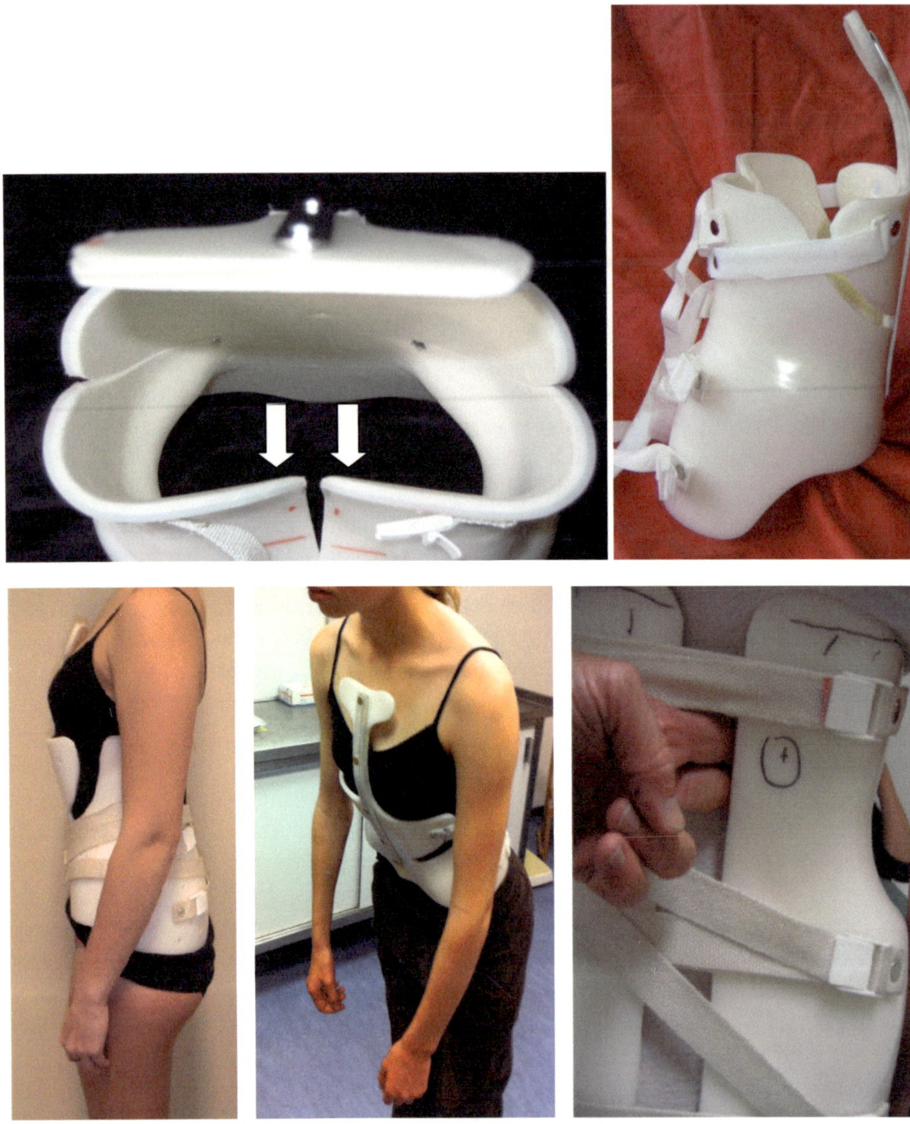

Fig. 17. Some aspects of Thoracolumbar Lordotic Intervention in a brace. Clockwise: A TLI brace seen from above with its backward bended sternal support. The places where pressure is applied on the paraspinal musculature at the thoracolumbar joint are symmetric and the same for all deformities (arrows); A TLI brace in lateral view. The short construction leaves a lot of freedom to move, except in flexion. a 15 year old girl wearing a TLI brace. The natural and cosmetic well accepted sagittal contour and normal balance are shown.; A girl with scoliosis in a TLI brace bending a little forward to show the extension that persist in the spine that leaves the sternum free.: By automatic further extension of the torso while wearing a TLI brace, at all controls the correction in lordosis can be augmented, whilst the upper and lower rims can be shortened with a positive effect on compliance. On the right the extra space after the first two months of wearing. The space willed be filled up and the upper side shortened and bended backwards.

A functional interrelationship between curves in more than one plane was already shown in a study on bracing (van Rhijn,2002) In literature the sagittal contour of the spine in scoliosis is gaining more attention in the last decade because of severe problems that can be present in adulthood (Glassman et al.,2005).

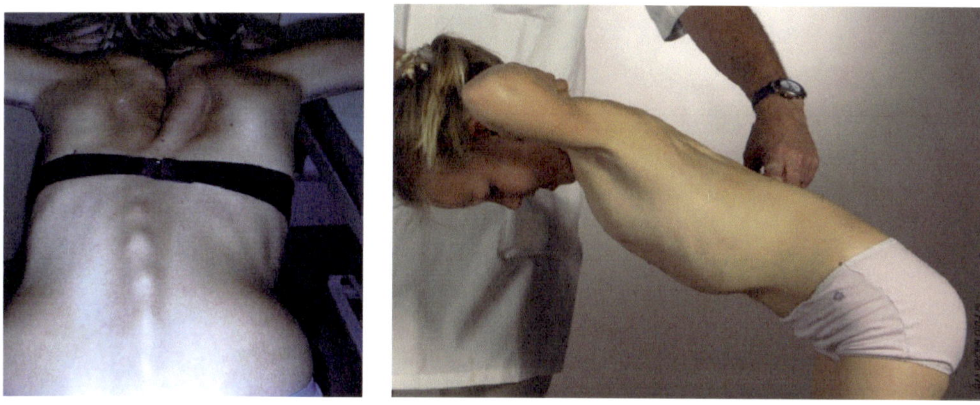

Fig. 18. The dynamic hypokyphosis in the thoracic spine above a thoracolumbar kyphosis. On the left a very well trained gymnastic girl of 16 after a (original, not TLI) Boston brace treatment for her scoliosis in a scoop test. The major asymmetric adaptations in muscular function and strength can be seen. On the right an 11 year old girl with a right sided thoracic scoliosis coming up from bending with the hands in the neck (scoop test) to achieve extension. Also here the hypokyphotic, almost lordotic spine at the level of the gibbus above the still kyphotic thoracolumbar spine is seen. In all children with deformations this scoop test shows a typical type of unrolling or coming up, with staged extension of the thoracic and lumbar spine.

7. Conclusions

Revitalization and combining older or dispersed knowledge on the causes of spinal deformities and on growth itself can bring an end to the "black box" or *Idiopathy*. Spinal growth can be seen as the result of a combination of neuro-osseous growth regulation in a very complex but understandable architecture of the loco motor system of all vertebrates. Three dimensional deformations are the result if any dyscongruency occurs between these two complete different types of growth in the neuro-osseous relationship. In scoliosis understanding of the meaning of the ever present torsional forces in the vertebrates and its special features in men is helpful. It seems that overlooking the work of Jansen, Roth and others kept the vision on the actual processes in the "black box" blurred.

In treating deformities with TLI principles we found an effective strategy in which the earliest etiologic moments and changes in functional anatomy of deformations is addressed. It applies a complete controlled lordosis, so normal growth forces and the proper function of the spine erecting muscles are being brought back in their anatomical tracts. And it prevents flexion, the rapidly increased and most prevailing "posture" in modern life of children. Much of these interventions can be done in a complete active way too by people themselves, guided by teachers, gymnasts or therapists that put development towards a good posture on the first place in their techniques.

This conjoined knowledge can also direct to new efforts in focused and dedicated research from unexpected etiologic view. New and possible better pathways can be developed for better preventive and conservative measurements in spinal deformities with progression during growth. Efforts to let children reach, from the start of their locomotion, a more optimal posture will increase the sustainability of the locomotor system as a whole and the durability of its functional parts.

8. Acknowledgements

The widow, Mrs Rothova, and sons of Milan Roth gave full support and consent to bring his legacy further on when his personal enthusiasm after first contacts ended by his sudden death.

The late Jan Munneke, orthotist in Arnhem, gave his best years and efforts in the first concepts, ameliorations and final use of TLI bracing.

The medical photographers Michel and Cathy Wijn, working at the Rijnstate Hospital in Arnhem were responsible for the most clinical pictures.

9. References

Andry N. (1741) in Orthopaedia or the art of preventing and correcting deformities in children, transl.1843, 2 volumes, London, Millar, Publisher.

Chu WC, Man GC, LamWW, YeungBH, Chau WW NgBK, Lam,T.P.; LeeKM, ChengJC, (2008) Morphological and functional electrophysiological evidence of relative spinal cord tethering in adolescent idiopathic scoliosis. Spine: 33;6(673-680)

Cobb JR (1958): Scoliosis- Quo Vadis? J Bone Joint Surg Am.; 40:507-510.

Dickson RA (1988): The aetiology of spinal deformations. Lancet: May21; 1(8595); 1151-5

Gelbke JH (1883) German translation of Lewis A. Sayre: Spondylitis and scoliosis of the spine and their treatment by suspension and plaster of Paris. Leipzig. F.C.Vogel, Publisher

Gesscher D.van. (1792) Aanmerkingen over de Wanstaltigheden der Ruggengraat. Amsterdam.J.B.Elwe Publisher.

Glasman S, Berven S, Bridwell K, Horton M, Dimar J (2005) Correlation of Radiographic Parameters and Clinical Symptoms in Adult Scoliosis. Spine 30: 6:682-688.

Gordon JE (1991) Structures or why things don't fall down. Pelican books 1978, reprinted in Penguin books.ISBN-13:978-0-14-013628.

Gracovetsky S, Farfan H. (1986) The optimum spine. Spine Jul; 11(6):543-73.

Hohmann G,Hackenbroch M &Lindemann K : (1956) Handbuch der Orthopaedie, vol I and II, 6vol.Stuttgart Georg Thieme Verlag (Extended and revised publication of the Handbuch der Orthopaedischen Chirurgie 1907 by G.Joachimsthal,editor, A.Lorenz, A. Hoffa, A.Schanz, W.Schulthess, F.Lange and others.)

Jansen M. (1912) The Physiologic Scoliosis and its Cause (in Dutch), Leiden, E.J.Brill, publisher.

Loon PJM van, Kühbauch BAG & Thunnissen FB. (2008a) Forced Lordosis on the Thoracolumbar Junction Can Correct Coronal Plane Deformity in Adolescents With Double Major Curve Pattern Idiopathic Scoliosis. Spine33; 7(797-801)

Loon PJM van, Rhijn LW van (2008b); The central cord-nervous roots complex and the formation and deformation of the spine; The scientific work on systematic body growth by Milan Roth of Brno (1926-2006). Stud Health Technol Inform; 140:170-86.

Loon PJM van (2008c), Clinical detectable tension in the growing body: new and revisited signs in clinical examination in children with postural problems and spinal deformities. Restoration of lordosis on the thoracolumbar junction can correct sagittal and coronal plane deformity; a new (revisited) linked approach on the treatment and etiology of adolescent spinal deformities. Stud Health Technol Inform; 140:52-8.

Loon PJM van et al., (2011.) A new brace treatment similar for adolescent scoliosis and kyphosis based on restoration of thoracolumbar lordosis. Radiological and subjective clinical results after one year of treatment. Eur.SpineJ. (n.d. submitted).

Negrini S, Minozzi S, Bettany-Saltikov J, Zaina F, Chockalingam N, Grivas TB, Kotwicki T, Maruyama T, Romano M & Vasiliadis ES, (2010)Braces for Idiopathic Scoliosis in Adolescents. Spine 35; 13(1285-1293)

Mauroy JC de Weiss HR, Aulisa AG, Aulisa L, Brox JI, Durmala J, Fusco C, Grivas TB, Hermus J, Kotwicki T, Le Blay G, Lebel A, Marcotte L, Negrini S, Neuhaus L, Neuhaus T, Pizzetti P, Revzina L, Torres B, Loon PJM van, Vasiliadis E, Villagrasa M, Werkman M, Wernicka M, Wong MS & Zaina F (2010) 7th SOSORT consensus paper: conservative treatment of idiopathic & Scheuermann's kyphosis. Scoliosis May 5:9

Ni H, , Zhu X, He S, Yang C, Wang C, Zhao Y, Wu D, Xu J, & Li M, (2010): An Increased Kyphosis of the Thoracolumbar Junction is Correlated to More Axial Vertebral Rotation in Thoracolumbar/Lumbar Adolescent Idiopathic Scoliosis. Spine 35; 33(1334-1338)

Rhijn LW van, Plasmans CM, Veraart BE. Changes in curve pattern after brace treatment for idiopathic scoliosis. Acta Orthop Scand 2002; 73:277–81.

Roth, M (1968), Idiopathic scoliosis caused by a short spinal cord. Acta Radiologica Diagnosis Vol. 7 p. 257-271.

Roth, M. (1969), Models of vertebro-neural relations, Acta Radiologica Diagnosis. Vol. 9 (51 55)

Roth, M (1981), Idiopathic scoliosis and Scheuermann "disease": Essentially identical manifestation of neuron-vertebral growth disproportion. Radiol. Diagn. 22 (1981), H.3, 380-391

Roth M. (1985) Neurovertebral and Osteoneural Growth Relations. A concept of normal and pathological development of the skeleton. First ed. Brno, Cech Republique.: ed. J.E.Purkyne University Brno, Medical Faculty;

Roth M, (1986) Cranio-cervical growth collision: another explanation of the Arnold Chiari malformation and of basilar impression. Neuroradiology: 28:187-194.

Weiss HR; Maier-Hennes A. (2008) Specific exercises in the treatment of scoliosis--differential indication. Stud Health Technol Inform, 135; 170-193

Wang WJ, Yeung HY; Chu W CW, Tang, NLS ,Lee KM, Qiu Y, Burwell RG, Cheng JCY Ed (Orth7) (2011), Top Theories for the Ethiopathogenesis of Adolescent Idiopathic Scoliosis. J.of Pediatric Orth1 Suppl. (S14-S2)

Zahner L, Puder JJ, Roth R, Schmid M, Guldimann R, Pühse U, Knöpfli M, Braun-Fahrländer C, Marti B & Kriemler(2006):A school-based physical activity program to improve health and fitness in children aged 6-13 years ("Kinder-Sportstudie KISS"): study design of a randomized controlled trial BMC Public Health. Jun 6; 6:147.

Long-Term Outcome of Surgical Treatment in Adolescent Idiopathic Scoliosis

Franz Josef Mueller[1], Herbert Gluch[2] and Cornelius Wimmer[3]
[1]*Clinic for Orthopedic and Trauma Surgery, Hospital Barmherzige Brueder, Regensburg,*
[2,3]*Department for Spine Surgery and Scoliosis Centre, Clinic Schoen, Vogtareuth, Germany*

1. Introduction

For the surgical treatment of adolescent idiopathic scoliosis various anterior and posterior procedures and instrumentations were developed. With regard to posterior procedures, two different well-known instrumentations must be distinguished:

With the development of the Harrington rod (Harrington, 1962) a long-segment rod and hook instrumentation was available for the first time, which became the worldwide standard procedure for many years in the surgical treatment of adolescent idiopathic scoliosis. According to a retrospective meta-analysis, Harrington rods were used in more than 85% of such cases between 1958 and 1993 (Haher et al., 1995). With this instrumentation, frontal correction was achieved primarily by the distraction and elongation of the concave side, and by the compression of the convex side of the curve. The disadvantage of this method was the flattening of the spinal profile (Humke et al., 1995), with less improvement of the rib hump deformity (Aaro & Dahlborn, 1982; Weatherley et al., 1987). Moreover, there have been reports of high revision rates with the complete removal of the instrumentation due to chronic complaints of the lumbar spine (Padua et al., 2001). The instrumentation has also required postoperatively external stabilisation for about 6 to 12 months with a plaster cast or an orthesis in order to avoid the loss of initial curve correction (Danielsson et al., 2001; Dickson & Harrington, 1973; Harrington, 1962; Mariconda et al., 2005).

With the development and introduction of a novel double-rod instrumentation by Cotrel and Dubousset (Cotrel & Dubousset, 1984) about 25 years later, the disadvantages of the Harrington rod seemed to be eliminated. Early results with a small number of patients showed that the instrumentation not only provided better lateral and frontal curve correction, but also a significant correction of vertebral rotation and thus a marked reduction in the cosmetic rib hump deformity (Cundy et al., 1990). Moreover, the instrumentation gives greater primary stability so that postoperative management with an external orthesis was no longer required. On the other side, the surgical procedure requires much greater surgical skill with a long learning curve, especially due to the correct placement of the multiple laminar hooks and the subsequent insertion of the transpedicular screws.

Several other instrumentations (e.g. Luque instrumentation, Lea Plaza frame) (Luque, 1982; Lea Plaza et al., 2004) were introduced and - due to various problems - abandoned, and none of these was broadly used for a long period of time. Apart from that, the authors of this chapter conducted literature research (Pubmed) and did not succeed in finding any long-term results for any of the above-mentioned instrumentations.

Different anterior and posterior instrumentations, including minimally invasive or thoracoscopic approaches, were introduced within the last 10 years (Ameri et al., 2008; Asher et al., 2004; Halm et al., 2000; Liljenqvist et al., 2006; Lonner et al., 2006; Reddi et al., 2008; Remes et al., 2004).

Today, transpedicular mono- or poly-axial titanium screws, with different fixation systems e.g. over the top or side loading systems, are mainly used for posterior procedures in order to fuse less vertebral segments and to achieve an increasing curve correction rate with stronger primary stability. For the spine surgeon, however, the surgical principles still remain the same: correction by instrumentation and solid fusion by spondylodesis.

However, what are the concerns and expectations of the patients before and after surgery?

For this reason, 91 adolescent patients and their parents were independently asked to complete a questionnaire regarding their concerns of upcoming scoliosis surgery in a multicentre cross-sectional study (Bridwell et al., 2000). Neurological deficits were the greatest concern of both patients and parents, and the most important expectation and main reason for undergoing surgery was to reduce future pain and disability as an adult.

The short-term results within 2 years postoperatively demonstrated that pain, general self-image, function from back condition and level of activity improved statistically significantly compared with the preoperative status, but without correlation between the magnitude of curve correction and outcome scores in validated questionnaires (Merola et al., 2002).

However, until 10 years ago, there was no standardised questionnaire available to evaluate the outcome of surgically treated patients for adolescent idiopathic scoliosis, despite the fact that (life) satisfaction and self-esteem are important qualities in social science and daily life.

On the other side, adolescent idiopathic scoliosis by itself has namely a significant negative impact on quality of life and psychological functioning (Kahanovitz & Weiser, 1989). Moreover, a study reported that scoliosis is a risk factor for depression, no matter what treatment the patients has received, and findings from other studies have indicated that idiopathic scoliosis may have a negative effect on one`s psychological state, development of friendships, and ability to adapt socially (Payne et al., 1997).

Surgical outcomes have traditionally been based on radiographic measures e.g. degree of correction and complications rates. Relatively few studies have had addressed patient-focussed measures. However, all these studies did not use a standardised and validated outcome questionnaire. Therefore, the Scoliosis Research Society charged an outcome committee with the development of a patient-focussed outcome questionnaire to assess the impact of the surgical treatment of adolescent idiopathic scoliosis. This initially developed and validated instrument (Haher et al., 1999) consisted of 24 questions – therefore named SRS-24 - divided into 7 equally weighted domains, which are: pain, general self-image, postoperative self-image, postoperative function, function from back condition, general level of activity, and satisfaction. All responses were rated on a 5 point scale with 5 being the optimal response. Although the SRS-24 is simple, practical, and easy to administer (Merola et al., 2002), there were several concerns that it had low internal consistency for some domains. Asher et al. modified it and created the SRS-22, which has 5 domains: function/activity, pain, self-image/appearance, mental health, and satisfaction with management (Asher et al., 2003). The SRS-22 has now become a widely used outcome instrument for evaluating adolescent idiopathic scoliosis, and has been properly validated (Bridwell et al., 2005).

On the other hand, both questionnaires (SRS-24; SRS-22) do not extensively assess mental health and have only very few items related to life satisfaction and self-esteem (Zhang et al., 2011).

No controlled study, at least not in the short-, mid- or long-term period, was found in a systematic PubMed search by Weiss to reveal evidence to support the hypothesis that the effects of surgery as a treatment option for adolescent idiopathic scoliosis is superior to natural history (Weiss, 2008).

Therefore, the author - senior consultant of the well-known and highly esteemed Spinal Deformity Rehabilitation centre in Bad Sorbernheim, Germany - concluded that the indication for the surgical correction of adolescent idiopathic scoliosis is limited to cosmetic reasons in severe cases, but the author did not define and discuss the term "severe" in detail.

Now, the long-term results of two of the authors' studies investigating posterior instrumentation and spondylodesis in patients with adolescent idiopathic scoliosis are presented. One of the two studies was published recently (Mueller & Gluch, 2009). Furthermore, original papers (exclusively) presenting other long-term results will be compiled in a chronological manner and reviewed critically, without making claims of being complete.

2. Long-term outcome with the Harrington rod

2.1 Background of the Harrington rod

In 1962 - partially even in 1960 during a lecture at the Annual Meeting of the American Orthopaedic Association - Paul R. Harrington published a paper, in which he was the first to introduce a long rigid instrumentation for the dorsal correction of scoliosis (Harrington, 1962). Up to that date (since 1914), only spondylodesis methods without instrumentation were known, based on a scientific publication from 1924 comprising 59 patients (Hibbs, 1924).

Harrington developed a stainless steel posterior rod system, which used 2 rods and hooks in the frontal spinal plane to create distraction as well as compression in the area of the curvature. In his original landmark paper he described the development and the utilisation of this instrumentation, which started as early as in 1947 and which was completed only in 1960, due to different problems with the instrumentation that required multiple modifications. At that time, the instrumentation had only been used in a few patients (1949-1954: 19 patients; 1955-1960: 49 patients) with scoliosis secondary to poliomyelitis. After the completion of this development phase, 68 patients were treated with the final rod system in 1960. However, even at that time, there was only little experience with the treatment of patients suffering from adolescent idiopathic scoliosis (Harrington, 1962).

Over time, almost 1,500 scoliosis patients were treated with the Harrington rod between 1961 and 1972, but further modifications of the instrumentation had to be implemented between 1960 and 1972 (Harrington & Dickson, 1973). At that time, the initial long-term results after a follow-up period of at least 5 years showed an unexpected high rate of loss of correction, despite additional spondylodesis (Harrington & Dickson, 1973).

2.2 Literature review regarding the Harrington rod

Although the Harrington rod was worldwide the most frequently used for the surgical correction of adolescent idiopathic scoliosis for more than 2 decades (Haher et al., 1995), the overall long-term results are scanty and are often limited to specific questions. This might be due to the fact that many of these instrumentations were removed after only a few years, routinely or because of complications (Padua et al., 2001).

2011 A recently published retrospective Japanese study (Akazawa et al., 2011) conducted patient follow-up (questionnaire) on only 66 out of 256 patients (25.8%) with adolescent idiopathic scoliosis after a period of 21 to 47 years (mean 31.5 years) post surgery. Mean age at the time of surgery was 14.8 years (range 10 to 19 years). In 51/66 cases, a Harrington rod was used for correction, with a variety of anterior and posterior systems being used for the other patients. The average Cobb angle was 69.5° (preoperatively) and 37.5° (postoperatively), respectively, equivalent to a correction of 46%. No radiological follow-up was conducted at the time of data collection, and it was not documented whether the instrumentations were still *in situ* at that time, or if removal had been performed. Furthermore, this study does not contain any information regarding scoliosis curvature or any complication analyses. A significantly worse function and worse self-image (as determined using the SRS-22) was observed in patients when compared to an age-matched control group, but no differences were reported regarding pain and mental health scales. Furthermore, there were no significant differences in the Roland Morris Disability Questionnaire; the mean value was 1.8 points.

The authors from the University Hospital in Chiba, Japan, concluded that surgery had no demonstrable adverse effects on pain or mental health in their patients, although they did have a significantly lower function and lower self-image than healthy controls.

2005 After a minimum of 20 years (range 20 to 27 years) post surgery, Mariconda from the University Hospital Naples, Italy, retrospectively tried to evaluate the outcome of 62 patients treated with a single Harrington rod between 1976 and 1981 (Mariconda et al., 2005). All patients were fused by autologous bone grafts, and postoperatively they wore a plaster cast for a minimum of 6 months, followed by a plastic brace for an additional 6 months. For different reasons, only 16 out of 62 patients (26%) participated in the clinic and radiographic study: At follow-up, the Cobb angle of the main curve still showed an average correction rate of 41%, and the average SRS-24 score was 101 (78-110) out of a maximum of 120 points.

Compared to a non-scoliosis control group, the only significant difference was aesthetic discomfort, reported by 10 out of 16 patients and only 2 out of 24 controls. No further significant differences in the individual domain scores were observed. Therefore, the authors considered Harrington fusion as a procedure that produces a long lasting high degree of self-reported postoperative satisfaction.

2003 A further study from Helsinki, Finland, investigated 78 out of 98 patients (80%) with adolescent idiopathic scoliosis and Harrington rod instrumentation with a follow-up of 20.8

years postoperatively (Helenius et al., 2003). However, all the rods were removed routinely only 2 years after index surgery, if there was no pseudarthrosis. Preoperatively, there was an average thoracic Cobb angle of 53°; at the time of follow-up the average thoracic curve was 45° and the correction rate was only 15% at the time of follow-up. The frontal lumbar correction was only 14%. Frontal decompensation (> 20 mm) was found in 9 out of 78 patients (12%). There was an overall complication rate of 12% but acute or late deep infection was not documented in any patient. A reason for this might have been the complete removal of the implants, which naturally avoids the attachment of bacteria to the implant. The average SRS questionnaire score was 97 points, but 10 patients (13%) complained of back pain often or very often. Individual items of the SRS questionnaire such as patient satisfaction were not presented.

2002 In 2002, a German study group from Muenster (Goetze et al., 2002) published the quality of life of 82 out of 104 patients treated with Harrington rods between 1979 and 1989. The aim was, to analyse long-term health-related quality of life and low back pain with a minimum of 10 years follow-up. After an average of 16.7 years (range 11 to 22 years) post surgery, quality of life was measured with the Short Form-36 health profile (Ware & Sherbourne, 1992). Low back pain was assessed using the Roland-Morris Questionnaire (Fairbank et al., 1980), and the radiological parameters were analysed longitudinally.

The mean Cobb angle in right thoracic scoliosis was 63.1° (range, 40–110°) before surgery and 30.6° (range, 14–70°) after surgery. The average primary correction was 51.5%. In double major curves, the right thoracic curve was corrected from 61° to 36.9° (39.5% correction) and the lumbar curve from 55° to 33.5° (39.1%). In double thoracic curves the right thoracic curve was corrected from 61° to 30.3° (50.3%) and the left high thoracic curve was corrected from 38.5° to 29.5° (23.4%). At 5 years, the mean Cobb angles were not significantly different from those at one year post surgery.

In comparison with an age-matched healthy population, there was no significant difference in the physical Short Form-36 scale, but surgically treated patients showed significantly lower scores in the psychological Short Form-36 scale. Vitality, general mental health, and role activities because of emotional problems were significantly different from those of the age-matched population. 65 out of 82 patients (79%) reported no or occasional back pain in the Roland-Morris Questionnaire. 5 patients (6.1%) reported chronic back pain. Neither patient age at the time of surgery nor the time of the follow-up, type of scoliosis, or extent of fusion were associated with health-related quality of life or pain. The size of the pre- and postoperative curves and pre- and postoperative rib cage deformities did not correlate with the data of the Short Form-36 scale and the Roland-Morris Questionnaire.

Therefore, the authors concluded that, in comparison with the age-matched population, the long-term effect of surgery does not affect the physical quality of life. The psychological health status, however, has been significantly impaired. Neither the type of curve, nor the size of scoliosis or rib cage deformity influences the data.

It was a considerable weakness of this study that the complication and/or surgical revisions rates were not presented.

2001 Until 2001, no results on the outcome in terms of validated health-related quality of life were presented for patients treated for AIS. For the first time, Danielsson et al. from

Gothenburg, Sweden, published a consecutive series of patients treated between 1968 and 1977 by using Harrington rods, and an additional brace treatment group (Milwaukee or Boston brace) (Danielsson et al., 2001). 146 of the surgical treated patients were followed for a period of at least 20 years (mean 23.3 years) after the completion of the treatment before the patients reached 21 years of age. Moreover, an age- and sex-matched control group of 100 persons was randomly selected and underwent the same examinations.

The health-related quality of life results showed no differences in terms of sociodemographic data (e.g. marriage or childbearing) between the three groups. The surgical treatment and brace treatment groups had a slightly, but significantly reduced, physical function using the SF-36 (Ware & Sherbourne, 1992) subscales as well as the Oswestry Disability Back Pain Questionnaire (Fairbank et al., 1980) compared to the healthy controls (100 patients). No correlation was found between the outcome scores and curve size after treatment, curve type, total treatment time or age at completed treatment. In conclusion, patients treated for AIS were found to have approximately the same health-related quality of life as the general population.

It must be emphasised that the publication of Danielsson et al. has been an excellent - although retrospective - long-term investigation on AIS treatment, and there are no other crucial aspects to criticise.

2001 In the same year, Padua et al. from Rome, Italy, published a follow-up of only 70 out of a total of 184 patients (38%) with a Harrington rod (Padua et al., 2001). The average follow-up was 23.7 years. In 48 out of 70 patients (68.8%) the Harrington rod had already been removed for a wide range of reasons: 10 times (14%) because of late surgical site pain, 3 times because of implant fracture, 5 times because of the worsening of the curve and 30 times for causes that were not specified in detail. Radiologically, the average preoperative Cobb angle was 58.8°, and immediately postoperatively the average was 22.8°. At the follow-up, the average Cobb angle was 43.4°, which corresponds to a loss of 20.6° or 47.9% of the initial correction. The reasons for this remain unclear: no pseudarthrosis was seen in this study and patients without a Harrington rod did not show a significantly greater loss of correction than those with the instrumentation still *in situ*. The clinical outcome was recorded with the SF-36 (Ware & Sherbourne, 1992), and the overall outcome was similar to that of a normal population. However, on further questioning, only 46 patients (66%) were satisfied with the operation overall and only 17 patients (24%) rated it as excellent or good with regard to aesthetic aspects.

2000 One year before, Cook et al. from the University hospital in Kansas, Canada, investigated 64 patients over an average postoperative period of 142 months (range 24 to 192 months) with an isolated inquiry for the revision rate compared to 2 other instrumentations (Cook et al., 2000). 12 out of 64 patients (19%) with a Harrington rod had to be re-operated, on average 55 months (range 20 to 97 months) post surgery. The most frequent indication was pseudarthrosis (5 out of 12; 8%), followed by late surgical site pain (4 out of 64; 6%).

1995 In 1995, Connolly et al. from Ontario, Canada (Connolly et al, 1995) were able to follow-up on 83 patients with AIS by means of a questionnaire, with radiological imaging in only 55 of these patients (66%), on average 12 years after Harrington rod instrumentation. The questionnaire yielded an excellent or good result for 55 of 83 patients (66%), and 28 patients (34%) assessed the result as fair or poor. 14 patients

(17%) did not think that the goals of the initial operation had been accomplished. 76% of the patients also complained of lumbar back pain, and this result was thus markedly worse compared to the control group. A total of 18 patients (22%) also required surgical revision for various reasons.

1995 Humke (Humke et al., 1995) investigated 63 out of 72 patients (86%) with adolescent idiopathic scoliosis treated between 1968 and 1977 at the Schulthess Hospital at Zuerich, Switzerland. All operations were performed by the senior author of the study. Fusion included 10.5 segments on average, but the fusion technique was not explained in the publication. Re-examination included clinical and radiological assessments after a mean period of 12.3 years post surgery compared to Cotrel-Dubousset instrumentation. All patients underwent additional brace treatment lasting 8 months on average (range 6 to 11 months). Preoperatively, the average Cobb angle of the main curve was 67.8°, with postoperative correction to 33°. At the follow-up, there was a high loss of correction of 20.7% compared to the correction achieved postoperatively. 40% of the patients also had a clinical flat back, but this was not associated with clinical back pain. However, lateral radiological imaging was not conducted. Subjectively 86% of the patients were satisfied or very satisfied with the outcome of the operation but 10% of the patients complained of severe lumbar back pain.

1990 The authors (Dickson et al., 1990) from Houston, Texas, USA, sent a questionnaire to 206 consecutive patients who were operated on for idiopathic scoliosis by Paul R. Harrington between 1961 and 1963. 83% of the patients responded to the questionnaire, which consisted of five sections: demographic data, activities of daily living, back symptoms (pain and fatigue), a history of personal and family health, and a personal assessment of the back. 111 out of 206 patients also sent recent radiographs. A control group, comprising 100 individuals who did not have scoliosis, was given the same questionnaire.

The results showed, that patients in the study group had more pain in the interscapular and thoracolumbar region compared with the control group, but there was no difference with respect to pain in the lumbosacral area of the low back. Neither pain nor fatigue was related to the type of curve, the preoperative degree of curvature, the degree of curvature as seen in the most recent radiograph, the extent of fusion into the lumbar spine, or the presence of a broken rod. 21 years after surgery, the patients were functioning quite well compared with the control subjects.

1983 As early as in 1983, Cochran et al. (Gothenburg, Sweden) were the first to publish medium- to long-term results of 95 out of 100 patients (Cochran et al., 1983): 52 of these patients were treated with two rods between 1968 and 1973, and 48 patients were treated with only one rod between 1973 and 1975. Fusion was performed in patients of the first group only in a second procedure one week post surgery, and all patients received an additional Milwaukee Corset post surgery.

At least 5 years (average: 9 years) post surgery, radiological findings showed a correction rate of 50% for the main curvature, although there was a significant lateral flattening of the lumbar spine. The patients did not show physical impairment or an increase of back pain when compared to a control group of 85 healthy persons.

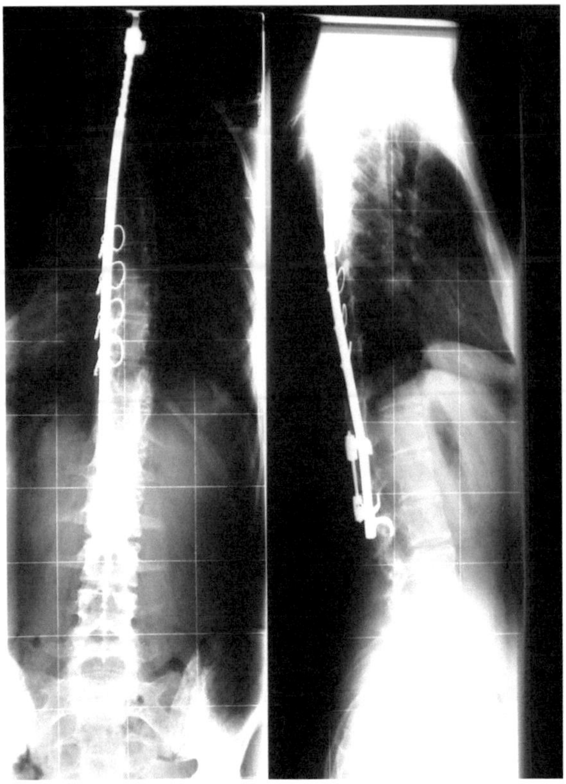

Fig. 1. X-ray of Harrington rod instrumentation with additional wires

A	B	C	D	E	F
2011	Akazawa	66	31	SRS-22: no adverse effects on pain or mental health	significant lower function and self image
2005	Mariconda	24	23	SRS-24: high degree of self-reported satisfaction	aesthetic discomfort
2003	Helenius	78	21	SRS: 97 points	
2002	Goetze	82	17	SF-36: surgery does not affect physical quality of life	psychological health status is significantly impaired
2001	Danielson	146	23	SF-36: approximately same quality of life as the general population	slightly reduced physical function
2001	Padua	70	24	overall outcome similar to the normal population	only 66% were satisfied with the surgery
1995	Connolly	83	12	66% with excellent or good results	34% assessed the result as fair or poor
1995	Humke	63	12	86% were satisfied with the outcome	10% patients complained of severe lumbar back pain
1990	Dickson	171	21	patients were functioning quite well	more pain in the interscapular and thoracolumbar region
1983	Cochran	95	9	no reduced activity, no back pain	significant reduction of lumbar lordosis

Table 1.

Overall summaries of the different studies on the Harrington rod

A: year of publication
B: author's name
C: number of patients
D: mean of follow-up in years
E: positive conclusions
F: negative conclusions

3. Long-term outcome of Cotrel-Dubousset (CD) instrumentation

3.1 Background to CD instrumentation

In 1984, Cotrel Y und Dubousset J - two orthopaedic surgeons - published a paper in the French language, in which they presented their new dorsal implant for scoliosis treatment for the first time (Cotrel & Dubousset, 1984). Theoretically, this instrumentation should provide a better coronal deformity correction than the Harrington rod. However, the axial correction or derotation potential is entirely attributable to the improvement in apical translation (Takahashi et al., 1997) and, therefore, has not been as effective as initially hoped. Moreover, the instrumentation requires greater surgical skill with extended surgical time and higher blood loss than a Harrington procedure. So far, very few long-term results have been published for the CD instrumentation although it has been available worldwide as a device now for over 25 years.

Some outcome studies were reviewed that did not meet our criteria for long-term outcome noted above but were considered, especially with regard to late deep infection and late surgical site pain, as we have seen in our own study patients with CD instrumentation.

3.2 Authors' study results on CD instrumentation

Between March 1990 and September 1992, a total of 40 consecutive patients with adolescent idiopathic scoliosis underwent surgical correction for adolescent idiopathic scoliosis with Cotrel-Dubouset instrumentation (Sofamor). This is a double rod system made of steel, which allows segmental fixation through laminar hooks and/or conical pedicle screws. During this period, no other posterior procedure was employed for the surgical treatment of adolescent idiopathic scoliosis. Before this period, we used Harrington rods and Luque instrumentation for this indication, while after the period, only instrumentation made of titanium alloy was used.

The indication for surgery was the progression of the scoliosis and/or a main curve of more than 45° in the frontal plane. The exclusion criteria were spinal abnormalities, e.g. wedge-shaped vertebrae, or previous surgical procedures such as Ascani rod or anterior correction spondylodesis. Anterior release to mobilise a rigid main curve was not an exclusion criterion.

Additional procedures or measures such as rib osteotomy or thoracoplasty were not performed in any of the 40 patients. For preparation and mobilisation for the operation, all of the patients carried out Cotrel self-extension over a period of 2 to 3 weeks and halo extension was not applied to any patient. Immediately preoperatively and if necessary intraoperatively, all the patients were given intravenous cephalosporin as prophylactic antibiotic.

The surgical procedure, after the exposure of the spine, involved the mobilisation of the scoliosis initially by the resection of the spinous processes, decortication of the laminae, facet joint cleaning and division of the ligamentum flavum on the concave side of the curvature. This was followed by the correction of the scoliosis by inserting the hooks and pedicle screws with loading of the two anatomically shaped vertical rods with rotation *in situ* with additional compression or distraction of segments as needed.

No spines were instrumented and fused to the sacrum. Two transverse connectors were placed cranially and caudally between the two vertical rods in all of the patients. A wake-up test was performed to check the intraoperative neurology after insertion of the vertical rod on the concave side; neurophysiological monitoring was not employed. For spondylodesis only homologous bone material reduced to chips was employed. All patients received autologous blood with or without cell saver, no patient received blood products that were not autologous. All patients were mobilised in principle from the 2nd or 3rd postoperative day without a corset.

For the study, the demographic data of all 40 patients were initially recorded from the medical files: age at the time of surgery and sex, operation time, blood loss and documented complications. All pre- and postoperative spinal radiographs in both planes (with the patients standing on cassettes that were 36 inches long) were then analysed with regard to the following parameters: curve patterns were classified by the method based on King-Moe (King et al., 1983) and Scoliosis research society terminology; measurement of the frontal main and secondary curves using the Cobb method (Cobb, 1948); number and height of the fused vertebra and number of hooks and pedicle screws employed.

Following the evaluation of the demographic and radiological data in 2005, it was attempted to invite the patients for a follow-up; however, it was only possible to contact a few patients, others refused clinical radiological follow-up for different reasons, and it was not possible to collect clinical data from more than 14/40 (35%) patients.

Results

The demographic data included 40 patients (28 women, 12 men), with an average age at the time of surgery of 16.0 years (range: 13 years to 21 years). Posterior fusion with the CD instrumentation was performed in all cases. Additionally, 3 out of 40 (7.5%) patients had anterior release preoperatively because of a severe main thoracic curve (average 81°). The average blood loss was 2770 ml, and average operation time was 325 min. Fusion with the CD instrumentation included 13.4 vertebrae (range 8 to 16) on average. The two rods were fixed by the hybrid technique, a combination of hooks and pedicle screws, with an average of 8 hooks and 4 screws per patient. A total of 325 hooks and 161 pedicle screws were inserted in 40 patients. The pedicle screws were inserted mainly in the lumbar region of the instrumentation.

According to the SRS terminology there were 23 right thoracic, 10 double major curves, 4 thoracolumbar, and 3 left thoracic curves. According to the King-Moe classification [12], 17 patients had type II curves; 7 patients type III, and 8 patients type IV curves.

There was no direct or indirect operative mortality. Furthermore, there was no permanent neurological complication. In one case, surgical correction was stopped incompletely because of massive bleeding, and then the correction was successfully concluded 14 days later.

According to the medical files, 21 out of 40 patients (52.5%) received one or more operative revisions, for a total of 23 surgical revisions:

Within the first 30 days post surgery, 3 out of 40 patients (7.5%) received early operative revision for the dislocation of hooks or rods.

At an average of 45.7 months (range 11 to 142 months), 19 out of 40 patients (47.5%; including 2 patients with early revision) received late operative revisions.

At this occasion, we documented the revision rate of the highest significance (9 out of 16 procedures; 56%), not in the first year of introduction (1990) but rather for 1992, the third and last year of application. Despite thorough data analysis, we could not find any explanations for this.

The reasons were late infection (10 out of 40 patients; 25%) with the development of fistulae (7 cases) or putrid secretion (3 cases), which was resolved with the complete removal of instrumentation after all. We documented 5 out of 7 fistulae at the distal end of the instrumentation. The average time until revision was 35.5 months (range 14 to 56 months) after CD instrumentation. There were no bacteriological findings of any pathogens after a maximum time of cultivation of 48 hours.

Furthermore, complete implant removal was necessary in 8 out of 40 patients (20%) for late operate site pain (LOSP). No infections or non-unions were detected intraoperatively, but there was a partial implant loosening in the caudal section of the implant in 6 cases, including corrosion in 2 out of 6 cases and broken cranial transverse connectors in 2 other cases. The average time until removal of instrumentation was 62.7 months (range 18 to 146 months) postoperatively.

Moreover, one more patient received partial device removal for prominent instrumentation 11 months postoperatively.

Altogether, only 22 out of 40 CD instrumentations (55%) were still in situ at the time of follow up.

Results for SRS-24

14 out of 40 patients (35%) completed the SRS-24 questionnaire after a mean of 11.3 years postoperatively. In the SRS-24 questionnaire, the total score averaged 93.3 points out of a maximum 120 points (min. 71 to max. 106 points) at the follow-up. The analysis of the questionnaire showed no significant differences between the 5 patients with instrumentation still in situ (average 96.4 points) and the 9 patients after the removal of the instrumentation (average 91.5 points).

Conclusions

In summary, and for the first time, we documented a very high surgical revision rate for CD instrumentation in the treatment of adolescent idiopathic scoliosis after long-term follow-up. The reasons for this high rate of revisions due to fistulae, infection, and late surgical site pain remain unclear.

3.3 Literature review to CD instrumentation

2007 In 2007, Boss et al. retrospectively investigated 54 consecutive patients who underwent CD instrumentation for right thoracic scoliosis at the University Hospital in Iowa, USA, between 1986 and 1991 (Boss et al., 2007). The CD was applied exclusively only with hooks by the senior author, and the patients had mobilisation without the use of a brace. The overall follow-up rate was 96% at an average of 79 months postoperatively, however the vast majority of patients could not be located or brought back for a 10 year follow-up, therefore only 38 out of 54 patients (70%) completed a self-administered - but not validated - questionnaire, and only 14 out of 54 patients (26%) had a follow-up of more than 10 years.

Radiologically, there were 18 King type 2, 19 Type 3, 5 type 4, 3 type 5 and 9 double major frontal curves. The average coronal Cobb angle of the primary thoracic curve was 55° preoperatively, 17° immediately postoperatively, and 22° at the latest follow-up. The lumbar curve (secondary or double major) averaged 40° preoperatively, 21° postoperatively and 23° at the latest follow-up. In 7 cases there was a loss of correction of the major curve of more than 10°, in which the authors concluded that this was due to various reasons. The results reflected that all the patients were doing well and had no complaints with regard to work or sporting activities. Moreover, there were no apparent non-unions, infections or neurological complications. Only one patient needed the partial removal of the instrumentation due to an irritated bursa over a prominent hardware.

In summary, the authors from the Iowa University Hospital, USA, concluded that CD provides encouraging clinical and radiographic results at an average follow-up of 7 to 9 years. Moreover, satisfaction, functional status and subjective cosmetic improvements were high.

2007 In the same year, a study group from Oslo, Norway, published their single centre results of CD instrumentation 10 years after surgery (Bjerkreim et al., 2007). The study included a total of the first 100 consecutive patients all with a single primary curve treated between 1989 and 1995. The average number of segments fused was 9.3. All the patients were mobilised without a brace. After 2 years of prospective follow-up, the correction rate of the primary curve was still 64% without a significant loss of correction and solid fusion, but within this period 5 out of 100 instrumentations (5%) were completely removed for suspected infection, without any evidence for bacteria. All wounds healed primarily after the removal of the instrumentation. Pseudarthrosis was not detected in any of the 100 patients.

Eventually, 10 years after surgery a total of 86 out of 100 patients (86%) answered a questionnaire mailed to the patients: 97% considered back function as excellent, good or fair, and 96% would have done the operation again. Scores for EuroQol (EuroQol; 1990) and Oswestry Disability Index (Fairbank et al., 1980) were within the normal range. However, 45% of the patients had consulted a physician or received physiotherapy for back pain during the last year before the follow-up.

2006 Weigert et al. conducted a study to assess the outcome after treatment for adolescent idiopathic scoliosis by means of the SRS-24 questionnaire (Weigert et al., 2006). 118 patients from a single centre, treated between 1987 and 1997, were included. 44 patients were treated with a Boston Brace only, 41 had surgery above all with CD instrumentation, and 33 were treated with a brace and surgery. At the follow-up, the re-operation rate was 21.6% (16 patients) for different reasons, especially due to abscess and fistula (5 patients). Patients with surgical complications had a significantly lower level of satisfaction, all other domain scores were unaffected by this factor and were similar to the scores of patients without complications.

The authors' overall conclusion of this study indicates that adolescent idiopathic scoliosis thrive after completed treatment, and the different treatment modalities do not clearly differ with respect to total SRS 24 outcome scores. Moreover, the Boston brace treatment does not permanently impair quality of life, whether applied alone or before surgery, and that combined treatment does not need to be regarded as a double burden with long-lasting negative effects on quality of life.

2003 In 2003, Helenius et al. investigated 57 out of 71 patients (80%) with AIS and CD instrumentation over a mean period of 13.0 years post surgery (Helenius et al., 2003). Preoperatively, the average frontal thoracic Cobb angle was 55°. At the time of the follow-up, the average thoracic curve was 32° so that the correction rate was 42%. The frontal lumbar curve showed an average correction of 32% at the time of the follow-up and frontal decompensation (> 20 mm) was found in 7% of the patients. The documented complications were one case of acute (1.7%) and 3 cases (5.3%) of late deep infection, but prophylactic antibiotics (single shot) were not given. Clinically the average SRS score was 97 points and 6 patients (11%) reported back pain often or very often.

2003 Bago et al. from Barcelona, Spain, presented a survivorship analysis of CD instrumenation treated in the surgical treatment of idiopathic scoliosis (Bago et al., 2003). Reoperation, usually the removal of instrumentation, had to be performed in 23 of 110 patients (21%) a mean of 56.7 months post surgery. The reason for the majority of reoperations was late infection (10 patients; 9%), followed by mechanical failure (6 patients), LOSP (4 patients) and acute infection (3 patients).

2000 Cook et al. investigated 49 patients a mean of 105 months post surgery with regard to the isolated question of the revision rate (Cook et al., 2000). 12 out of 49 patients (24%) had to be re-operated on 41 months (range 20 to 71 months) following index surgery. The indications were late surgical site pain (6 out of 49 patients, 12%), prominently or improperly placed implant (2 patients), pseudarthrosis (1 patient) and late deep infection (1 patient).

1999 In 1999, Clark and Shufflebarger from Miami, USA, retrospectively investigated 917 out of total 1,247 patients with CD instrumentation especially for late deep infection (Clark & Shufflebarger, 1999). A total of 22 patients were documented. The initial symptom was a fistula or a fluctuant swelling an average of 3.1 years post surgery (1.2 - 8.5 years). In specimens from these patients cultured only 72 hours, 1 out of 10 was positive. Of those cultured for 7-10 days (the last 12) 11 were positive, usually for low-virulence skin organisms. After surgery, patients received antibiotics parenterally for 48 hours and orally for 7 days. In all cases, complete instrumentation removal was done well. The authors concluded, that late-appearing infection can be treated with instrumentation removal, primary skin closure, and short-term oral antibiotics. Moreover, the infections affect soft tissue, and not the bone.

1998 In 1998, Lenke et al. evaluated the radiographic results of CD instrumentation in 76 patients who had been surgically treated in their department and who were followed for an average period of 6 years (Lenke et al., 1998). Comparison of radiographs showed that no patient had lost any correction in the frontal plane at the levels with instrumentation, and 75 out of 76 patients had no change in the thoracic or lumbar sagittal alignment at the levels with or without instrumentation. Only 1 patient received surgical revision for the loss of correction, and no further complication was reported. 63 out of 76 patients (85%) responded to a non-validated questionnaire assessing the clinical status. The authors from the University Hospital St. Louis, Missouri, USA, reported that the outcome was favourable with regard to function, cosmetic appearance, and general satisfaction with the surgical result. 24 out of 76 patients (38%) reported occasional pain in the spine, but 62 out of 63 patients (98%) would have the operation again.

1997 Takahashi et al. performed a study focusing on postoperative changes in the lumbar spine in 30 patients who had been treated with CD instrumentation (Takahashi et al., 1997). They reported that the prevalence of low back pain increased from 3% before surgery to 20% during the follow-up. However, in none of the patients was the pain so severe that specific treatment was required. From their data, the authors concluded that the overall clinical and radiographic results were satisfactory, but the unfused lumbar segments requires careful surveillance.

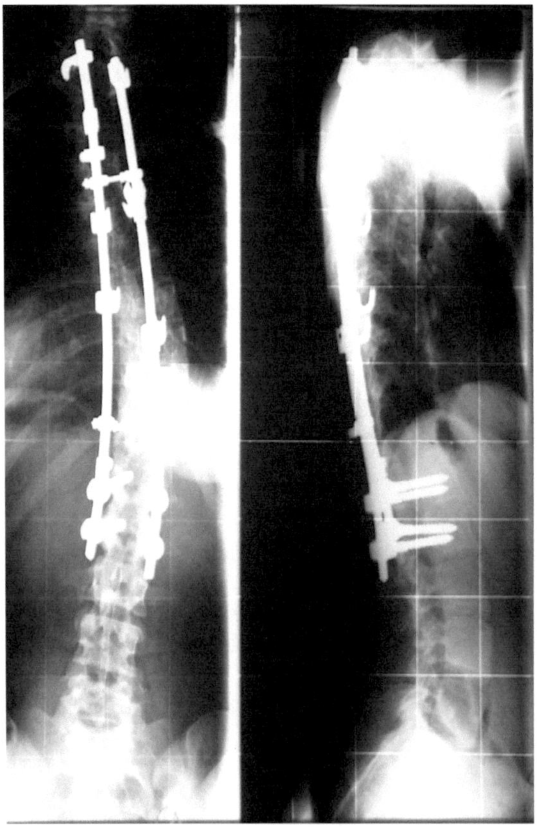

Fig. 2. X-rays of CD instrumentation with hooks and pedicle screws

A	B	C	D	E	F
2007	Boss	38	7	satisfaction, functional status and subjective cosmetic improvement was high	none
2007	Bjerkreim	86	10	scores for EuroQol were within the normal range	45% had back pain within the last year
2006	Weigert	41	>2	SRS-24: fair or better in all domains	re-operation rate was 21.6%
2003	Helenius	57	13	SRS: 97 points	11% reported back pain often or very often
2003	Bago	110	5	?	re-operation rate was 21%
2000	Cook	49	9	?	re-operation rate was 24%
1998	Lenke	76	6	outcome was favourable	38% reported occasional pain in the spine
1997	Takahashi	30	6	the overall clinical results were satisfactory	20% prevalence of low back pain

Table 2.

Overall summaries of the different studies on the CD instrumentation

A: year of publication
B: author's name
C: number of patients
D: mean of follow-up in years
E: positive conclusions
F: negative conclusions

4. Long-term outcome of other instrumentation technologies

4.1 Authors' study results

In the scoliosis centre of the Behandlungszentrum Vogtareuth, Germany, a double-rod system made of titanium alloy has been used since 1993 for the surgical correction of scoliosis, which also allows three-dimensional correction through segmental hooks and/or transpedicular screws (System WSI Titan, Peter Brehm Chirurgie Mechanik, 91084 Weisendorf, Germany). With regard to long-segment implants made of titanium in the treatment of AIS, to our knowledge there are so far no radiological and clinical long-term results of at least 10 years on average in the Pubmed literature.

The aim of our study was, therefore, to examine the efficacy and safety of this titanium instrumentation in AIS and to compare the results achieved with the two standard procedures referred to above. Our hypothesis was that titanium achieves the same or better long-term results in the surgical treatment of AIS compared to the data in the literature with regard to the Harrington rod or the CD instrumentation.

Between January 1993 and March 1996, a total of 50 patients with AIS had surgical correction with the titanium WSI (**W**irbel**s**äulen**i**mplantat; the German language for the spine implant).

This is a double rod system made of pure titanium (rods) with a diameter of 6 or 7mm, which allows segmental fixation through lamina hooks and/or conical pedicle screws (TiAl6V4) (Figure 1).

The indication for operation was the progression of scoliosis and/or a main curve of more than 45 degrees in the frontal plane. During the study period, no other posterior procedure was employed for the surgical treatment of AIS. The exclusion criteria were spinal abnormalities, e.g. wedge-shaped vertebra, or previous surgical procedures such as Ascani rod or anterior correction spondylodesis. Anterior release to mobilise a rigid main curve was not an exclusion criterion. Additional procedures or measures such as rib osteotomy or thoracoplasty were not performed in any of the 50 patients. For preparation and mobilisation for the operation, all of the patients carried out Cotrel self-extension over a period of 2 to 3 weeks, and halo extension was not applied to any patient. Immediately preoperatively - and if necessary intraoperatively - all patients were given intravenous cephalosporin as prophylactic antibiotic. Nearly all the surgical procedures were performed by the senior author (H.G.). The surgical procedure, after the exposure of the spine, involved the mobilisation of the scoliosis initially by the resection of the spinous processes, decortication of the laminae, facet joint cleaning and the division of the ligamentum flavum on the concave side of the curvature. This was followed by the correction of the scoliosis by inserting the hooks and pedicle screws with the loading of the two anatomically shaped vertical rods with rotation *in situ* with additional compression or distraction of segments as needed. No spines were instrumented and fused to the sacrum or the fifth lumbar vertebra. A transverse connector was placed cranially and caudally between the two vertical rods in all of the patients. A wake-up test was performed to check intraoperative neurology after the insertion of the vertical rod on the concave side; neurophysiological monitoring was not employed. For spondylodesis, only local bone material reduced to chips was employed. An iliac crest autograft or homologous bone was not used in any patient. All patients received autologous blood with or without cell saver, no patient received blood products that were not autologous. All patients were mobilised in principle from the 2nd or 3rd postoperative day without a corset.

For the study, the demographic data of all 50 patients were initially recorded from the medical files: age at the time of surgery and sex, operation time, blood loss and documented complications. All pre- and postoperative spinal radiographs in both planes (with the patients standing on cassettes that were 36 inches long) were then analysed with regard to the following parameters: curve patterns were classified by the method based on King-Moe (King et al., 1983) and the Scoliosis research society terminology; measurement of the frontal main and secondary curves using the Cobb method (Cobb, 1948) number and height of the fused vertebra and number of hooks and pedicle screws employed.

Frontal balance, determined on the basis of the horizontal distance, in millimetres, from the centre of the C7 vertebral body to the centre of the sacrum. Imbalance was defined as a horizontal distance of > 20 mm. Apical vertebral translation was defined as the distance, in millimetres, between the plumbline and the mid-portion of the vertebral body at the apex of the curve. The sagittal thoracic kyphosis angle was measured between T5 and T12 and the lordosis angle between L1 and S1, also using Cobb's method[6]. Attention was also paid to radiological complications, such as rod fracture, pedicle screw fracture, or hook dislocation. Because of the relatively low accuracy of the measurements, the radiological measurement of vertebral rotation or clinical measurement of ribcage projection was omitted. CT scans were not performed routinely, neither pre- nor postoperatively.

Following the evaluation of the demographic and radiological data between January 2005 and August 2005, the patients were invited by telephone to attend the follow-up, and the above-described radiological examinations were repeated and compared with previous films. The patients were also given a questionnaire from the Scoliosis Research Society with 24 questions (SRS 24),[20] translated into German, which measures the quality of life of scoliosis patients. The SRS 24 questionnaire is a disease-specific, reliable, and validated questionnaire used to assess outcomes in AIS. The questionnaire includes 24 questions, and the maximum possible score is 120 points, indicating that the patient is highly satisfied and asymptomatic. The questions represent seven major patient-based outcome domains; The responses are rated on a scale of 1 to 5, with 5 being the optimal response. The domains included: pain (7 items, max 35 points), general self-image (3 items, 15 points), function from back condition (3 items, 15 points), general level of activity (3 items, 15 points), postoperative self-image (3 items, 15 points), postoperative function (2 items, 10 points) and satisfaction (3 items, 15 points).

The demographic data included 50 patients (44 women, 6 men), with an average age at the time of surgery of 16 years and 6 months (range 12 years and 5 months to 21 years and 8 months). The mean follow-up was 121.7 months or 10.14 years (± 14.1 months, range 101 to 151 months). 49 of the 50 patients (98%) accepted the invitation to follow-up; only one patient was living abroad and could not be contacted for the questionnaire, but the demographic data and the pre- and postoperative radiological results and those at the time of the last follow-up were included. Posterior fusion with the titanium instrumentation was performed in all cases. Additionally, 9 of 50 patients had anterior release preoperatively because of a severe main thoracic curve (average 81°, range 71° to 111°). Average blood loss was 1980 ml (range 600 - 4500 ml), and average operation time was 270 min (range 140 to 410 min). Fusion with the WSI titanium included 10.0 (range 6 to 13) vertebrae on average. The average cephalic level of fusion was T 5.2 and the average caudal level of fusion was L 2.3. The two rods were fixed with a combination of hooks and pedicle screws only, with an average of 8.9 hooks and 4.2 screws per patient. A total of 424 hooks and 209 pedicle screws were inserted in 50 patients. The pedicle screws were inserted mainly in the lumbar region of the instrumentation. According to SRS terminology, there were 30 thoracic, 16 double, 2 thoracolumbar and 2 lumbar curves. According to the King classification, there were 2 patients with type I curves, 25 patients with type II curves, 9 patients with type III curves, 7 patients with type IV curves and 3 patients with type V curves. 4 patients could not be classified according to the King system.

SPSS Version 8 software for Windows was used for the statistical analysis, and the P values of ≤ 0.05 were considered significant. Descriptive statistics were used to determine means, standard deviations (SD), and ranges. Comparisons between variables were performed using a Student's t test and the Kruskal-Wallis test.

Results

In the frontal plane, the mean preoperative thoracic curve was 62.4 degrees (range 32° to 111°; ± 14.1°). Postoperatively, the thoracic curve was 26.9 degrees (range 8° to 58 °; ± 9.8°), equivalent to a correction rate of 56.9%. At the most recent follow-up evaluation, the Cobb angle of the thoracic curve was 31.0 degrees (range 8° to 58 °; ± 11.2°), equivalent to a final correction rate of 50.3%. The mean preoperative lumbar curve was 43.5 degrees (range 18° to 82°; ± 14.9°). Postoperatively, the lumbar curve was 16.3 degrees (range 2° to 36°; ± 9.9°), equivalent to a correction rate of 62.5%. At the most recent follow-up evaluation, the Cobb angle of the lumbar curve was 21.3 degrees (range 2° to 55 °; ± 13.3°), equivalent to a final correction rate of 51.0%. Average frontal balance as determined by mediolateral offset of the C7 vertebral body centre in relation to CSVL was 15.4 mm ± 12.4 preoperatively and 10.8 ± 9.7 mm at the most recent follow-up. 16 of 50 patients (32%) showed preoperative C7 offset of more than 20 mm. At the most recent follow-up, 5 of 50 patients (10%) showed frontal imbalance: 3 out of these 5 patients had preoperative imbalance and 2 patients showed preoperative regular frontal balance. Apical translation (apex of thoracic curve to CSVL) measured 51.7 mm ± 26.2 preoperatively, 18.7 mm ± 14.7 postoperatively, and 25.3 mm ± 11.9 at the final follow-up, equivalent to a final correction rate of 51.1%

In the sagittal plane, the average preoperative thoracic kyphosis angle (T5 to T12) curve was 19.8 degrees (range 2°- 63°, ± 14.5°). At the most recent follow-up, the thoracic kyphosis angle measured 25.8 ± 12.3 degrees. 4 patients had thoracic hyperkyphosis of more than 40 degrees preoperatively, and all of these patients still showed thoracic hyperkyphosis at the most recent follow-up.

3 out of 28 patients (10.7%) with normal preoperative thoracic kyphosis developed minor hyperkyphosis of more than 40 degrees at the most recent follow-up (35 to 51°; 25 to 46°; 26 to 45°). No one with preoperative flat back (18 patients with less than 10° thoracic kyphosis) showed hyperkyphosis at the most recent follow-up. Moreover, the average preoperative lumbar lordosis angle (L1 to S1) curve was 56.1 degrees (range 32°- 90°, ± 12.8°). At the most recent follow-up, the lumbar lordosis angle measured 57.9 ± 9.8 degrees. 7 of 50 patients showed preoperative lumbar hyperlordosis of more than 70 degrees; at the most recent follow-up, 2 out of these 7 patients showed normal lordosis (between 40 and 70 degrees) and 5 patients had still hyperlordosis. No one with normal preoperative lumbar lordosis showed hyperlordosis of more than 70 degrees at the most recent follow-up.

There was no direct or indirect surgical mortality, and there were no permanent neurological complications. According to the medical files, 7 re-operations had to be performed: one patient developed incomplete postoperative paraparesis of the lower limb, so the implant had to be removed and the correction was immediately reverted on the first postoperative day. After complete neurological recovery, posterior re-instrumentation was performed 3 weeks later; at the time of follow-up the implant is *in situ*. We also saw one acute deep infection 3 weeks postoperatively with the detection of Staphylococcus aureus. The infection was cured by means of surgical debridement with the placement of a temporary suction/irrigation drain and targeted antibiotic therapy; the implant did not have to be removed and was likewise still *in situ* at the time of follow-up. Because of a loosened pedicle screw in the distal fusion region, a revision of the pedicle screw was performed 3 weeks postoperatively, and the implant was likewise *in situ* at the time of follow-up. In one patient, there was a distal loss of correction below the instrumentation at the level of L1, retrospectively due to an excessively short distal fusion, which did not include the caudal final vertebra of the curve. In this case, the extension of the posterior instrumentation as far as L3 was performed 22 months postoperatively, after an additional anterior release. Here, too, the implant was still *in situ*. Complete implant removal was performed in one patient 43 months postoperatively because of persistent back pain in the region of the instrumentation (LOSP). Intraoperatively, there was slight corrosion and there was no evidence of infection or pseudarthrosis. Re-instrumentation had to be performed in 2 patients 73 and 102 months postoperatively, respectively, because of radiological evidence of pseudarthrosis with loosening of the implant and loss of correction. In these two patients, the implant is also still *in situ* at the time of the follow-up. The complete re-operation rate is 14% (7 out of 50 patients). It must be emphasised that we did not see any late deep infection in any patient, and only one implant had been completely removed at the time of follow-up. We also recorded the following complications, which did not require revision: 8 patients had an asymptomatic hook dislocation, in each case in the distal region of the instrumentation. In 2 further patients there was a dislocation of the vertical rod, and in 4 further patients the last radiological follow-up showed an asymptomatic fracture of the vertical rod without a significant distraction of the fracture site as possible evidence of pseudarthrosis. One case of haemothorax was documented, which required a chest drain for several days. There was no case of pedicle screw fatigue fracture or fracture of a transverse connector rod.

In the SRS-24 questionnaire, the total score averaged 95.8 points out of a maximum of 120 points (min. 60 to max. 110 points, SD± 8.8) at the final follow-up. In the questionnaire, 48 out of 49 patients (98%) were highly or fairly satisfied (scores of 4 or 5) with the result of the back treatment; only one patient was somewhat dissatisfied. 42 out of 49 patients (86%) reported never or rarely having back pain (score of 4 or 5) at rest. Only 3 out of 49 (6.1%) patients had back pain often or very often. Overall 44 out of 49 patients (90%) would definitely (36 patients with a score of 5 points) or probably (8 patients with a score of 4 points) undergo the same treatment again. Statistical analysis yielded the following results: 25 patients had a distal fusion segment from T12 to L2 inclusive, 24 patients had a distal fusion segment between L3 and L4 (L5 and sacrum were not fused). Both groups showed a nearly identical average SRS score (96.5 versus 95.0 points) with no significant difference (t-test 0.59). 20 patients had fusion of more than 11 vertebrae, 20 patients had fusion of 9 or 10 vertebrae, and 9 patients had fusion of less than 9 vertebrae. The three groups showed an average SRS score of 97.8 points versus 95.6 versus 91.6 points, respectively, with no significant difference. Within the individual classifications (SRS, King), no significant differences were found with regard to the subjective outcome. And there was no significant difference in the outcomes between the 6 male and 43 female patients in the study (average score 97.7 versus 95.5 points).

Conclusions

All together, this study presents the first long-term results with a titanium instrumentation for the treatment of AIS. 49 out of 50 patients (98%) were clinically followed-up on over a mean period of 10.14 years post surgery via questionnaire and radiological imaging. Re-operation for all reasons was 14%: it was 2% for LOSP and 4% for pseudarthrosis. No permanent neurological deficits and no late infections were observed. The instrumentation shows stability; the loss of correction at the frontal thoracic and lumbar curve is low, with a correction rate of 50.3% and 51.0% at the most recent follow-up. In the frontal plane, only 2 patients developed decompensation and 3 patients showed proximal junctional hyperkyphosis in the sagittal plane at follow-up. No screw fracture and no transverse connector fracture were detected. The survival rate of the implant is very high; 98% of the implants are still *in situ*. 98% of the patients were very or fairly satisfied with the result; 86% of the patients never or rarely have back pain at rest.

Year of publication	Authors	Instrumentation	No. of patients	Re-operation rate %
2009	Mueller	WSI	0/50	0
2008	Rihn	?	6/236	2.5
2005	Hahn	USS	5/67	7.5
2004	Remes	USS	4/55	7.2
2004	Remes	CD	3/57	5.3
2003	Bago	CD	10/113	8.8
2003	Helenius	CD	3/57	5.3
1999	Clark	CD	21/917	2.3
1995	Richards	TSHR	10/149	6.7

Table 3. Re-operation rates due to late infection in the literature.

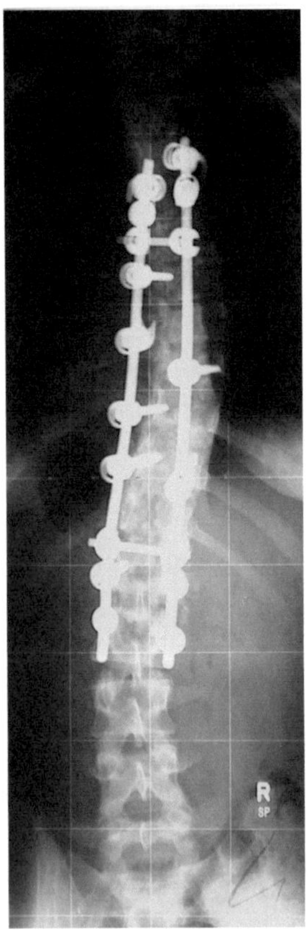

Fig. 3. X-ray of titanium instrumentation with hooks and pedicle screws.

4.2 Review of other posterior instrumentations

2011 In a prospective, multicentre cohort study with data from 6 scoliosis centres in the USA, the outcome of 745 surgical patients was evaluated 2 years after surgery (Carreon et al., 2011). There were 622 female and 123 male patients with a mean age of 14.2 years and a mean Cobb angle of 54°. The result showed a statistically significant difference between paired preoperative and 2 year postoperative SRS-22 domain scores, but there were low to moderate associations between the change in any of the domain scores and patients satisfaction with the treatment. Moreover, there was no statistically significant correlation between the 2-year postoperative SRS satisfaction score and the amount of curve correction.

The authors conclude that this may be because of the ceiling effect in the satisfaction domain, the lack of responsiveness of the SRS-22 to measure clinically relevant changes in activity, pain and mental health or a true lack of change in these domains.

(2007) In 2007, Benli et al. published their results on a posterior implant, the so-called Texas Scottish Rite Hospital System (TSHR), which is an instrumentation similar to the CD.

In their study (Benli et al, 2007), the surgical results of 109 idiopathic scoliosis patients, treated between 1991 and 1994 were evaluated. The mean follow-up period was 137 months, with a minimum of 10 years post surgery. The mean age of patients at the time of surgery was 14.4 years. Postoperatively, no cast or brace was utilised. The initial correction rate of the major curve was 64%, with a correction loss of 10.3° at the last follow-up. About 10 out of 109 patients (9.2%) were considered to have pseudarthrosis: 4 patients with instrumentation failure and 6 patients with a correction loss over 15° at the frontal plane. These 10 patients underwent re-operation. Overall, the average scores of the SRS-22 questionnaire for general self-image, function, mental status, pain, and satisfaction with the treatment were 3.8, 3.6, 4.0, 3.6, and 4.6, respectively, at the last follow-up. The pain scores were not correlated with the curve types, final Cobb angles, or the amount of correction loss.

The authors' therefore, concluded that the instrumentation is efficient for the correction of frontal and sagittal plane deformities and trunk balance resulting in a better quality of life.

2001 In 2001, Parsch et al. reported about the effect of multisegmental spinal fusion on the long-term functional and radiological outcome compared to patients whose spine had not been fused, and to a control group (Parsch et al., 2001). They studied 68 patients with AIS (34 with and 34 without surgery, respectively) who had been followed-up for a minimum of 5 years after treatment. An age and gender matched control group of 34 patients was also recruited. The study was based on a non-validated questionnaire introduced by Connolly in 1995, an individual assessment of chronic back pain using a numerical rating scale and an evaluation of radiographs.

The results of the spinal score showed no significant difference between fused and unfused patients. However, compared with the healthy control group, a significant lower score was demonstrated for both scoliosis groups. They concluded that multisegmental spinal fusion does not have an adverse effect on the long-term functional outcome, or on the frequency and severity of back pain in patients with AIS compared with unfused patients. However, patients with AIS have a worse long-term spinal function, and a greater frequency and severity of back pain when compared with healthy age-matched controls.

It is a critical aspect that only a small number of patients and data, respectively, were collected from as many as 8 hospitals. Furthermore, the authors failed to provide precise empirical data with regard to treatment measures, such as the type of instrumentations or the possible application of corset treatment in non-surgical patients. In addition, given a follow-up time of 5 years, the results cannot be considered long-term results.

5. Long-term outcome of anterior instrumentation

5.1 Background to anterior instrumentation

Open anterior spinal instrumentation with fusion for adolescent idiopathic scoliosis has its origins with Dwyer and Zielke (Dywer et al., 1969; Zielke et al., 1976), who developed anterior instrumentation for thoracolumbar and lumbar scoliosis. The approach offers the ability to fuse a small number of vertebral segments, thereby protecting more lumbar motion segments. Moreover, anterior correction can theoretically achieve a higher correction rate in the coronal plane. On the other side, if there is substantial growth in the adolescent spine, anterior fusion can lead to hyperkyphosis.

5.2 Review on anterior instrumentation

2010 Lately, Kelly et al. published a retrospective review on the long-term clinical and radiographic outcomes of open anterior spinal fusion with instrumentation for thoracolumbar and lumbar curves. During an 11-year period between 1984 and 1995, overall only 31 patients underwent anterior instrumentation and fusion with 3 different systems (Dwyer, TSRH, and Zielke) at one single centre (the University Hospital Memphis, USA) performed by the senior author only (Kelly et al., 2010).

18 out of 3 patients (58%) were still available for review with an average follow-up of nearly 19 years (range 12 to 22 years). The instrumented thoracolumbar curves were corrected from an average of 49° before to 19° after surgery and 25° at long-term follow-up. The uninstrumented thoracic curves were corrected from an average of 34° before surgery, to 25° at follow-up and 24° at a long-term follow-up. No progression occurred in the uninstrumented thoracic curve. Based on the SRS-30 questionnaire and the Oswestry Disability Index, most patients had good function scores and acceptable pain levels. The SRS-30 score was 98 out of a maximum of 115 points. The surgical satisfaction score was 9.3/10, and most patients stated that they were pleased with the result and would have the same procedure again. Instrumentation failure was identified in 2 patients, but without the detection of pseudarthrosis. Changes of early degenerative disc disease on plain radiographs and MRI were identified in most patients but had no correlation with SRS and Oswestry data.

Therefore, the authors concluded that anterior surgery offers good long-term functional outcomes.

1997 More than 10 years earlier, Otani et al. from Tokyo, Japan, represented the long-term follow-up results after open anterior instrumentation for the first time (Otani et al., 1997). The study represented a retrospective follow-up of an average period of 14.6 years. 134 patients with idiopathic scoliosis were treated between 1973 and 1993, and 53 out of 134 patients (39%) were followed for a minimum of 10 years. Dwyer instrumentation was used in 17 and Zielke in 36 cases, respectively. The curve was thoracic in 16, thoracolumbar in 27 and lumbar in 10. The average preoperative Cobb angle was 64°. The average angle at follow-up was 21° with 62% of the average correction maintained (61%/Dwyer and 65%/Zielke).

The authors reflected that most patients were satisfied subjectively and, therefore, they recommend this type of operation.

6. Conclusions

Summarising, the following statements regarding long-term results in the surgical treatment of adolescent idiopathic scoliosis can be made:

Operative correction and stabilisation of scoliosis using instrumentation started with the development, utilisation, and worldwide propagation of a rod and hook system and, 50 years ago, Harrington PR was the first to publish a scientific paper on this in 1962.

The development of the Harrington rod was based on the analyses of scoliosis in poliomyelitis patients, rather than on adolescent idiopathic scoliosis.

Frontal corrections using the Harrington rod required the application of an additional corset, which had to be worn for 6 to 12 months after surgery, for external immobilisation in order to avoid loss of correction.

Most of the scientific publications regarding the long-term results on the surgical treatment of adolescent idiopathic scoliosis investigated this instrumentation.

All of these studies are characterised by low levels of evidence (evidence level 3 and 4), small numbers of patients, and a high loss to follow-up.

In the medium and long term, many Harrington rods were removed with only insufficient data and without providing precise reasons for this.

Radiological findings have shown a mostly significant loss of correction and a flattening of the spinal profile.

Quality of life does not directly correlate with radiological parameters such as correction rate or length of fusion.

However, there is a long-term tendency of patients suffering from increased back pain.

In addition, there is a tendency suggesting that shorter spondylodeses and instrumentations, respectively, result in clinically improved outcome.

A few so-called cohort studies mainly showed a clinically high quality of life after Harrington rod correction when compared to healthy populations.

25 years ago, Cotrel and Dubousset were the first to publish research on a segment-stabilising rod system, which was designed to eliminate the disadvantages of the Harrington rod; in particular, it did not require corset treatment over several months, due to its high primary stability.

Proprietary long-term results after correction using CD instrumentations also show a high complication rate, particularly fistulae and infections.

The few retrospective long-term studies (evidence level 3 and 4) showed a significant higher correction rate and a lower loss of correction over time in favour of the CD system when compared to the Harrington rod.

Until now, no significant differences between the Harrington rod and the CD system have been observed with regard to the clinical long-term outcome.

Based on rapid advancements that have been achieved in implant design during the last 10 to 20 years, the Harrington rod - which was the implant of choice - has been gradually abandoned and has been considered obsolete in the meantime.

Long-term results for newer instrumentations in larger patient populations are currently missing. The question of whether improved clinical results can be achieved despite a lower number of fused segments, remains currently unanswered.

After an average follow-up of 10 years, our own study using a new generation titanium instrumentation showed at least clinically and radiologically equivalent results for the first 50 consecutive patients when compared to both of the instrumentations mentioned above.

And all instrumentations were still *in situ* at the time of the follow-up.

The term "long-term follow-up" has not been defined until now. Since patients - based on their young age - require a long follow-up period even at the beginning of the treatment, we suggest follow-up periods of at least 10 or even 20 years after the completion of the treatment, particularly when considering the data of our own studies.

However, one must not expect final results in adolescent idiopathic scoliosis, due to lifelong clinical and radiological changes of the scoliotic vertebral column - with or without instrumentations.

It remains a hypothetical question, if and when patients after surgical correction are equivalent to so-called healthy populations.

Results from randomised prospective studies are still missing.

We will see in the future, whether currently available, clinically evaluated tools such as the SRS Questionaire, SF-36, or other health-related questionnaires are sufficient to assess the quality of life in scoliosis patients, or if these questionnaires will be modified or replaced within the next few years.

Last but not least, a randomised prospective multicentre study with three levels (natural course versus corset treatment only versus surgical procedure) is ethically justified and urgently required face to currently available data.

7. References

Aaro, S. & Dahlborn, M. (1982). The effect of Harrington instrumentation on the longitudinal axis rotation of the apical vertebra and on the spinal and rib-cage deformity in idiopathic scoliosis studied by computer tomography. Spine, Vol. 7, No. 5, (September/October 1982), pp. 456-462, ISSN 0362-2436

Ameri , E. ; Behtash, H. ; Mobini, B. ; Omidi-Kashani, F. & Momeni, B. (2008). Radiographic outcome of surgical treatment of adolescent idiopathic scoliosis in males versus females. *Scoliosis,* Vol. 3, No. 12, (September 6, 2008), ISSN 1748-7161

Asher; M.; Min Lai, S. ; Burton, D. & Manna, B. (2003) Discrimination validitiy of the Scoliosis Research Society-22 patient questionnaire : relationship to idiopathic scoliosis curve pattern and curve size. *Spine,* Vol. 28, No. 1, (January 1, 2003), pp. 74-77, ISSN 0362-2436

Asher, M.; Lai, SM. ; Burton, D. ; Manna, B. & Cooper, A. (2004). Safety and efficacy of Isola instrumentation and arthrodesis for adolescent idiopathic scoliosis. Two- to 12-year follow up. *Spine,* Vol. 29, No. 18, (September 15, 2004), pp. 2013-2023, ISSN 0362-2436

Bago, J.; Ramirez, M.; Pellise, F. & Villanueva, C. (2003). Survivorship analysis of Cotrel-Dubousset instrumentation in idiopathic scoliosis. *European Spine Journal,* Vol. 12, No. 4, (June 21, 2003), pp. 435-439, ISSN 0940-6719

Benli, IT.; Ates, B.; Akalin, S.; Citak, M.; Kaya, A. & Alanay, A. (2007). Minimum 10 years follow up surgical results of adolescent idiopathic scoliosis patients treated with TSRH instrumentation. *European Spine Journal,* Vol. 16, No. 3, (March 2007), pp. 381-391, ISSN 0940-6719

Bjerkreim, I. ; Steen, H. & Brox, JI. (2007). Idiopathic scoliosis treated with Cotrel-Dubousset instrumentation. Evaluation 10 years after surgery. *Spine,* Vol. 32, No. 19, (September 1, 2007), pp. 2103-2110, ISSN 0362-2436

Boss, N. ; Dolan, LA. & Weinstein, SL. (2007). Long term clinical and radiographic results of Cotrel-Dubousset instrumentation of right thoracic adolescent scoliosis. *Iowa Orthopedic Journal,* Vol. 27, pp. 40-46

Bridwell, KH.; Shufflebarger, HL. ; Lenke, LG.; Lowe, TG. ; Betz, RR. & Bassett, GS. (2000) Parents' and patients' preference and concerns in idiopathic adolescent scoliosis : a cross-sectional preoperative analysis. *Spine,* Vol. 25, No. 18, (September 15, 2000), pp. 2392-2399, ISSN 0362-2436

Bridwell, KH.; Cats-Baril, W.; Harrast, J.; Berven, S.; Glassman, S.; Farcy, JP.; Horton, WC.; Lenke, LG.; Baldus, C. & Radake, T. (2005) The validity of the SRS-22 instrument in an adult spinal deformity population compared with the Oswestry and SF-12: a study of response distribution, concurrent validity, internal consistency and reliability. *Spine,* Vol. 30, No. 4, (February 15, 2005), pp. 455-461, ISSN 0362-2436

Carreon, LY.; Sanders, JO.; Diab, M.; Sturm, PF.; Sucato, DJ.; the Spinal Deformity Study Group. (2011). Patient satisfaction after surgical correction of adolescent idopathic scoliosis. *Spine,* Vol. 36, No. 12, (May 20, 2011), pp. 965-968, ISSN 0362-2436

Clark, CE. & Shufflebarger, HL. (1999). Late-developing infection in instrumented idiopathic scoliosis. *Spine,* Vol. 24, No. 18, (September 15, 1999), pp. 1909-1912, ISSN 0362-2436

Cobb, JR. (1948). Outline for the study of scoliosis. In: Instructional Course Lectures, The American Academy of Orthopaedic Surgeons. Vol. 5, pp. 261-275. Ann Arbor, J. W. Edward, 1948

Cochran, T.; Irstam, L. & Nachemson, A. (1983). Long term anatomic and functional changes in patients with adolescent idiopathic scoliosis treated by Harrington rod fusion. *Spine,* Vol. 8, No. 6, (September 1983), pp. 576-584, ISSN 0362-2436

Connolly, PJ.; Von Schroeder, HP.; Johnson, GE. & Kostuik, JP. (1995). Adolescent idiopathic scoliosis. Long-term effect of instrumentation extending to the lumbar spine. *The Journal of Bone and Joint Surgery American,* Vol. 77, No. 8, (August 1995), pp. 1210-1216, ISSN 1535-1386

Cook, S.; Asher, M.; Lai, SM. & Shobe J. (2000). Reoperation after primary posterior instrumentation and fusion for idiopathic scoliosis. *Spine*, Vol. 25, No. 4, (February 2000), pp. 463-468, ISSN 0362-2436

Cotrel, Y. & Dubousset, J. (1984). Nouvelle technique d`ostheosynthèse rachidienne sègmentaire par voie postèrieure. *Rev Chir Orthop Reparatrice Appar Mot,* Vol. 70, No. 6, pp. 489-495

Cundy, PJ.; Paterson, DC.; Hillier, TM.; Sutherland, AD.; Stephen, JP. & Foster, BK. (1990). Cotrel-Dubousset instrumentation and vertebral rotation in adolescent idiopathic scoliosis. *The Journal of Bone and Joint Surgery British,* Vol. 72, No. 4, (July 1990), pp. 670-674, ISSN 0301-620X

Danielsson, AJ.; Wiklund, I.; Pehrsson, K. & Nachemson, AL. (2001). Health-related quality of life in patients with adolescent idiopathic scoliosis: a matched follow-up at least 20 years after treatment with brace or surgery. *European Spine Journal,* Vol. 10, No. 4, (August 2001), pp. 278-288, ISSN 0940-6719

Dickson, JH. & Harrington, PR. (1973). An eleven-year clinical investigation of Harrington instrumentation. A preliminary report of 578 cases. *Clinical Orthopaedics and Related Research,* Vol. 93, No. 6, (June 1973), pp. 113-130, ISSN 0009-921X

Dickson, JH.; Erwin, WD. & Rossi, D. (1990). Harrington instrumentation and arthrodesis for idiopathic scoliosis. A twenty-one-year follow up. *The Journal of Bone and Joint Surgery American,* Vol. 72, No. 5, (June 1, 1990), pp. 678-683, ISSN 1535-1386

Dwyer, AF.; Newton, NC. & Sherwood, AA. (1969). An anterior approach to scoliosis. A preliminary report. *Clinical Orthopaedics and Related Research,* Vol. 62, No. 1; (January/February, 1969), pp. 192-202, ISSN 0009-921X

EuroQol Group. (1990). EuroQol: a new facility for the measurement of health related quality of life. *Health Policy,* Vol. 16, No. 3, (December 1990), pp. 199-208, ISSN 0168-8510

Fairbank, JC.; Couper, J.; Davis, JB. & O`Brien, JP. (1980). The Oswestry low back pain disablitiy questionnaire. *Physiotherapy,* Vol. 66, No. 8, (August, 1980), pp. 271-273, ISSN 0031-9406

Goetze, C.; Liljenqvist, UR.; Slomka, A.; Goetze, HG. & Steinbeck, J. (2002). Quality of life and back pain: Outcome 16.7 years after Harrington instrumentation. *Spine,* Vol. 27, No. 13, (July 1, 2002), pp. 1456-1463, ISSN 0362-2436

Haher, TR.; Merola, A.; Zipnick, RI.; Gorup, J.; Mannor, D. & Orchowski, J. (1995). Meta-analysis of surgical outcome in adolescent idiopathic scoliosis. A 35-year English literature review of 11,000 patients. *Spine,* Vol. 20, No. 14, (July 1995), pp. 1575-1584, ISSN 0362-2436

Haher, TR.; Gorup, JM.; Shin, TM.; Homel, P.; Merola, AA.; Grogan, DP.; Pugh, L.; Lowe, TG. & Murray; M. (1999). Results of the Scoliosis Research Society instrument for evaluation of surgical outcome in adolescent idiopathic scoliosis: a multicenter study of 244 patients. *Spine,* Vol. 24, No. 14, (July 15, 1999), pp. 1435-1440, ISSN 0362-2436

Hahn, F.; Zbinden, R. & Min, K. (2005). Late implant infections caused by Propionibacterium acnes in scoliosis surgery. *European Spine Journal,* Vol. 14, No. 8, (October 2005), pp. 783-788, ISSN 0940-6719

Halm, H.; Niemeyer, T.; Link, T. & Liljenqvist, U. (2000). Segmental pedicle screw instrumentation in idiopathic thoracolumbar and lumbar scoliosis. *European Spine Journal,* Vol. 9, No. 3, (June, 2000), pp.191-197, ISSN 0940-6719

Harrington, PR. (1962). Treatment of scoliosis. Correction and internal fixation by spine instrumentation. *Journal of Bone Joint Surgery Am,* Vol. 44, No. 6, (June 1962), pp. 591-610, ISSN 1535-1368

Helenius, I.; Remes,V.; Yrjönen, T.; Ylikoski, M.; Schlenzka, D.; Helenius, M. & Poussa, M. (2003) Harrington and Cotrel-Dubousset instrumentation in adolescent idiopathic scoliosis. Long-term functional and radiographic outcomes. *The Journal of Bone Joint Surgery American,* Vol. 85, No. 12, (December 2003), pp. 2303-2309, ISSN 1535-1368

Hibbs, RA. (1924). A report of fifty-nine cases of scoliosis treated by the fusion operation. *The Journal of Bone Joint Surgery American,* Vol. 6, No. 1, (January 1, 1924) pp. 3-34, ISSN 1535-1368

Humke, T.; Grob, D.; Scheier, H. & Siegrist, H. (1995). Cotrel-Dubousset and Harrington Instrumentation in idiopathic scoliosis: a comparison of long-term results. *European Spine Journal,* Vol. 4, No. 5, (October 1995), pp. 280-283, ISSN 0940-6719

Kahanovitz, N. & Weiser, S. (1989). The psychological impact of idiopathic scoliosis on the adolescent female. A preliminary multi-center study. *Spine,* Vol. 14, No. 5, (May 1989), pp. 483-485, ISSN 0362-2436

Kelly, DM.; McCarthy, RE.; McCullough, FL. & Kelly, HR. (2010). Long-term outcomes of anterior spinal fusion with instrumentation for thoracolumbar and lumbar curves in adolescent scoliosis. *Spine,* Vol. 35, No. 2, (January 15, 2010), pp. 194-198, ISSN 0362-2436

King, HA.; Moe, JH.; Bradford, DS. & Winter, RB. (1983). The selection of fusion levels in thoracic idiopathic scoliosis. *The Journal of Bone and Joint Surgery American,* Vol. 65, No. 9, (December 1983), pp. 1302-1313, ISSN 1535-1368

Lea Plaza, CA.; Karsaclian, M. & Rocca, C. (2004). Segmental scoliosis correlation: use of the Lea Plaza frame. *Spine,* Vol. 29, No. 4, (February 15, 2004), pp. 398-404, ISSN 0362-2436

Lenke, LG. ; Bridwell, KH. ; Blanke, K. ; Baldus, C. & Weston, J. (1998). Radiographic results of arthrodesis with Cotrel-Dubousset instrumentation for the treatment of adolescent idiopathic scoliosis. A five to ten-year follow-up study. *The Journal of Bone and Joint Surgery American,* Vol. 80, No. 6, (June 1998), pp. 807-814, ISSN 1535-1368

Liljenqvist, UR.; Bullmann, V.; Schulte, TL.; Hackenberg, L. & Halm, HF. (2006). Anterior dual rod instrumentation in idiopathic thoracic scoliosis. *European Spine Journal,* Vol. 15, No. 7; (July 2006), pp. 1118-1127, ISSN 0940-6719

Lonner, BS.; Kondrachov, D.; Siddiqi, F.; Hayes, V. & Scharf, C. (2006). Thoracoscopic spinal fusion compared with posterior spinal fusion for the treatment of thoracic adolescent idiopathic scoliosis. *The Journal of Bone Joint Surgery American,* Vol. 88, No. 5, (May 2006), pp. 1022-1034, ISSN 1535-1368

Luque, ER. (1982). Segmental spinal instrumentation for correction of scoliosis. *Clinical Orthopaedics and Related Research,* Vol. 163, No. 3, (March 1982), pp. 192-198, ISSN 0009-921X

Mariconda, M.; Galasso, O.; Barca, P. & Milano, C. (2005). Minimum 20-year follow-up results of Harrington rod fusion for idiopathic scoliosis. *European Spine Journal,* Vol. 14, No. 9, (November 2005), pp. 854-861, ISSN 0940-6719

Merola, AA.; Haher, TR.; Brkaric, M.; Panagopoulos, G.; Mathur, S.; Kohani, O.; Lowe, TG.; Lenke, LG.; Wenger, DR.; Newton, PO.; Clements, DH III. & Betz, RR. (2002). A multicenter study of adolescent idiopathic scoliosis using the Scoliosis Research Society (SRS) outcome instrument. *Spine,* Vol. 27, No. 18, (September 15, 2002), pp. 2046-2051, ISSN 0362-2436

Mueller, FJ. & Gluch, H. (2009) Adolescent idiopathic scoliosis (AIS) treated with arthrodesis and posterior instrumentation: 8 to 12 years follow up without late infection. *Scoliosis,* Vol. 4, No. 16, ISSN 1748-7161

Otani, K.; Saito, M. & Sibasaki K. (1997). Anterior instrumentation in idiopathic scoliosis: a minimum follow-up of 10 years. *International Orthopaedics,* Vol. 21, No. 1, (January 1997), pp. 4-8, ISSN 0341-2695

Padua, R.; Padua, S.; Aulisa, L.; Ceccarelli, E.; Padua, L.; Romanini, E.; Zanoli, G. & Campi, A. (2001). Patient outcomes after Harrington instrumentation for idiopathic scoliosis: a 15- to 28- year evaluation. *Spine,* Vol. 26, No. 11, (June 1, 2001), pp. 1268-1273, ISSN 0362-2436

Parsch, D.; Gaertner, V.; Brocai, DR. & Carstens, C. (2001). The effect of spinal fusion on the long-term outcome of idiopathic scoliosis. A case-control study. *The Journal of Bone and Joint Surgery British,* Vol. 83, No. 8, (November 2001), pp. 1133-1136, ISSN 0301-6207

Payne, WK III.; Ogilvie, JW.; Resnick, MD.; Kane, RL.; Transfeldt, EE. & Blum, RW. (1997) Does scoliosis have a psychological impact and does gender make a difference? *Spine,* Vol. 22, No. 12, (June 1997), pp. 1380-1384, ISSN 0362-2436

Reddi, V.; Clarke, DV. & Arlet, V. (2008). Anterior thoracoscopic instrumentation in adolescent idiopathic scoliosis: a systematic review. *Spine,* Vol. 33, No. 18, (August 15, 2008), pp. 1986-1994, ISSN 0362-2436

Remes, V.; Helenius, I.; Schlenzka, D.; Yrjönen, T.; Ylikoski, M. & Poussa, M. (2004). Cotrel-Dubousset (CD) or Universal Spine System (USS) instrumentation in adolescent idiopathic scoliosis (AIS): comparison of midterm clinical, functional, and radiologic outcomes. *Spine,* Vol. 29, No. 18, (September 15, 2004), pp. 2024-2030, ISSN 0362-2436

Richards, BS. (1995). Delayed infections following posterior spinal instrumentation for the treatment of idiopathic scoliosis. *The Journal of Bone of Joint Surgery American,* Vol. 77, No. 4, (April 1995), pp. 524-529, ISSN 1535-1368

Rihn, JA.; Lee, JY. & Ward, WT. (2008). Infection after the surgical treatment of adolescent idiopathic scoliosis. *Spine,* Vol. 33, No. 3, (February 1, 2008), pp. 289-294, ISSN 0362-2436

Takahashi, S.; Delecrin, J. & Passuti, N. (1997) Changes in the unfused lumbar spine in patients with idiopathic scoliosis. A 5- to 9-year assessment after cotrel-dubousset instrumentation. *Spine,* Vol. 22, No. 5, (March 1, 1997), pp. 517-523, ISSN 0362-2436

Ware, JE Jr. & Sherbourne, CD. (1992) The MOS 36-item short-form health survey (SF-36). I. Conceptual framework and item selection. *Medical Care,* Vol. 30, No. 6, (June 1992), pp. 473-483, ISSN 0025-7079

Weatherley, CR.; Draycott, V.; O' Brien, JF.; Benson, DR.; Gapalakishnan, KG.; Evans, JH. & O`Brien, JP. (1987). The rib deformity in adolescent idiopathic scoliosis : A prospective study to evaluate changes after Harrington distraction and posterior fusion. *The Journal of Bone and Joint Surgery British,* Vol. 69, No. 2, (March 1987), pp. 179-182, ISSN 0940-6719

Weigert, KP.; Nygaard, LM.; Christensen, FB.; Hansen, ES. & Bünger, C. (2006) Outcome in adolescent idiopathic scoliosis after brace treatment and surgery assessed by means of the Scoliosis Research Society instrument 24. *European Spine Journal,* Vol. 15, No. 7, (July 15, 2006), pp. 1108-1117, ISSN

Weiss, HR. (2008). Adolescent idiopathic scoliosis (AIS) – an indication for surgery ? A systematic review of the literature. *Disability and Rehabilitation,* Vol. 30, No. 10, (January 2008) pp. 799-807, ISSN 0963-8288

Wimmer, C. & Gluch, H. (1998). Aseptic loosening after CD instrumentation in the treatment of scoliosis: A report about eight cases. *Journal of Spinal Disorders & Techniques,* Vol. 11, No. 5, (October 1998), pp. 440-443, ISSN 1536-0652

Zhang, J.; He, D.; Gao, J.; Yu, X.; Sun, H.; Chen, Z. & Li, M. (2011). Changes in life satisfaction and self-esteem in patients with adolescent idiopathic scoliosis with and without surgical intervention. *Spine,* Vol. 36 ; No. 9, (April 20, 2011), pp. 741-745, ISSN 0362-2436

Zielke, K.; Stunkat, R. & Beajean F. (1976). Ventrale derotations-spondylodesis. *Archiv für Orthopädische und Unfall-Chirurgie,* Vol. 85, No. 3, (August 1976), pp. 257-277 (Article in the German language)

15

Complications in Scoliosis Surgery

Femenias Rosselló Juan Miguel and Llabrés Comamala Marcelino
Department of Orthopaedic Surgery and Traumatology
Hospital Son Espases
Palma de Mallorca,
Spain

1. Introduction

The surgical treatment of all types of scoliosis pursues correction of the deformity, get a solid spinal fusion and balance the trunk in the sagittal and coronal plane. For this it is necessary to perform technically demanding surgery, long lasting, with great exposure of the surgical field, high blood loss and ultimately extremely aggressive. No doubt we can say that scoliosis surgery is one of the more complex interventions that are performed in orthopedic surgery. This makes complications of these surgeries not uncommon and potentially very serious.

Constant improvement of fixation systems, evolution of anesthesiology techniques as well as the Intensive Care Services have helped to reduce and better manage the complications that may arise from these surgeries, but it is also true that for these same causes more complex patients go after surgery.

The purpose of this chapter will be to conduct a review of the literature published complications from the surgery of scoliosis develop and deepen their study.

2. General

Scoliosis is defined as a three-dimensional deformity of the spine as torsion about its longitudinal axis. Lateral tilt occurs in the frontal plane resulting in a curve. The deformity must be accompanied by vertebral rotation. Vertebral body rotates toward the convexity, while the spinous processes rotate toward the concavity. When the curve in the frontal plane is not accompanied by rotation we speak of scoliotic attitude, which is never a permanent deformity.

The transmission of loads in scoliosis is not uniform. The asymmetry of the pressures on the vertebrae because of its tilt and rotation determines a wedge with its vertex in the concavity and its base in the convexity.

When ossification of the wedge vertebrae is completed and ligament and disc deformity is fixed, we talk of a structured curve, which is stiff and difficult to modify by gravity action or traction maneuvers.

In order to systematize the etiology, course and prognosis of scoliotic deformities, the Scoliosis Research Society has developed a universally accepted classification.

2.1 Idiopathic scoliosis

Constitute over 80% of all scoliosis and its cause is unknown. It is more common in girls by a ratio of 7:1. Depending on the age in which it is diagnosed is divided into three types:

- Infantile idiopathic scoliosis: from birth to 3 years old.
- Juvenile idiopathic scoliosis: between 4 and 9 years.
- Adolescent idiopathic scoliosis: from 10 years and skeletal maturity.

2.2 Congenital scoliosis

Vertebral deformities caused by birth. They can be caused by defects of formation (hemivertebra) or segmentation defects.

2.3 Neuromuscular scoliosis

Are due to primary neurological alterations or muscle disorders that cause loss of control of the trunk because of weakness or paralysis.

- Neuropathic. Due to upper motor neuron affectation (cerebral palsy is the most common) or lower motor neuron affectation (polio, spinal muscular atrophy, etc).
- myopathic. Secondary to muscular dystrophy (the most common is Duchenne muscular dystrophy), arthrogryposis, congenital hypotonia, and so on.

2.4 Other

Secondary to connective tissue diseases, neurofibromatosis, traumatic or intra or extradural spinal tumours, etc...

Although in all cases of scoliosis surgery can occur both intra-and postoperative complications, there are multiple factors that increase the risk of such complications.

Neurological and connective tissue diseases scoliosis are often associated with congenital heart disease and with severe restrictions on the patient's respiratory vital capacity. This fact, coupled with the high blood loss that occurs during surgery can lead to severe hemodynamic failure.

Adult scoliosis is defined as the occurrence of scoliosis deformity after the patient has reached skeletal maturity. Surgical treatment of scoliosis in the adult has a much higher rate of complications when compared to the correction of the same type of deformity in the adolescent. Some factors that contribute to this higher rate of complications are:

- Important bleeding because of the difficult subperiosteal detachment of the muscles of the rear column.
- Higher structural stiffness of the curves.
- Less rigid anchoring of the instrumentation due to osteoporosis of the bone.
- Increased difficulty to accomplish fusion in the elderly patients.

- Appearance of medical complications during and after the intervention due to the greater duration of the same , the increased risk of infection and the risk of deep vein thrombosis and pulmonary sequelae.
- Patient's nutritional depletion following major spinal reconstruction that makes necessary optimize the patient's nutritional status.

Although all types of complications can occur in scoliosis of any etiology, in healthy subjects with idiopathic scoliosis, the incidence of complications can't be as high as in patients with neuromuscular diseases. In a systematic review of the literature in PubMed on the rate of complications in scoliosis surgery (Rudolf Weiss & Goodall, 2008) the rate of complications for the different causes was specified (Table I). This study found that those fusions extended to the pelvis in idiopathic scoliosis showed higher complication rate (73%).

	Studies	Average rate	Range
Neuromuscular Scoliosis	22	35% SD(21)	0-89%
Adult Scoliosis	11	44% SD(24)	10-78%
Idiopathic Scoliosis	11	20% SD (22)	0-73%
Early Onset Scoliosis	1	48%	
Congenital Scoliosis	4	14% SD (23)	0-48%
Congenital Heart Disease	1	27%	

Table 1. Hans Rudolf Weiss & Deborah Goodall. Scoliosis 2008. Complications rate for the different causes of scoliosis.

Therefore, it is imperative to have a thorough knowledge of the preoperative characteristics of each patient to know the possible complications that may arise during or after surgery.

3. Preoperative assessment of patients with scoliosis

Complications in the surgical treatment of scoliosis can occur in all patients, but are especially important in patients with neuromuscular diseases. Because of this a comprehensive assessment of all patients that will be operated on for scoliosis must be made preoperatively, but especially in neurological patients because in these cases the deformity of the spine may be associated with, in some cases, respiratory function and heart alterations. These changes, along with the pathology of the disease itself, cause of the deformity (for example deformities secondary to neuromuscular disease) are risk factors that modify the anesthetic-surgical prognosis of patients with scoliosis.

Respiratory disturbances, cardiovascular abnormalities and multiple changes experienced by patients with scoliosis secondary to neurological diseases are a very important risk factor in patients about to undergo surgery for scoliosis.

It is essential to have a thorough understanding of the characteristics of each patient regarding the etiology of the scoliosis to know the possible complications that may arise, with particular attention to nutritional status, assessment of respiratory and cardiovascular function and neurological status preoperatively.

3.1 Nutritional status

It is necessary to make an assessment of patient's nutritional status prior to surgery. In neurological patients is very common that nutritional status is poor and therefore they are at increased risk of infections and wound dehiscence. It is very important to optimize the nutritional status of the patient before surgery, although in these cases is very difficult. It may be necessary to place a feeding jejunostomy tube when it is insufficient by mouth. In the postoperative period it may be useful the administration of parenteral-nutrition.

3.2 Respiratory function

It is known that respiratory restriction in idiopathic scoliosis is low, except in high-grade scoliosis.

It is important to note that respiratory function is mainly affected in thoracic scoliosis. There is a direct relationship between impaired lung function test and the magnitude of the thoracic curve. It has been observed that significant changes in lung function are found when the deformity curves have a Cobb angle greater than 70-80°. In these cases, diaphragm function is impaired, so respiratory function depends on a greater degree of accessory muscles.

In major thoracic scoliosis, the deformity alters the position of the ribs decreasing the anteroposterior diameter of the chest producing a defect of coupling between the respiratory muscles and rib cage which results in a decreased mobility of the chest and a loss of respiratory mechanics ability to adapt to rapid respiratory changes (Colomina & Godet 2005).

This alteration in respiratory mechanics results in a restrictive pattern. This involves a small lung volume, increased work of breathing, high energy costs, hypoxemia, respiratory acidosis by hypoventilation, inadequate ventilatory response to hypoxic stimulus, pulmonary hypertension, limitation of the development of lung parenchyma and anomalous relationship between lung function and respiratory muscle mechanics (Molina et al., 2003).

The prognosis of scoliosis secondary to neuromuscular disease is worse than idiopathic scoliosis, and in fewer years it will evolve into respiratory failure. Curves over 30 degrees can have a severe respiratory impairment as it happens in muscular dystrophies.

The causes that influence respiratory disturbances in patients with neuromuscular diseases have been studied (Colomina & Godet 2005).

- A disturbance in the central control of breathing
- Myopathies and nerve damage in these patients have the effect of an alteration of muscle function. The loss of respiratory muscle strength has a direct effect on respiratory function.

The deterioration of respiratory function is progressive and depends on the loss of respiratory muscle strength, which may affect both the inspiration and the expiration. It is shown that in Duchenne muscular dystrophy vital capacity decreases by 8% per year (Galaska et al., 1992).

Abnormalities of respiratory function may also be aggravated by joining the alteration of the defense mechanisms of the airway, with loss of laryngeal and pharyngeal reflexes, which along with muscle weakness will condition an ineffective cough and lung facility, and anomalous relationship between lung function and respiratory muscle mechanics.

The relationship between the magnitude of the thoracic curve and a lower respiratory vital capacity is amply demonstrated in idiopathic scoliosis, but in neuromuscular scoliosis this relationship is not as clear, as we have seen, there are a multitude of factors that influence in the impairment of respiratory function.

It has been shown that scoliosis surgery produces immediate and transient decrease in vital capacity (CV) of up to 40% in almost all patients undergoing surgery (Koumbourlis, 2006). The reasons for this decline are many, including the duration of the operation, the patient positioning and surgical trauma to various muscle groups (especially when it has practiced a thoracotomy). Given that the CV is usually much lower than normal before surgery, any further reduction can easily lead to respiratory failure. This risk is significantly higher in patients with neuromuscular scoliosis for reasons already explained.

As a result of this, during the preanesthetic visit a thorough assessment of respiratory function by physical examination, detailed previous history, and specific additional examination (respiratory function tests, arterial blood gases) must be conducted. In many neurological patients can be very difficult to perform pulmonary function tests, so it is very important the opinion and experience of the patient's usual pulmonologist.

3.3 Cardiovascular function

As the alteration of respiratory function, cardiovascular abnormalities occur primarily in thoracic scoliosis. In large deformities of the thoracic spine there is an alteration of the position and function of the mediastinal structures affecting the pericardium and great vessels and may mimic constrictive pericarditis, pulmonary hypertension and right ventricular failure (Colomina & Godet 2005).

Congenital scoliosis is often associated with primary heart disease or cardiac conduction disorders. This is due to the embryonic disorder that causes the appearance of this type of scoliosis. In Marfan syndrome is frequent valvular disease, especially mitral valve. Friederich's ataxia is often associated with hypertrophic cardiomyopathy and arrhythmias. They may also have dilated cardiomyopathy because of myocardial degeneration in the muscular dystrophies. Other malformations that are frequently associated with congenital scoliosis are tetralogy of Fallot, transposition of great arteries, ductus, etc..

To rule out the existence of these cardiac abnormalities is necessary to conduct a systematic cardiological examination with ECG and echocardiography, especially in the preoperative exam in patients with congenital scoliosis.

3.4 Neurological status

Congenital scoliosis has an incidence of up to 40% of intraspinal abnormalities. Some of these abnormalities are lipomas, benign fatty tumors of the spinal canal, scar tissue within the spinal canal, osteocartilaginous bone spicules that can cause an diastematomyelia, and so on.

A thorough clinical examination of neurological status of the patient and cranial and complete spine MRI are essential in the preoperative evaluation of patients with congenital and neuromuscular scoliosis.

4. Classification of the complications of scoliosis surgery

The appearance of complications in scoliosis surgery itself or derived from it is not uncommon for many reasons already discussed. It is very difficult to systematize and collect all the complications of scoliosis surgery described in the literature. Some authors classify them according to severity. Others depending on the time of appearance (intraoperative, immediately after surgery or belated). We will follow the scheme proposed by Hawes in 2005, modified.

- Vascular and visceral injuries.
- Hemodynamic complications.
- Neurological complications.
- Gastrointestinal complications.
- Infections.
- Failure of instrumentation and nonunion.
- Decompensation and increased deformity.
- Pathology of adjacent level.
- Other complications.

4.1 Vascular and visceral

Scoliosis surgery often requires anterior approach of the column involving laborious dissection of visceral and vascular structures in contact with the spine.

Although vascular and visceral injuries occur more frequently in the anterior approach they can also occur in other situations. In the posterior approach of the thoracic spine, pleural damage may occur. If so, it is advisable placing a pleural drainage tube. It's also been described in the literature gluteal artery injury caused by removing large amounts of graft from the iliac crest.

The placement of pedicle screws can also cause vascular and visceral injuries. This technique is not free from risks due to the close anatomical relationship between the spine and the aorta and other major retroperitoneal structures. The risk of misplacement of pedicle screws is increased in scoliosis surgery, especially of high magnitude, compared to other surgeries of the spine due to anatomical changes caused by vertebral rotation. Vascular injuries may occur during insertion of pedicle screws or deferred usually presented as pseudoaneurysms. All such injuries occur as a result of injury of the anterior or lateral cortical of the pedicle. Exceptionally injuries can also occur during surgery pedicle screw removal. Our team has published a case of gonadal and renal vein injury and duodenal ulcers during the attempt of removal of a malpositioned pedicle screw in an adult scoliosis. There was a violent migration of the screw toward the anterior part of the vertebral body, coming to stay in the abdominal cavity. It was necessary to turn the patient in the supine position, a laparotomy to locate the screw at the root of the mesentery and then extraction of the screw and reparation of vascular and duodenum lesions were performed (Femenias et al., 2009).

4.2 Hemodynamic complications

As already mentioned in the introduction of this chapter, scoliosis surgery is surgery of long duration, with great exposure and high blood loss. If this high blood loss is not properly answered it can lead to hemodynamic failure. To minimize blood loss is very important a meticulous surgical technique with respect to hemostasis and frequent hemostatic plugs during skeletonization, but there are circumstances that may aggravate the bleeding.

Patients with neurofibromatosis present hyper vascularization around neurofibromas, patients with coagulopathy or cardiac malformations also have a high risk of bleeding.

All the situations already described along with the need to curettage large bone areas or the need of vertebral osteotomies can produce excessive bleeding leading to severe hemodynamic failure and even death of the patient.

The decrease in respiratory vital capacity occurs especially in severe scoliosis and neuromuscular scoliosis with the appearance of atelectasis due mainly to severe pain after surgery, the chest tightness and weakening of the defense mechanisms of the air way, with loss of laryngeal and pharyngeal reflexes and muscle weakness together cause hypoxemia. This situation of hypoxemia along with the excessive bleeding that can result from factors already discussed certainly leads to hemodynamic instability.

Another situation that can lead to hemodynamic failure is intraoperative hypothermia as it can trigger an arrhythmia and myocardial depression. It is important to prevent hypothermia, the patient must be adequately covered in the unexposed areas, warming the skin and administering all fluids with temperature.

The advancement of endoscopic techniques has its impact on the evolution of surgical treatment and the lower incidence of hemodynamic complications. The advent of thoracoscopy has greatly decreased the need for thoracotomy to ease the thoracic spine. With this technique, surgical aggression is much lower, reducing analgesic requirements, bleeding and respiratory affectation.

In these patients during the surgical procedure, the controlled hypotension and self transfusion techniques are very important for greater hemodynamic stability, blood loss savings and reduction of the number of blood units for transfusion.

4.3 Neurological complications

Neurological injuries are perhaps the most feared injuries in scoliosis surgery, with devastating results for the patient and his family.

To monitor and try to combat the onset of these complications is very important neurological intraoperative monitoring through the awaking test and electrophysiological monitoring with evoked potentials. Neurophysiological monitoring in spine surgery should be considered mandatory not only for surgical reasons but also due to the adjuvant techniques used such as controlled arterial hypotension.

Probably the most traditional method used to monitor neurological function test is Stagnara awakening. This test is performed after completion of the reduction maneuvers for scoliosis, and the goal is to reduce the level and depth of anesthesia to achieve a state of waking of the patient enough to move his limbs. Once the test is finished, a level of deep anesthesia is obtained to allow completion of the intervention (Vauzelle et al., 1973). However it is known that this test has many limitations among which the failure to prevent possible early injury, is not sensitive enough to small fluctuations of medullary function and that evaluates only the anterior spinal cord.

Lonstein group in a 1980 study placed the incidence of neurological injury from 3.7 to 6.9%. With the advent of intraoperative neurophysiological monitoring techniques spine surgeons have reduced the incidence figures to 0.5% and now is possible to detect alterations in the function of the spinal cord at an early stage so the surgeon can correct the situation before irreversible damage occurs. Neurophysiological monitoring of somatosensory PES and motor PEM evoked potentials is done by analyzing the latency and amplitude of the response to the stimulus caused. The PES analyzes the integrity of the posterior way from the peripheral nerves to the cerebral cortex. The PEM is the result of stimulating the cortex or the medulla and collecting the response in the peripheral nerves or muscles directly innervated by these nerves. Keep in mind that these potentials may be affected by hypothermia and hypoxia.

The causes that can produce these neurological complications may be due to reduced vascular blood flow, metabolic or mechanical direct contusion or stretching. Depending on the cause, the injuries can range from mild root injury to paraplegia and quadriplegia (Hawes, 2005). In rare cases it may also present as a cauda equina syndrome when working distally to L3. It also may occur infrequently dural tears when performing the way for the insertion of sublaminar hooks (Fig. 1).

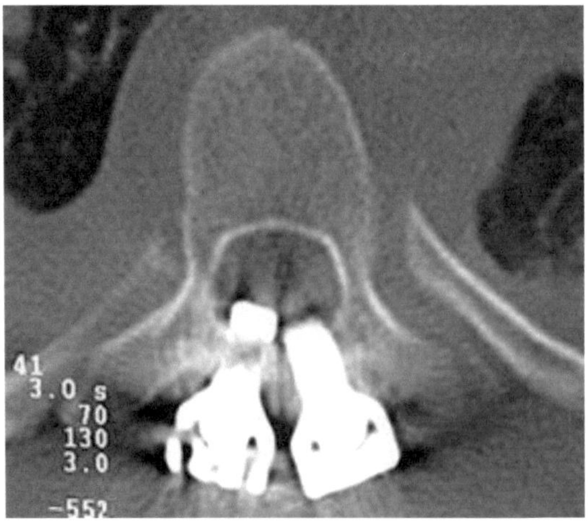

Fig. 1. CT Scan showing the intimate connection between sublaminar hooks and the spinal cord.

The critical point to cause spinal cord injury during surgery is when derotation and distraction maneuvers of the spine are performed to correct scoliosis. There is risk of generating excessive traction and cause spinal cord damage due to tension changes in the vessels supplying the spinal cord which can alter blood flow and produce a spinal cord dysfunction. Direct contusion is also a very important cause of neurologic injury. There are published cases of bone graft migration into the spinal canal, penetration of instrumentation into the spinal canal, compressive phenomena because of hematomas and nerve compression by the components of the implants.

The type of instrumentation used also has a direct relationship to neurological damage. During the Harrington instrumentation era, incidence was lower than the highly invasive instrumentation such as Luque and variants. With increasing use of pedicle screws root injuries have increased. The pedicle screw may violate the medial pedicle wall and invade the spinal canal or break the lateral wall (Fig. 2). It is important intraoperative radiographic control to ensure correct placement of pedicle screws as well as stimulating each screw to rule changes in the neurophysiological recording. If there's a suspicion that a screw may cause nerve irritation it should be removed or relocated.

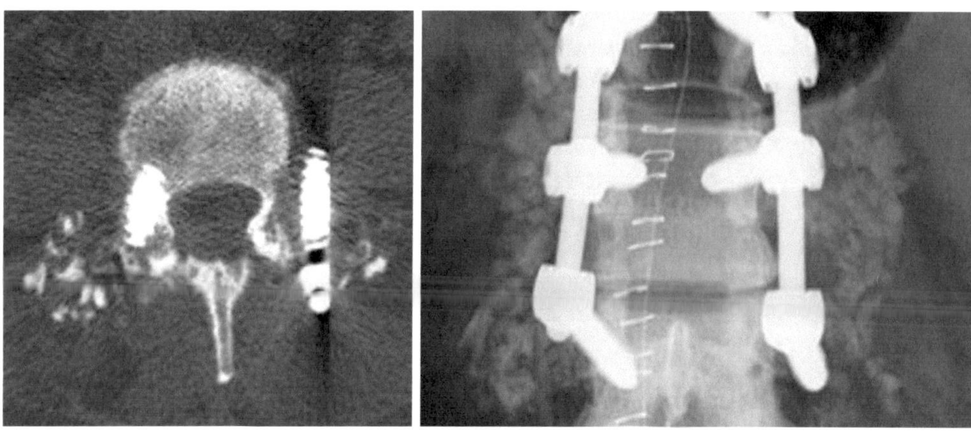

Fig. 2. Radiographic and CT image showing the extrapedicular position of the screw.

When a neurological disorder at the time of awakening test or a change in the amplitude or latency of the SSEP is noted, the correction should be decreased until the patient move his limbs normally and / or recovers potentials.

It can happen that a patient in the postoperative period does not present any neurological problems but afterwards develops paralysis within a few hours. In this case is very important to check blood pressure. If there is a problem of hypotension is important to correct it because as blood pressure increases improves the paralysis. If not, patient must be taken to the operating room immediately to cut the bars or revoke the instrumentation.

4.4 Gastrointestinal complications

Digestive complications are not uncommon in scoliosis surgery. It can be found in the literature paralytic ileus, stress ulcers, pancreatitis and superior mesenteric artery syndrome.

Postoperative ileus is frequently present in the instrumentation of the spine and scoliosis surgery in particular. When distraction mechanisms to reduce scoliosis are performed, peritoneum suffers a mechanism of traction and along with the use of opioids produces an intestinal paralysis.

Stress ulcers, like all major surgery can occur after surgery for scoliosis. It is important the administration of gastric protectors to prevent this complication.

Pancreatitis appears as a postoperative complication of scoliosis surgery in children and young adults. Etiology is unknown but is related to the patient's position, anemia, anesthetic agents, metabolic factors and autonomic nervous system abnormalities that could affect pancreatic secretion. It should be suspected with the appearance of vomiting and abdominal pain. If there's suspicion, blood test should be requested to evaluate amylase and lipase levels in serum. The evolution is usually favorable with prolonged postoperative fasting and parenteral nutritional support if required.

The syndrome of the superior mesenteric artery (SAMS) is produced by a closure of the exit angle of the superior mesenteric artery from the aorta that causes extrinsic compression of the third portion of duodenum. This is attributed to excessive stretching of the spine or extrinsic compression with corrective casts. The symptoms are rather nonspecific. These patients may present in postoperative nausea, permanent bilious vomiting, pain and bloating. To confirm the diagnosis, abdominal radiography showing gastric and first portions of the duodenum dilatation should be taken. Also intestinal transit study with the presence of obstruction of the contrast at the second or third portion of the duodenum where it intersects with the spine is defining. Medical treatment with fluid therapy, parenteral nutrition and nasogastric tube is usually the solution. In extreme cases, given the failure of medical treatment, a duodenojejunostomy should be practiced. Almost all cases reported in the literature are related to the implementation of Harrington device. Currently, its occurrence is exceptional.

4.5 Infectious complications

Infection rates in scoliosis surgery range between 2 and 6% (Hilibrand et al., 2003). There are multiple risk factors that influence in the occurrence of postoperative infections. The prolonged duration of surgery, severe blood loss, morbid obesity, scoliosis requiring multiple procedures or stages, malnutrition, etc.

In a report from the Scoliosis Research Society Morbidity and Mortality Committee (Smith et al., 2011) the reported rate of postoperative spine infection in scoliosis surgery is analyzed including subdiagnosis, patient age, spinal level, primary versus revision surgery, and surgical approaches to determine the corresponding rates of infection and to assess for potential factors associated with the occurrence of infection.

It is very important, in cases with high risk of infection, to optimize the patient's ability to heal following surgery for scoliosis, especially with adequate nutritional replacement.

We recommend a lymphocyte count greater than 1500 cells/mm3 and an albumin level greater than 3.4 g / dL to make the risk of infection due to immunodeficiency in these patients not too high.

The general recommendation for antibiotc prophylaxis is to administrate first generation cephalosporin 20 to 30 minutes before surgery and then 3 doses postoperatively. If one keeps the antibiotic longer it may appear resistance to the antibiotic.

The recommendation for using first-generation cephalosporins is because it provides broad coverage against Staphylococcus aureus and Staphylococcus epidermidis which are the organisms that are isolated more frequently in infections in scoliosis surgery. Cefazolin is a first generation cephalosporin and is recommended as first choice because it reaches peak serum level and does so during the first 20 minutes after administration and has a long half-life compared to other first-generation cephalosporins.

Infections in surgery of scoliosis can occur immediately after surgery or late. Early infections occur during the first 7-10 days of postoperative period and present with fever, wound erythema, pain and drainage. If you perform a blood test is usually seen a rise in Erythrocyte Sedimentation Rate (ESR) and C-reactive protein (CRP).

In case of occurrence of an early infection cures of the wound are recommended daily, making crops for specific antibiotic treatment and, if not resolved, it requires a wide surgical debridement with copious irrigation of the wound, removal of slough and closing the surgical wound leaving drainage. In these cases, the instrumentation should not be removed. Then, once you have the antibiogram result, specific intravenous antibiotics should be instituted according to it.

In late infections after a symptom-free period, patients begin with localized inflammation of the wound, pus out and the presence of sinus tracts. In these cases the surgical strategy consists of debridement and cleaning as in early infection and it may be necessary to remove the implants if loosening is proved.

It may sometimes happen that a debridement is not enough and is needed repeated debridement of the wound until the resolution of the infection.

If that is associated with extensive skin necrosis or severe wound dehiscence which makes impossible to close, it may be necessary surgical mobilization of the muscle and skin for closure or, in more advanced cases, plastic surgery techniques consisting of flaps or expanders.

4.6 Instrumentation bugs and nonunions

To correct and stabilize scoliosis correction accomplished, spinal instrumentation is essential. A fault in the instrumentation inevitably entails the development of pain and loss of correction obtained.

Implant failures may occur due to poor location of the same or by having to resist excessive tension to hold the achieved correction of scoliosis

We have seen how the pedicle screws placed outside the pedicle can cause neurological symptoms or vascular compression, but besides that these screws have less gripping force and compromise the stability of the reduction. Pedicle hooks can also migrate if not properly hooked on the pedicle. Laminar hooks under excessive kyphosis pressure can dislodge because a fracture of the lamina and, like it happens with screws, compromise mounting stability especially if the bars are placed with excessive tension. In all these cases, if stability is compromised or if the bar produces a protrusion on the skin that bothers the patient, the implant must be repositioned.

In the long term, instrumentation failure can occur as we have seen because the emergence of infections. Another cause of failure of the instrumentation is the debris of particles of the implants. This particle release stimulates autoimmune responses that result in deterioration of bone quality and in loosening of the implants. These inflammatory responses to metallic instrumentation can occur independently or associated with infection (Fig. 3).

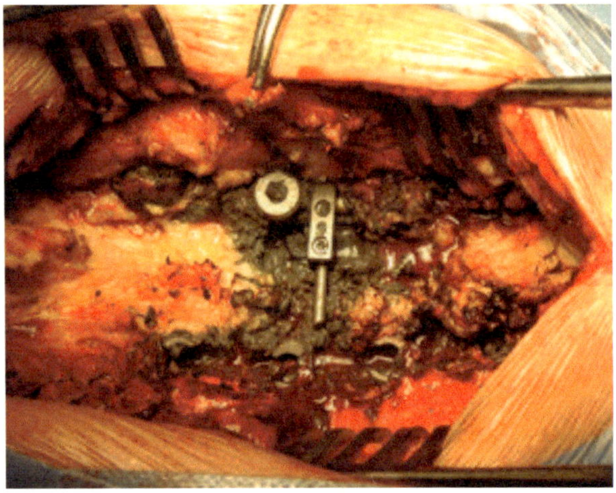

Fig. 3. Image of metallosis due to particle debris.

Although it may seem paradoxical, fewer mobilizations and material failure were seen in the past. This is because fewer implants were used as anchor points in the column and most stringent postoperative containment methods were adopted, such as casting and prolonged rest. Today, thanks to the improved quality of implants and to changes in evolution in the quality of life of society these uncomfortable patient immobilization systems will not be faced and the trend is towards to an early rehabilitation and a quick return to the normal daily activity. In general terms, and to try to prevent these failures of the material, we recommend limiting the sport until 6 months after surgery and, if mentioned sport requires contact or lifting this limitation can be extended to the year.

The late failure of the instrumentation is often associated with nonunion. The nonunion indicates a failure in the aim of the intervention since no solid spinal fusion is achieved. The consequence is that the instrumentation must assume all the forces and suffers permanent micromotion coming to be insufficient, so it results in material failure and rupture of the implants. The form of expression is the appearance of pain and progression of the deformity.

There are local, general and technique causes that increase the risk of developing pseudarthrosis. Locally there are areas of the spine more predisposed to defects such as lumbosacral areas (Edwards et al., 2004). Among the general causes we can enumerate old age, malnutrition and nicotine use which affect in a higher incidence of nonunion and postoperative infections. With regard to technical considerations, the existence of previous laminectomy or dysraphism limits the field to make a good fusion.

Advances in instrumentation and fusion techniques have produced a steady decline in the rate of nonunion. In adolescent idiopathic scoliosis nonunion rate is approximately 0,5-1% (Hicks et al., 2010). However, this percentage is higher in neuromuscular scoliosis (Reames et al., 2011).

If a nonunion is diagnosed, it must be repaired by defect curettage and new bone grafting or it may be necessary to perform an anterior approach to ensure a circumferential fusion.

4.7 Increase decompensation and sagittal deformity

The alteration of the sagittal profile is a major problem when there is a reduction of scoliosis. Classically it was very common when using Harrington stems acting on distraction which did not correct the vertebral rotation. The result was a loss of lumbar lordosis due to the correction of the sagittal lumbar plane (flat back syndrome). This fixed sagittal imbalance syndrome is characterized by progressive lumbosacral pain, forward bending of the trunk, inability to maintain an upright position and a serious aesthetic alteration. In extreme cases it could lead to obstructive lung problems.

When we started correcting scoliosis by rotation of the vertebral bodies the incidence of flat back decreased significantly but other causes of imbalance appeared, such as the selective application of fusion in special cases trying to preserve lumbar curves that should be fused to avoid long arthrodesis . In these cases, due to poor planning, it can occur progression of the non-fused curve resulting in high imbalances of the trunk.

The use of anterior mountings can also cause an alteration of the sagittal profile as it is known to have a recognized kyphosis effect. Surgeon must know very well the anterior instrumentation indications and try to avoid them in case of thoracic kyphosis above 40º.

Another source of imbalance is crankshaft phenomenon (Dubousset et al., 1989). Occurs after posterior spinal fusion in immature patients (Risser less than 1 and less than 10 years) and is attributed to the constant growth of the vertebral body in the anterior part which takes the posterior fixed structures as the axis of rotation. The consequence is an increase in the angular value of the curve and an increase in the thoracic hump. The thoracic hump deteriorates mainly due to the fact the surgical treatment improves the central axis, that is the spinal curve, but it is not affecting the deleterious forces acting on the thorax, wich probably lead to the deformity (Grivas et al., 2008). In these very immature patients is advisable to perform surgery involving anterior and posterior fusion to prevent this phenomenon.

4.8 Pathology of adjacent levels

The appearance of disc and intervertebral joints degeneration above or below the instrumentation is a common complication of scoliosis surgery, especially if there is a sagittal imbalance. Some of the patients experiencing this problem may require revision surgery to perform an extension of the arthrodesis.

Another adjacent level pathology described in the literature is the occurrence of acute vertebral fractures at the end of long instrumentation after spinal deformities surgery. These fractures are especially common in adult scoliosis due to the high rate of osteoporosis that can present these patients. It has been reported the incidence of this event in 4.9% (O'Leary et al., 2009). These fractures may be accompanied by severe neurological deficits.

4.9 Other complications

There are many other complications been reported in patients undergoing scoliosis surgery. Many of these complications are common to any other major surgery. The syndrome of inappropriate secretion of antidiuretic hormone, cholelithiasis, cervical pain, recurrent meningitis, renal failure due to ureteral compression by the implants, blindness caused by occlusion of the central retinal artery, thromboembolism, urinary infections, etc..

Many of the complications we have discussed, in extreme cases can lead to the most serious complication which is patient's death. The incidence of death as a complication of scoliosis surgery in healthy patients is less than 1%. Life expectancy in patients undergoing neuromuscular scoliosis with complex pathologies dramatically decreases.

5. Conclusions

Spinal deformities are a problem that affects a heterogeneous group of patients. The surgery required to correct or stabilize these deformities is in all cases very demanding and aggressive for the patient and has frequent complications with different incidence depending on the etiology of scoliosis.

It is very important, when there is an indication of surgery for scoliosis, to inform the patient and the family of the objectives pursued with this surgery, but also be very objective and clear about the complexity of the surgery, alert about the high incidence of complications that can appear during surgery and record it by making an informed consent for the surgery.

6. References

Barois A. Les problèmes respiratoires des scolioses graves. *Bull Acad Natl Med* 1999;183(4):721-730.

Bradford DS, Kay BKB & Hu SS. Adult scoliosis: surgical indications, operative management, complications and aoutcomes. *Spine* 1999;24:2617-2629.

Colomina MJ & Godet C. Anestesia para la cirugía de la escoliosis. Estudio preoperatorio y selección de pacientes de riesgo en la cirugía de las deformidades raquídeas. *Rev. Esp. Anestesiol. Reanim.* 2005;52:24-43.

Crowther MA, Webb PJ & Eyre-Brook IA. Superior mesenteric artery syndrome following surgery for scoliosis. *Spine* 2002;27(24):E528-533.

Dubousset J, Schufflebarger HL & Herring JA. The crankshaft phenomenon. *J Pediatr Orthop* 1989; 9:541-550.

Edwards CC, Bridwell KH, Patel A, Rinella AS, Berra A & Lenke LG. Long adult deformity fusions to L5 and the sacrum. A matched cohort analysis. *Spine* 2004;29:1996-2005.

Gaine WJ, Andrew SM, Chadwick P, Cooke E, Williamson F & Bradley R. Late operative site pain with Isola posterior instrumentation requiring implant removal: infection or metal reaction. *Spine* 2001, 26:583-587.

Galasko CSB, Delaney C & Morris P. Spinal stabilisation in Duchenne muscular dystrophy. *Journal of Bone and Joint Surgery. British Volume* 1992;74(2):210-211.

Grivas TB, Dangas S, Polyzois BD & Samelis P. The double rib contour sign (DRCS) in lateral spinal radiographs: aetiologic implications for scoliosis. Stud Health Inform. 2002;88:38-43.

Grivas TB, Vasiliadis ES, Mihas C, Triantafyllopoulos G & Kaspiris A. Trunk asymmetry in juveniles. Scoliosis 2008 Sep 23;3:13.

Hawes M. Impact of spine surgery on sign and symptoms of spinal deformity. *Pediatric Rehabilitation* 2006;9(4):318-339.

Hicks JM, Singla A, Shen FH & Arlet V. Complications of pedicle screw fixation in scoliosis surgery. A systematic review. Spine 2010;35(11):E465-E470.

Hilibrand AS, Quartararo LG & Moulton MJ. 2004. Infecciones de la columna vertebral. In: *Orthopaedic Knowledge Update Spine Spanish Edition*, Kenneth J. Koval, 625-635, AAOS, B-50.672-2003. Spain.

Koumbourlis AC. Scoliosis and the respiratory system. *Paediatr Respir Rev.* 2006 Jun;7(2):152-60.

Laplaza FJ, Widmann RF, Fealy S, Moustafellos E, Illueca M & Burke S et al. Pancreatitis after surgery in adolescent idiopathic scoliosis: incidence and risk factors. *J Pediatr Orthop* 2002;22(1):80-83.

Lonstein JE, Winter RB,Moe JH, Bradford DS, Chou SN & Pinto WC. Neurologic deficits secondary to spinal deformity . A review of the literature and report of 43 cases. *Spine* 1980;5(4):331-355.

Molina A, Ramírez M, García-Casas O, Puig LL, Cáceres-Palou E, Gea J & Bagó J. New approaches to the surgical treatment of severe thoracic cage diseases with respiratory repercussions. *Arch Bronconeumol* 2003; 39:507-513.

O'Leary PT, Bridwell KH, Lenke LG, Good CR, Pichelmann MA, Buchowski JM.; Kim YJ & Flynn J. Risk factors and outcomes for catastrophic failures at the top of long pedicle screw constructs. *Spine* 2009;34:2134-2139.

Reames DL, Smith JS, Fu K-MG, Polly Jr DW, Ames CP, Berven SH, Perra JH, Glassman SD, McCarthy RE, Knapp Jr RD, Heary R, Shaffrey CI & Scoliosis Research Society Morbidity and Mortality Committee. Complications in the surgical treatment of 19,360 cases of pediatric scoliosis. Spine 2011;36(18):1484-1491.

Rihn JA, Lee JY & Ward WT. Infection after the surgical treatment of adolescent idiopatic scoliosis. Spine 2008; 33(3):289-294.

Smith JS, Shaffrey CI, Sansur CA, Berven SH, Fu K-MG, Broadstone PA, Choma TJ, Goytan MJ, Noordeen HH, Knapp Jr RD, Hart RA, Donaldson III WF, Polly Jr DW, Perra JH & Boachie-Adjei O. Rates of infection after spine surgery based on 108,419 procedures. A Report from the Scoliosis Research Society Morbidity and Mortality Committee. Spine 2011;36(7):556-563.

Taylor BA & Webb PJ et al. Delayed postoperative paraplegia with hypotension in adult revision scoliosis surgery. *Spine* 19:470-474, 1994.

Tsirikos AI, Chang WN, Dabney KW, Miller F & Glutting J. Life expectancy in pediatric patients with cerebral palsy and neuromuscular scoliosis who underwent spinal fusion. *Dev Med Child Neurol*. 2003 Oct; 45(10):677-82.

Vauzelle C, Stagnara P & Jouvinroux P. Functional monitoring of spinal cord activity during spinal surgery. *Clin Orthop* 1973;93:173-78.

Weiss HR & Goodall D. Rate of complications in scoliosis surgery. A systematic review of the Pub Med literature. *Scoliosis* 2008,3:9.

Section 4

Health Related Quality of Life in Idiopathic Scoliosis

16

Health Related Quality of Life in Adolescents with Idiopathic Scoliosis

Elisabetta D'Agata and Carles Pérez-Testor
Research Group of Couple and Family/Ramon LLull University
Spain

1. Introduction

The great number of articles about Health Related Quality of Life (HRQOL) in adolescents with Idiopathic Scoliosis (AIS) as well as the creation of measuring instruments indicates the emerging interest present in the health world, at the moment.

This work has come into being as a reflection between two researchers from Barcelona (Spain): Elisabetta D'Agata and Carles Pérez Testor. Besides, they both have collaborated with Manolo Rigo, director of E. Salvà Institute.

The present study is meant to deepen the concept of HRQOL and to understand how it is used, its strong and weak points.

Besides, the authors intend to complement the medical model with the *psychological* one, in a bio-psycho-social framework. They consider that the integration of the two perspectives could help to better understand AIS, in order to open the way to new research avenues. They hope that these reflections can have a practical impact on the process of *humanizing* health.

The present study is organized into four parts: at the beginning, the authors explore the historical origin of the HRQOL construct and its definition correlating it to the concepts of body image, stress and family function. The second part is about the impact of the scoliosis diagnosis and conservative treatment on the patient. The third part is a brief description of the measuring instruments and the last one discusses authors' contribution to the field.

2. Health related quality of life in adolescence

Happiness and wellbeing have been important themes of reflection since the ancient Greek philosophers' time. Nowadays, they have been considered the origins of the present concept of Quality of Life (QoL).

The QoL had its origin in the USA after the Second World War, when the Country was concerned to build up a Welfare State. The idea at first was that the QoL correlated with the possessions of material goods. However, with the progressive economic development of the 1970s, the concept changed and opened the way to social themes. In the 1980s, as sickness evolved from „severe" to „chronic" thanks to the technological and pharmaceutical improvements, the new concept of HRQOL began to be employed.

Its definition came from the *World Health Organization*'s statement (1948), that "health is a state of complete physical, mental and social well-being, and not just the absence of disease". This concept has influenced a progressive process of understanding *health* in a subjective way, not only considered as a "state" or a "functional capacity" of patients (*biomedical model*), but also as the patients' perception and the personal representation of the disease (*bio-psycho-social* model) (Galán Rodriguez et al., 2000).

Thus, in 1995 the Group of the *World Health Organization* dealing with the QOL (WHOQOL) developed a definition of HRQOL. Since then it has been considered as a **multidimensional construct** that includes the patient's perception and the different levels of his life (physical, emotional, interpersonal, etc.); this new model emphasizes the **dynamic temporal dimension** (depending on age, patient's life stage and phase of the disease), and stresses the importance of **cultural factors** in a **subjective process of self-evaluation**.

Furthermore, this concept implies the presence of positive aspects (*quality*) in people's life and not only the absence of negative ones. As a consequence, it breaks with the former ideology of intervening only in case of troubles while it embraces a preventive principle: it justifies intervention **before** problems are present (Casas, 2000).

At the same time, in the 80s some publications about children HRQOL (CHRQOL) appeared in literature, although in smaller proportion than in studies related to adult population (Quiceno & Vinaccia, 2008). Until recently, children were considered patients without power. In the research field, the younger they were, the more the researchers relied on their parents into account (Andelman et al., 1999). Moreover, Frisén (2007) considered not to evaluate adolescents with the same parameters used for adults. In the specific case of adolescence, HRQOL study has to include such aspects as physical maturation and body image, peer relationships, intimacy, sexuality and autonomy.

However, in the past the concepts of HRQOL and CHRQOL were criticized for the lack of a clear, robust, consensus-based theoretical framework (Pane et al., 2006), for confusing the QoL just with health (Verdugo et al., 2006), and for the lack of definitions as these concepts were considered „self-evident" (Andelman et al., 1999).

Nowadays, despite these limitations, the above stated concepts seem very important as they underline the emergence of the *bio-psycho-social paradigm* into the health field. It expresses a huge epistemological shift: it is a systemic model, which integrates bio-physiological systems with mental levels. According to this model, the disease arises as an interference in the systems' interaction while a single system may not be considered responsible for it. (Solano, 2001).

Considering the widespread debate and its interdisciplinary aspects, the authors intend to investigate some psychological dimensions, choosing three main concepts correlated with adolescent HRQOL: **body image**, **stress** and **family.**

2.1 Body image

Body image is considered relevant when a body falls ill.

At the beginning, body image was only studied by neurologists in cases of brain damages, then, neurologist Paul Schilder (1886-1940) widened the perspective through psychoanalysis and sociology.

However, an entity called *Body image* does not exist per se (Fisher, 1990); it is more accurately to define it as a multidimensional construct which includes the following three aspects (Raich, 2004): 1. a *perceptive* dimension, meaning the precision through which a person distinguishes size, weight and shape; 2. a *cognitive-affective* dimension, encompassing thoughts, feelings and values related to the body.; 3. a *behavioural* dimension, comprising inhibition, avoidance, obsessive checking, rituals, camouflage.

Body image has been studied in psychopathology, above all in the cases of eating disorders where its alteration is evident. However, it is a property belonging to the human being and it is *dynamic* in the life process, influenced by physiologic bodily changes. **Adolescence** is the period when the changes in body image are experienced with more intensity (Markey, 2010) because of the hormonal influences. Therefore puberty is considered a risk factor in terms of body dissatisfaction (Toro, 2010). Moreover, there are several intervening factors affecting body satisfaction as it is unrelated to the actual real weight or to the Body Mass Index, and it is more predictable in the case of a history of teasing, for example (Toro, 2010).

It has also been observed (Cahill & Mussap, 2007) that a protective factor for the body image is **self-esteem**. Self-esteem is considered the value that the person assigns to him/herself, in the process of self-evaluation (Rosenberg, 1965). But in the opposite direction, as in adolescence a great part of self-esteem is determined by body satisfaction, if the person does not accept his/her own body, it is difficult for him/her to accept the person living in it (Raich, 2004). For all these reasons, the influence of body satisfaction could have dramatic consequences during adolescence, such as poor self-esteem, depression, social anxiety, inhibition, sexual dysfunction, eating disorders, onset of cosmetic and surgical treatments, and so on (Salaberria et al., 2007).

Finally, in this context, it is important to underline that a disease may play an important role in body satisfaction, above all when it is an *acquired* disease, which could alter identity dramatically.

2.2 Stress

Stress has been studied in relation to HRQOL as it deteriorates the QoL (Schwartzmann, 2003). The concept of stress originated from the field of physics where it refers to those forces applied to an object which leads it to a breaking point (Buendia & Martinez, 1993). Similarly, McGrath (1970) defined it as an imbalance between environmental demands and individual responsiveness. The concept has been re-defined several times and has been changing over the time. At the moment, there are different definitions of stress, mainly divided into three categories: 1. *Stress* as a physiological, mainly hormonal, response to environmental demands (Selye, 1956); 2. *Stress* as a stimulus caused by the environment (Holmes & Rahe, 1967); 3. *Stress* as a relationship between the person and the environment (Lazarus & Folkman, 1984).

In this last theory, through a cognitive appraisal, the person has an active role in evaluating situations. Lazarus and Folkman (1984) called "coping strategies" the individual's cognitive and behavioural efforts aiming to minimize, reduce, tolerate and dominate environmental demands. Coping strategies could be divided synthetically into two groups: *approach* and *avoidance*. The first is an active strategy, orientated towards problem-solving and/or actively seeking support; the second is a passive strategy, involving denial of the situation and withdrawal from it (Seiffege-Krenke & Klessinger, 2000).

Stress and disease have a two-way relationship, as stress may have direct effects on health while the impact of a disease could generate stress.

Two of the most difficult phases in a state of disease are the diagnosis and the treatment (Espina & Ortega, 2003). In the acquired diseases, the diagnosis may provoke emotional responses of shock, anxiety, feelings of loss and grief in the patient (and in his/her family). In the course of the treatment, the patient and his family could become aware of the problem. They are in *mourning* for the lost functions and habits (Espina & Ortega, 2003). This process (Bowlby, 1983) consists of four phases: 1.*Numbness* (slumber and denial of reality); 2. *Searching and yearning* (anger, anxiety, fear, disorientation, etc.); 3. *Desperation* (apathy, absence of emotion, etc.); 4. *Acceptance* (self redefinition and life reorganization).

2.3 Family with an ill child

Any illness is not confined only to the patient's body, but has an impact on the whole family; similarly in the opposite direction, family may influence the course of the disease and/or rehabilitation. These connections are possible as the family is a system (Bronfenbrenner, 1976), a unique "body" (Cigoli & Scabini, 2006), a set of internal, social and generational relationships where their components influence one another.

With the disease, the entire family may feel a loss of identity as a "healthy family" and face a process very similar to the mourning one. In the initial phase, there is a state of confusion over the diagnosis while later a state of depression may follow. There are different possible stages of adaptation to the disease (Gómez & Flores, 1999). Usually the family may alter its structure with a reorganization of the roles, the creation of new alliances, coalition, changed hierarchy, isolation (Ferrari & Adami, 1997). Familiar relationships may sometimes change so much that, although they seem helpful, they become part of the problem as a maneuver of the complex family game (Ferrari & Adami, 1997).

A main caregiver, that culturally is the mother, appears. But the main caregiver can have a so close relationship with the patient (exclusive dyad) that the rest of the family can live feelings of jealousy, abandonment, and even potential couple problems; the main caregiver can also gain power as the patient loses it, but, on the other hand, the total and exclusive dedication leads her/him to exhaustion and isolation within the family (Espina & Ortega, 2003).

3. HRQOL in adolescents with idiopathic scoliosis

The peculiarity of having a scoliosis places the patient in an undefined region between illness and health, as a scoliosis is a spine deviation but also a deviation from normality, a feature that could be lived either as a deformity or not, depending on whether the posture stoops, the person has to wear a brace or to be operated, and generally how to deal with it.

It has been shown that scoliosis is a risk factor in adolescence and may produce psychosocial issues (Payne et al., 1997).

Moreover, the issue of a *poor body image* is an almost universal evidence found in studies of adolescent scoliosis (Tones et al.,2006), although it seems to the authors of the present study insufficiently investigated. Several researchers (Payne et al., 1997; Weinstein et al., 2008) observed that patients who develop a disease that alters their physical appearance during adolescence, such as scoliosis, arthritis, diabetes, psoriasis or other, have a poorer body image compared to patients with an acquired disease in childhood or adulthood. In adolescence, scoliosis may threat the integrity of body image and attack self-esteem; so, it could hinder the creation of a new image, with the appearance of feelings of insecurity and of inferiority (Saccomani et al., 1998). The research detected two levels about body image: on a conscious level, the 63% of patients minimized the impact of scoliosis on their body experience while, on an unconscious level, the 45% expressed anxiety about the experience of a bodily deterioration (Saccomani et al., 1998). In addition, considering a possible relationship between body image problems and eating disorders, Smith et al. (2008) observed that the 25% of the patients with scoliosis were severely underweight.

Besides, Forstenzer and Roye (1988) referred to the mourning process which the patient has to go through after the diagnosis of scoliosis. Like the patients, also parents live the mourning of the perfect and healthy daughter/son (Forstenzer & Roye, 1988). A further complication is present if these patients injured are daughters of mothers with scoliosis (Forstenzer & Roye, 1989). Consequently, a diagnosis of scoliosis may represent a double attack towards these mothers: in relation to their own imperfection and to their daughter's.

3.1 Conservative treatment

In literature there are contradictory results on the impact of brace in adolescent HRQL, due to a variety of factors present in the researches, such as the type of the ortheses, the daily use (part-time/full-time), cultural differences among patients (Cheung et al., 2007) or the measuring instruments used.

Surely, the kind of brace has a different impact on HRQOL: Milwaukee brace is considered the most stressful for its impact on the psychosocial area and back flexibility (Climent & Sánchez, 1999). Milwaukee-treated patients have a worse body image and worse experience with the hospital staff in comparison with the group of operated patients (Fällström, et al., 1986). However, low values in vitality and pshysical functioning have been observed also in adolescents treated with a modified Boston brace for a minimum of two years (Vasiliadis et al., 2006).

Since the beginning of the treatment and for six months later, in these patients, researchers have observed feelings of fear and anger (against the parents, the doctor, her/himself); in addition, denial is often used (Sapountzi-Krepia et al., 2006). Because of the feeling of being different, a lot of patients may develop a sense of shame. The fear that others can discover their "secret" may lead them to be more stressed, anxious, with a less positive attitude towards life and with feelings of body inferiority (Reichel & Schanz, 2003). As a consequence, the threat to body image and the social integration difficulty can guide the adolescent towards activities that isolate him/herself, developing the building of neurotic personality with depressive aspects, emotional coartation and relational difficulties (Saccomani et al., 1998). Although stress decreases during the first months of treatment, at the end of the treatment, a significative worsening in different areas (physical, emotional and social functioning, selfesteem, pain and body image) has been assessed (Vasiliadis and Grivas, 2008).

At the opposite, a Swedish study (Olafsson et al., 1999) concluded that brace treatment has no negative effect on the image of the teenager, although a half of the sample believed that brace may affect the muscles.

Psychological stress due to the treatment is a concern among professionals, as it is also negatively related to the compliance with the treatment (Olafsson et al., 1999, Burkhart & Sabaté, 2003). For these reasons, a shorter brace type or a part-time wearing modality were proposed. Indeed, a 64% of high-school teens do not wear the brace as they should or long enough to be effective (Vandal et al.,1999), and this can interfere with the treatment effectiveness (Yrjönen et al., 2007).

Generally the reported compliance is less than the admitted one and it does not increase when the patient is prescribed to wear the brace in a part-time modality respect to a full-time one (Takemitsu et al., 2004). However, compliance can be considered a dynamic behavior, which is reduced with the age (increasing among patients aged 11-14 and worsening in older adolescents) and in relation to the duration of treatment (Takemitsu et al., 2004). It improves after school and during the night, while it worsens during summertime and on weekends (Nicholson et al., 2003). In addition, Lindeman and Behm (1999) underlined a relationship with sex: non compliant girls were anxious and expected to fail in facing scoliosis; non compliant boys, in contrast, had high self-esteem and high expectation of success.

Finally, also about the long-term tratment effects there is not always consensus on results. The study carried out by Haefeli et al. (2006), in monitoring HRQOL, showed no differences comparing patients treated with braces, with a control group, after a period of time *between 10 and 60 years*. The patients of the study, reporting psychological problems due to scoliosis, had a low self-esteem problem related to the feeling of no appeal and relational problems. Despite the negative effect of the brace, this does not develop a psychopathology (MacLean et al., 1989).

However, another research (Freidel et al., 2002) does not confirm these results: brace-treated patients are more unhappy with their lives; they report more physical problems and score higher in depression compared to a control group. Despite these feelings of depression, they appreciate more positive events in their lives. Moreover, in *a 10-year-long study* after Boston treatment (Andersen et al., 2002), the 24% of patients who had worn a brace over the age of 16 had problems with the opposite sex, compared to the 7% of those who had started wearing the brace before they were 16; a difficulty in the sexual area was confirmed in another study with Milwaukee brace patients (Apter et al., 1978), who showed anxiety and rigidity. Finally, *22 years after* the treatment, there were no differences in relation to marriage and to the number of children among brace-treated patients and control group; only the mean age of brace-treated patients at their first child was higher (28 years) compared to the average (25.9) (Danielsson & Nachemson, 2001).

However, as the conservative treatment is long and affects the daily lives of almost asymptomatic patients, some psychological interventions have been implemented with the aims of sharing experiences, enhancing self-acceptance and learning strategies to manage social life. Different techniques of art therapy, relaxation and games have been used (Reichel & Schanz, 2003; Weiss, 2003), while in case of pain, groups of handling pain have been set up (Weiss, 2003).

4. HRQOL measuring instruments

Although health has always interested researchers, the HRQOL history is quite recent and as a result, a large amount of questions can arise (Climent et al., 2009). The problem is wider, as difficulties appear in the use of HRQOL measuring instruments either in the research or in the clinic fields.

In the AIS, the debate focuses on the possibility of using generic, specific and super-specific questionnaires (Climent et al., 2009).

4.1 Tools in AIS

Generic questionnaires are valid for the general asymptomatic population, widely used in epidemiological general studies (as in the case of health surveys); they are usually well validated but they lack of sensitivity to detect clinically important changes throughout the time or the treatment. Instead of a global measure of HRQOL, the most authors break down the concept in various domains; among these, there are still important discrepancies about the appropriate dimensions of the concept.

In the AIS, **Short Form Survey-36** (SF-36) and Short form-12 (SF-12) have been widely used.

SF-36 (Ware & Shebourne, 1992) consists of 36 items covering 8 dimensions: physical functioning; role limitations due to physical problems; bodily pain; general health perceptions; vitality; social functioning; role limitations due to emotional problems; mental health. This questionnaire, translated into 15 languages, has good psychometric properties, valued in more than 400 articles (Vilagut et al., 2005).

A limitation found in this type of assessment refers to the fact that it has been validated for the adults. To take more appropriate areas into account, the following two questionnaires have been used: the **Paediatric Outcomes Data Collection Instrument** (PODCI) and the **Child Health Questionnaire** (CHQ).

The PODCI, created by the Pediatric Orthopaedic Society of North America in the late nineties, aims at measuring paediatric orthopedic problems. It consists of three instruments: the pediatric questionnaire (for parents of children between the age of 2 and 11), the questionnaire for parents of teens (aged 13 and 18) and the questionnaire for adolescents (between 11 and 18) (Furlong et al., 2005).

The latter from the U.S.A is the CHQ, with three versions for parents (CHP-PF 28, CHP-PF50, CHP-PF98) to assess the HRQL of children aged 5-10 and a version (87 items) for adolescents (between the age of 10 and 18) (HealthActCHQ, 2010).

The **specific instruments** measure the impact of a particular disease and have a greater sensitivity to change (Clarke & Eiser, 2004).

The most widely used questionnaire remains the **Scoliosis Research Society-22** (SRS-22), developed in its first version in 1999 (SRS-24) by the Scoliosis Research Society (Haher et al.,

1999). At the moment, SRS-22 measures the HRQOL of patients with scoliosis, has 22 items and a structure of 5 factors: function/ activity (5 items), pain (5 items), self-image, appearance (5 items), mental health (5 items) and satisfaction with treatment (2 items). Each question has 5 possible answers, scored from 1 to 5. The higher the score is, the higher the quality of life of patients is. The results for the concurrent validity, using as criterion the SF-36 ($r \geq 0.70$ for 17 comparisons), internal consistency (Cronbach's $\alpha = 0.86$) and test-retest reliability ($\rho = 0.90$) are significant (Asher et al., 2003). The questionnaire was constructed and evaluated using patients undergoing surgery as samples.

The original English version has been translated and adapted into many languages. It has been suggested that SRS-22 would not work well with younger patients or the ones with mild scoliosis because these patients scores present a higher ceiling effect (Feis et al., 2005).

Another questionnaire is the **Quality of Life Profile for Spinal Disorders** (QLPSD) (Climent et al., 1995), previously created and less widespread than SRS-22. This instrument has good reliability (test-retest: $r = 0.91$, internal consistency: $\alpha = 0.88$) and construct validity. The questionnaire was specifically designed for adolescents only with IS, but then used for any kind of spinal deformities. Its final version consists of 21 items and 5 dimensions:function, sleep disturbances, pain, body image, trunk flexibility. There are currently three versions: Spanish, English and French.

Finally, there is **the Bad Sobernheim Stress Questionnaire (deformity)** (Weiss et al., 2006), a specific questionnaire that measures the stress particularly due to spinal deformity. The questionnaire consists of 8 items, evaluated from the highest stress (0) to no stress (3), so the final score indicates different stress levels: 0-8 for high stress, 9-16 for average stress, 17-24 for minimal stress. The questionnaire has good test-retest coefficient ($r = 0.95$), a good criterion validity ($r = 0.78$), while possibly due to the small number of items, Cronbach's α is less than 0.7. Currently, there are the German original version and the Polish validated one (Misterska et al.,2009).

Another specific questionnaire is **Oswestry Low Back Pain Disability Questionnaire** (Fairbank et al., 1980), which is used in cases of low back pain. It consists of 10 items. A similar scale is the **Roland-Morris Disability Questionnaire** (Roland & Morris, 1983) which consists of 24 items describing situations of pain.

The **superspecific instruments** can belong to two types: the ones which study only one HRQOL dimension and the others that consider a very specific clinic situation in AIS (Climent et al., 2009). **Walter Reed Visual Assessment Scale** (WRVAS) and **Trunk Asymmetry Perception Scale** (TAPS) belong to the first type.

The WRVAS was created to deepen into the relationship between body image and spinal deformity(Sanders et al., 2003). It is a visual test, composed of 7 items related to: 1. spinal deformity, 2. rib prominence, 3. lumbar prominence, 4. thoracic deformity, 5. trunk imbalance, 6. shoulders asymmetry and 7. scapular asymmetry. Each aspect is shown with 5 progressive levels of severity from the least (1) to the maximum (5). The result is the sum of 7 items. The images show a person from behind and thus the scales measure the subjective perception from how the others see the patient's back.The instrument is able to discriminate between patients who notice the deformity and those who do not. In addition, there is a high correlation between parents and patients' scores ($r=0.8$). The scale has an excellent reliability (internal consistency: Cronbach's α = 0.9), a good discriminant validity (using Cobb angle, r = 0.69) and a convergent one (using SRS-22, r =- 0.5). However, as the scale has some limitations (for example related to the lack of stratification of different curve patterns), another scale has been created: TAPS (Bago et al., 2010). The scale has a good reliability (Cronbach's α = 0.89, test-retest = 0.92) and validity (convergent validity, using the SRS-22: r = 0-45-0.52, discriminant validity, using Cobb degrees, r =- 0.55).

4.2 Tools for AIS conservative treatment

A super-specific questionnaire that measures HRQOL in brace-treated patients is the Greek questionnaire, **Brace Questionnaire** (BRQ) (Vasiliadis et al., 2006), which has the merit of measuring HRQOL in a very specific situation. This questionnaire consists of 34 Likert- scale items and can be used with people aged between 9 and 18. Minimum score is 20 and maximum is 100; higher scores indicate better HRQOL. The psychometric properties are good: high reliability (α = 0.82) and convergent validity (r ≥ 0.40). It measures 8 areas: general health perception, physical functioning, emotional functioning, self-esteem and aesthetics, vitality, school activity, bodily pain and social functioning. BrQ has been validated in Italian (Aulisa et al., 2010) and in Polish (Kinel, 2011).

Finally, a questionnaire derived from BSSQ (deformity) is the **BSSQ (mit Korsett)** which assesses the stress due to the brace impact (Weiss et al., 2006; Weiss et al., 2007). Like BSSQ (deformity), a maximum score of 24 indicates the lowest level of stress while 0 means the highest level of stress. The questionnaire has good psychometric properties: test-retest reliability is high (r = 0.88) as its internal consistency (α = 0.97), although there is not any validity measurement. It was translated and validated into Polish (Misterska et al., 2009), Spanish (D'Agata et al., 2010) and into Italian (Aulisa et al., 2010).

In an Italian study (Aulisa et al., 2010), BrQ had the highest capacity among SRS-22 and BSSQ (mit Korsett) in detecting changes in HRQOL in relation to the sex of patients, brace type and severity of curve. This finding could be related to the higher BRQ items number, allowing to explore more areas than the other instruments

Finally, it is worthy to mention an instrument which is a personality test. Although it does not belong to the HRQL ones, it can give an important contribution to the research. This test is called "Drawing a Person" (DAP) and it is a graphic and projective instrument. It has been studied by several authors (Goodenough, 1926; Machover, 1969; etc.). These authors have underlined that the non-conscious component is projected in the drawing: children project what they see and feel and what they can not verbalize (Hammer, 2005). According to Machover, the body with its visceral tensions and muscle tones is the battleground between needs and pressures. The drawing of a person refers to the body and this, in turn, represents his/her inner world. People with orthopedic problems have complex reactions to the images of their bodies, which are usually plastic and sensitive to diseases and cures (Machover, 1969).

5. Our contributions

The authors of this work are willing to show two researches presented with Dr. Rigo; the former, communicated in SOSORT Congress (2010), was about the psychological impact of a

Rehabilitation treatment; the latter, referred to the Spanish validation study of the Bad Sobernheim Stress Questionnaire (brace), was published in Scoliosis Journal (D'Agata et al., 2010). They present a further contribution which is a reflection relating to the professional help.

5.1 Psychological changes during one-month course in Barcelona Scoliosis Rehabilitation School (BSRS)

5.1.1 Background

The studies about physiotherapy effects on AIS HRQOL opened to interesting questions. A research in Bad Sobernheim Clinic found an increase in self-esteem and social skills (Weiss & Cherdron, 1994) as a result of a Schroth rehabilitation group program. The authors explained that patients learn they can actively influence their symptoms; as a consequence, self-esteem improves with a more positive attitude toward deformity. It has also been observed that patients who attribute responsibility for their musculoskeletal disorders to themselves are more likely to report an improvement in the results of physiotherapy (Larsson et al.,2010). Fox (2000) studied a circular relationship between physical activity and self-esteem, showing that regular exercise may increase self-perceived competence and body image. By contrast, adolescents with scoliosis, who do not practice physical activity, have a poorer body image, especially among boys (Dekel et al., 1996).

The mentioned research aims at studying the personality aspects of adolescents treated with a rehabilitation program as there are no researches in this sense.

5.1.2 Methods

The study was a pre-post, quasi-experimental design with the aim of assessing differences at an emotional level, before and after an intensive course of Rehabilitation.

The materials used were a Socio-demographic Questionnaire, created *ad hoc;* and the test of the **Drawing a Person**, according to which a person constantly expresses him/herself in drawing. There are examples of the use of this test in literature (Saccomani, et al., 1998).

Through this test, the authors assessed 5 emotional categories (aggressiveness, impulsiveness, insecurity, shyness and anxiety), sexual identity and defence mechanisms.

The sample was composed of 35 young people, 33 girls and 2 boys, aged 11 - 26 (M= 16, SD=4.2). Twenty-two of them were treated by bracing (11 part-time, 11 full time).

There was no control group.

The treatment consisted of one-month Rehabilitation, according to the protocol of Barcelona Scoliosis Rehabilitations School (BSRS), with a frequency of 5 days per week, 4 hours per day.

The setting had a group modality and was located in a private centre, E. Salvá Institute (Barcelona, Spain).

To analyze the nominal data, a non-parametric test (McNemar's test) was used.

5.1.3 Results

In pre-test and post-test, the sample showed a low level of aggressiveness (pre-test: 11%; post-test: 26%), of impulsiveness (pre-test:34%; post-test: 31%) and of insecurity (pre-test and post-test 43%). On the contrary, a high percentage of shyness (77%) and anxiety (83%) was assessed in the pre-test while in the post-test shyness decreased in a significant way (51%, p=0.035); anxiety maintained the same value.

About the sexual identity, before the treatment, the 66% of the sample drew a person of the same sex; in the post-test, the percentage of the sample who represented the same sex increased (86%) although not in a significant way (p=0.06).

Finally, at the beginning the 51% of the sample represented a blank outline without any treats (Figure 1) while in the post-test the percentage decreased (29%) in a significant manner (p=0.008) (Figure 2).

5.1.4 Discussion

From the results it is possible to observe that the rehabilitation program had an impact on the reduction of shyness, but not in anxiety. These data could be explicated, considering that the setting had a group modality. After one month this method activated a process of socialization, reducing the initial shyness, due to the first-day session. With regard to anxiety, it seemed that the treatment had no effect in reducing it.

An interesting datum was about the massive use of **evasion and withdrawal** mechanisms that had these *ghost* drawings as consequence. The extremely poor body representation is possibly related to the use of this mechanism, as the person is escaping from his/her own reality.

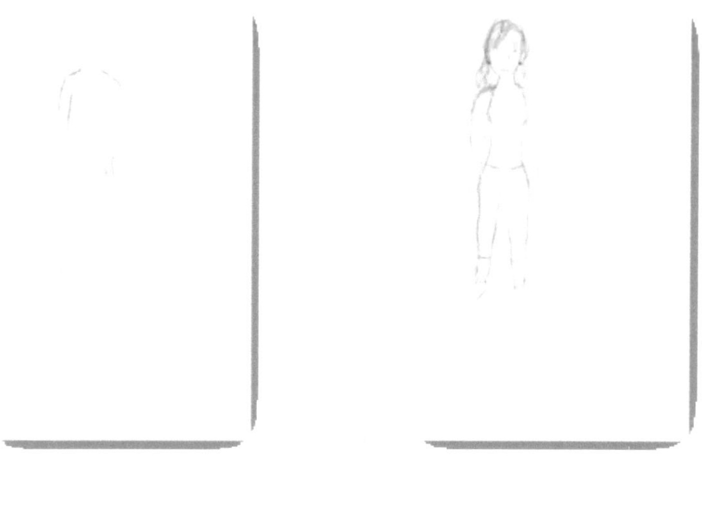

Fig. 1. 12-year-old girl's pre-test and post-test.

5.1.5 Conclusion

Further researches will aim at increasing the sample size to confirm these results. Besides, it would be interesting comparing different kinds of physiotherapy methods and different modalities (group/individual) to detect other impacts on a psychological level. Finally, to the rehabilitation treatment the authors would like to associate a specific psychological one, aiming at reducing anxiety.

5.2 Spanish validation of Bad Sobernheim Stress Questionnaire (BSSQ (brace).es)

The authors reported a synthesis of the research published in Scoliosis Journal (D'Agata, Pérez-Testor & Rigo, 2010).

5.2.1 Background

Owing to the recent attention among the clinicians towards the impact of brace on adolescent life, the aim of the present research was to validate into Spanish the German questionnaire Bad Sobernheim Stress Questionnaire (mit Korsett), applied to an adolescent population undergoing bracing treatment.

5.2.2 Methods

It has been followed the methodology used in trans-cultural adaptation (translations and back translation).

The sample consisted of 35 adolescents, in the 10-16 age range, with AIS, wearing Rigo System Chêneau Brace. Mean Cobb angle of the major curve was 35.42° (SD= 11.28°; Range: 20°-68°). Patients had been wearing the brace for 14 months (SD= 21) on average.

The setting was the private centre, E. Salvá Institute(Barcelona).

The materials used were a socio-demographic-data questionnaire, the SRS-22 and the Spanish version of BSSQ(brace).es.

The statistical analysis calculated the reliability (test-retest reliability and internal consistency) and its validity (convergent and construct validity).

5.2.3 Results

Average value was 11.7 (SD=4.8) in a score between 0 (maximum stress) and 24 (minimum stress); there were neither floor nor ceiling effect.

Test-retest reliability was satisfactory ($r=0.9$, $p<0.01$) as well as its internal consistency ($\alpha= 0.8$, $p < 0.001$).

The questionnaire demonstrated convergent validity with SRS-22 since the Pearson correlation coefficient was 0.7 ($p < 0.01$). Pearson correlation coefficient between BSSQ (brace).es and SRS-22 scales were the following: function 0.4 ($p = 0.05$), pain 0.4 ($p = 0.05$), Self Image 0.6 ($p = 0.01$), health mental 0.6 ($p = 0.01$) and satisfaction 0.5 ($p = 0.05$).

By undertaking an Exploratory Principal Components Analysis, they found out a latent structure based on two Components which explicate the variance at 60.8%.

5.2.4 Discussion

The statistic properties assessed were satisfactory. However, the structure of the concept below does not appear really clear, possibly due to the small number of patients. Nevertheless, it could be explicated considering Factor 1 as Presence of stress and Factor 2 as lack of stress.

Besides, the sample presented a medium level of stress produced by the brace. The authors chose SRS-22 for the negative correlation between stress and HRQOL. In addition, it was interesting to observe its correlation with BSSQ(brace).es, specifically those referred to SRS-22 subscales. The highest correlations were found with self- image and mental health. These statistical correlations indicated that the stress roused by brace is connected to the patient's body image and to suffering.

5.2.5 Conclusion

BSSQ (brace).es is a reliable and valid test that can be used in clinic as it is easy to employ.

5.3 Help relationship in AIS: a reflection

In literature some psychological interventions aimed at patients with scoliosis have been described (Reichel & Schanz, 2003; Walker, 2003; Weiss, 2003), as well as self-help groups among parents and adolescents (Hinrichsen et al., 1985). However, the authors consider that the psychologist's attention is not greatly addressed yet to this direction and they desire to promote their participation both in the research and in the clinic field.

In this paragraph they intend to point out the relevance of the help relationship by professionals in the area of scoliosis and the potentiality of a psychological work next to the essential work of the doctors and physical therapists.

5.3.1 The reasons for the help relationship

When a person gets sick, the problem is not limited only to one part of the body but the whole organism is weakened. It is not possible to consider the dimension of the *disease*, which means the physiological malfunction, without considering the *illness* that expresses the subjective dimension, the patient's inner experience (Kleinman, 1980). Considering the human being as a a psychological, social and spiritual structure, sickness is a fact that demolishes this "construction" and breaks the balance of life on all the levels (Cánovas, 2008).

In this sense, to highlight the dimension of the illness, it seems appropriate the message left at a forum on scoliosis (ISICO, 2010) by a teenager who writes: "Please help! I am a girl of 14 years old. I have scoliosis. Who can I contact? I think my life is useless. Sometimes I wish to kill me: but I think I will. Sorry "

The sick person claims care since suffering a process of global disintegration (Torralba, 1998). Understanding this destructuring process, it is important to help the patients re-build their world, using personal resources; so the task of caring has a relationship with the ones of *edifying* and re-building (Torralba,1998). It is impossible to cure the physical body, without considering all the other dimensions: it would be an incomplete work. The healing process involves a rethinking of values, behaviours, relationships with others and a style of living (Chadifour, 1994).

5.3.2 Characteristics of the helping relationship

The teenager with IS should be accompanied by an empathic attitude, which means "going down into the well of the other" and getting wet, getting involved. The only way to find the patient is sailing in the same boat, embarked on the same project, beside and not above (Planella, 2006).But for this, it is important to recognize the patient, calling him/her by his/her own name and giving voice, allowing its expression through words authentically.

The relationship with the physicians or physical therapists may be helpful, though the difference is that professionals such as psychologists and psychotherapists have a deeper understanding of the person and are equipped with a proper set of skills acquired through training and experiences.

5.3.3 Helping relationship phases

The helping relationship supports the patients in finding solutions to the problem that affects them. Difficulties may be of different natures and it is always important to take the family into account as the patient's system (Bronfenbrenner, 1976).

According to the phase in which the patient is, the issues presented will be different: in diagnosis, the difficulty may occur in accepting scoliosis; in the conservative treatment, in accepting the brace. Transversally to the two phases, a common task may help the patient and family to express their emotions (fear, aggression, guilt, rejection, etc.); to make him/her aware of his/her active role as *agent* and not patient, encouraging the progression of autonomy; to help accept a difficult situation, promoting self-care.

In the diagnostic phase, the psychologist makes an assessment of patients and their families, integrating his work with the physician's and physical therapist's. According to the specific needs of the patient and his family, a planning intervention can follow. The setting can be individual or familiar, according to each case. Professionals (doctor, physiotherapist and psychologist) work together to integrate their vision in a complex way.

Finally, answering to the question that an intervention like this could mean a psycho-pathologization of the stress, Buendía, Ruiz and Riquelme (1999) argued that intervention should be preventive. If stress is considered not as a disorder, but as a challenge which, if poorly resolved, can lead to disorders, a brief but in time intervention can help the "stressed person" to develop appropriate coping strategies to face with the situation.

6. Conclusions

6.1 General conclusions

With the present work the authors have tried to outline a theoretical framework on the issue of AIS HRQOL. Referring to scientific literature and from a psychological perspective they can conclude that:

- HRQOL is a multidimensional concept including the physical, psychological and social life of a human being (bio-psycho-social model). Teenage HRQL is different from the corresponding one for adults (Frisen, 2007).
- Body image is a multidimensional construct comprising the perceptual, cognitive-affective and behavioural dimensions (Raich, 2004). In AIS, the most universal evidence is the poverty of body image (Payne et al., 1997).
- With reference to conservative treatment, among the possible reactions described in the first months caused by brace, there are fear, anger, shame, and a high use of denial and isolation (Sapountzi-Krepia et al., 2006). *Compliance* is a dynamic behaviour (Takemisu et al., 2004).

Finally, the authors' contributions refer to different areas: the rehabilitation effects on HRQOL; the Spanish validation of the BSSQ(brace).es; a reflection on a system of professional help relationship in AIS.

6.2 Limitations of the study

The authors are aware that their reflections are limited and that the present study does not cover all the researches on HRQOL in AIS. The work they present is meant to be an attempt to detect coherent lines in the researches. Besides, they do not mention HRQOL in case of surgery, because it would take up much space for its importance. So they have decided to focus their attention completely on the experience of scoliosis and the conservative treatment.

6.3 Future researches

As psychology is new in AIS, there are several areas that should be explored. At this stage the authors select only four points:

1.Paying attention to HRQOL impacts of those rehabilitation treatments which exalt respiration and movement. Theory as mindfulness in psychology and the use of respiration have been studied for the preventive effect of depression, the increasing of awareness and of wellbeing (Brown & Ryan, 2003). 2. Studying the AIS family, its structure to find any common patterns. 3. Questioning about the effectiveness of the questionnaires used so far. The great challenge in AIS HRQOL measurements is to create a complex instrument specifically addressed to the essential aspects of adolescents' lives, to their conscious aspects of the body and to those who fail to reach consciousness.4. Deepening the relational aspects of adolescence: peer relationship and intimacy.

7. References

Andelman, R., Attkisson, C., Zima, B. & Rosenblatt, A. (1999). Quality of life of children: Toward conceptual clarity. In: *The use of psychological testing for treatment planning and outcomes assessment*, Maruisch, M., pp. 477-510, LEA, 0-8058-4330-2, London

Andersen, M., Andersen, G. R., Thomsen, K. & Christensen, S. (2002). Early weaning might reduce the psychological strain of Boston bracing: a study of 136 patients with adolescent idiopathic scoliosis at 3.5 years after termination of brace treatment. *Journal Of Pediatric Orthopaedics. Part B*, Vol.11, No.2, pp.96-99.

Apter, A., Morein, G., Munitz, H., Tyano, S., Maoz, B. & Wijsenbeek, H. (1978). The psychosocial sequelae of the Milwaukee brace in adolescent girls. *Clinical orthopaedics and related research,* Vol. 131, pp. 156-159.

Asher, M., Min Lai, S., Burton, D. & Manna, B. (2003). The reliability and concurrent validity of the scoliosis research society-22 patient questionnaire for idiopathic scoliosis. *Spine,* Vol. 28, No.1, pp. 63-69.

Aulisa, A., Guzzanti, V., Perisano, C., Marzetti, E., Specchia, A., Galli, M., Giordano, M. & Aulisa, L. (2010). Determination of quality of life in adolescents with idiopathic scoliosis subjected to conservative treatment. *Scoliosis,* Vol. 5, No. 21, pp. 1-7. Available from *www.scoliosisjournal.com*

Bago, J., Sanchez-Raya, J., Sanchez, F.J. & Climent, J.M. (2010). The Trunk Appearance Perception Scale (TAPS): a new tool to evaluate subjective impression of trunk deformity in patients with idiopathic scoliosis. *Scoliosis,* Vol. 5, No. 6, (March 2010), pp. 1-9. Available from *www.scoliosisjournal.com*

Bowlby, J. (1983). *La pérdida afectiva,* Paidós, ISBN: 950-12-4050-9, Buenos Aires

Bronfenbrenner, U. (1976). The ecology of human development: History and perspectives. *Psychologia Wychowawcza,* Vol. 19, No.5, pp. 537-549

Buendía, J., Ruiz, J. & Riquelme, A. (1999) Efectos del estrés familiar en niños y adolescentes. In: *Familia y psicología de la salud,* Buendía, J., pp.181-202, Pirámide, Madrid

Burkhart, P. & Sabaté, E. (2003). Adherence to long-term therapies: evidence for action. *Journal Of Nursing Scholarship,* Vol. 35, No.3, pp. 207-207.

Cahill, S. & Mussap, A. (2007). Emotional reactions following exposure to idealized bodies predict unhealthy body change attitudes and behaviors in women and men. *Journal of Psychosomatic Research, Vol.*62, No.6, (June 2007), pp. 631-639, 0022-3999

Cánova, M. (2008). La relación de ayuda en enfermería. Una lectura antropológica sobre la competencia relacional en el ejercicio de la profesión. Phd Thesis, University of Murcia

Casas, F. (2000). Indicadores sociales subjetivos y bienestar en la infancia y adolescencia. In: *Propuesta de un sistema de indicadores sobre bienestar infantil en España,* 25/09/2011, Available from: http://www.unicef.es

Chadifour, J. (1994). *La relación de ayuda en cuidados de enfermería. Una perspectiva holística y humanista,* SG editores, Barcelona

Cheung, K., Cheng, E., Chan, S., Yeung, K. & Luk, K. (2007). Outcome assessment of bracing in adolescent idiopathic scoliosis by the use of the SRS-22 questionnaire. *International orthopaedics,* Vol. 31, No. 4, pp. 507-511

Cigoli, V. & Scabini, E. (2006). *Family identity. Ties, symbols, and transitions,* Taylor, 0-8058-5231-X, New York

Clarke, S. & Eiser, C. (2004). The measurement of health-related quality of life (QOL) in paediatric clinical trials: a systematic review. *Health And Quality Of Life Outcomes,* Vol.2, pp.66-66

Climent, J. M. & Sánchez, J. (1999). Impact of the type of brace on the quality of life of Adolescents with Spine Deformities. *Spine,* Vol.24, No.18, pp.1903-1908.

Climent, J. M., Cholbi Llobell, F., Rodríguez Ruiz, C., Mulet Perry, S., Mendéjar Gómez, F. & Pradas Silvestre, J. (2009). La medida de la salud en la escoliosis. *Rehabilitación,* Vol.43, No.6, pp.299-305

Climent, J. M., Reig, A., Sánchez, J. & Roda, C. (1995). Construction and validation of a specific quality of life instrument for adolescents with spine deformities. *Spine,* Vol.20, No.18, pp. 2006-2011.

D'Agata, E., Pérez-Testor, C. & Rigo, M. (2010). Spanish validation of Bad Sobernheim Stress Questionnaire (BSSQ (brace).es) for adolescents with braces. Scoliosis, Vol. 5, No. 15 (July 2010)

Danielsson, A. & Nachemson, A. (2001). Childbearing, curve progression, and sexual function in women 22 years after treatment for adolescent idiopathic scoliosis: a case-control study. *Spine,* Vol. *26,* No.13, pp. 1449-1456.

Dekel, Y., Tenenbaum, G. & Kudar, K. (1997).An exploratory study on the relationship between postural deformities and body-image and self esteem in adolescents: the mediating role of physical activity. *International Journal of Sports Psychology,* Vol.27,pp. 183-196.

Espina, O. & Ortega, M. A. (2003). *Discapacidades físicas y sensoriales,* CCS, Madrid

Fairbank, J. C., Couper, J., Davies, J. B. & O'Brien, J. P. (1980). Oswestry Low Back Pain Disability Questionnaire. *Physiotherapy,* Vol.66, No.8, pp. 271-273.

Fällström, K., Cochran, T. & Nachemson, A. (1986). Long-term effects on personality development in patients with adolescent idiopathic scoliosis. Influence of type of treatment. *Spine,* Vol.11, No.7, pp.756-758.

Ferrari, A. & Adami, R. (1997). Cuerpo, familia e institución. In: *La palabra del cuerpo,* Onnis, L., pp. 198-205, Herder, 9788425419683, Barcelona

Fisher, S. (1990). The evolution of psychological concepts about the body. In: *Body Images,* Cash, T. & Pruzinsky, T., (pp. 3-20), The Guildford Press, New York

Forstenzer, F.& Roye, D. (1988). Some aspects of psychosocial sequelae to treatment of scoliosis in adolescent girls. *Loss, Grief & Care,* Vol.2, No.3-4, pp.53-58.

Forstenzer, F. & Roye, D. (1989). Psychological implications of genetic factors in scoliosis. *Loss, Grief & Care,* Vol. 3, No.3-4, pp.169-173.

Fox, K (2000). Self.-esteem, self perceptions and exercise. *International Journal of Sport Psychology,* Vol.31, No.2, (April-June 2000) pp. 228-240

Freidel, K., Petermann, F., Reichel, D., Steiner, A., Warschburger, P. & Weiss, H. R. (2002). Quality of life in women with idiopathic scoliosis. *Spine,* Vol.27, No.4, pp. E87 E91.

Frisén, A. (2007). Measuring health-related quality of life in adolescence. *Acta Paediatrica,* 96, 7, (July 2007), pp. 963-968, 0803-5253

Furlong, W., Barr, R. D., Feeny, D. & Yandow, S. (2005). Patient-focused measures of functional health status and health-related quality of life in pediatric orthopedics: a case study in measurement selection. *Health and Quality of Life Outcomes,* Vol.3, No.3, pp.1-15. Available from www.hqlo.com

Galán Rodriguez, A., Blanco Picabia, A. & Pérez San Gregorio, M. (2000). La Calidad de Vida en la Salud: un Análisis Conceptual. *Clínica y Salud: Revista de Psicología Clínica y Salud,* Vol.11, No.3, pp.309-328

Gómez, E. & Flores, R. (1999). Necesidades y demandas de las familias con menores discapacidados, *Minusvalías,* Vol. 120, pp.26-28.

Goodenough, F. (1926). *Test de inteligencia infantil por medio del dibujo de la figura humana,* Paidós, Buenos Aires

Haefeli, M., Elfering, A., Kilian, R., Min, K. & Boos, N. (2006). Nonoperative treatment for adolescent idiopathic scoliosis: a 10- to 60-year follow-up with special reference to health-related quality of life. *Spine,* Vol.31, No.3, pp. 355-366.

Haher, T. R., Gorup, J. M., Shin, T. M., Homel, P., Merola, A. A., Grogan, D. P., Pugh, L. et al. (1999). Results of the Scoliosis Research Society instrument for evaluation of surgical outcome in adolescent idiopathic scoliosis. A multicenter study of 244 patients. *Spine,* Vol.24, No.14, pp.1435-1440.

Hammer, E. (2005). *Tests proyectivos gráficos*. Paidós. Buenos Aires

HealthActCHQ (2010). In: *Surveys.CHQ: Child Health Questionnaire,* 2/2/2011, Available from http://www.healthact.com

Holmes, T. H. & Rahe, R. H. (1967). The social readjustment rating scale. *Journal of Psychosomatic Research,* Vol.11, No.2, (May, 2002),pp. 213-218

Isico Scoliosi (2011). In: *Il blog di Isico dedicato alla scoliosi,* 10/05/2011, available from www.scoliosi.org

Kinel,E., Kotwicki,T., Podolska, A. & Stryla W. (2011). Polish validation of Brace Questionnaire. *Proceedings of 8th Annual Meeting of the SOSORT 2011,* Barcelona, May 2011

Kleinman, A. (1980). *Patients and Healers in the Context of Culture,* University of California Press, 0-520-03706-5, Los Angeles

Larsson, M. E. H., Kreuter, M. & Nordholm, L. (2010). Is patient responsibility for managing musculoskeletal disorders related to self-reported better outcome of physiotherapy treatment? *Physiotherapy Theory And Practice,* Vol.26, No.5, pp.308-317.

Lazarus, R. & Folkman, S. (1984). *Stress, appraisal, and coping*. Springer Publishing Company, New York

Lindeman, M. & Behm, K. (1999). Cognitive strategies and self-esteem as predictors of brace-wear noncompliance in patients with idiopathic scoliosis and kyphosis, *Journal of pediatric orthopedics,* Vol.19, No.4,pp. 493-499.

Machover, K. (1969). *Il disegno della figura umana*. O.S., Firenze

MacLean, W. E., Green, N. E., Pierre, C. B. & Ray, D. C. (1989). Stress and coping with scoliosis: psychological effects on adolescents and their families. *Journal of pediatric orthopedics,* Vol.9, No.3, pp.257-261

McGrath, J. (1970). A conceptual formulation for research on stress. In *Social and psychological factor in stress,* McGrath, J., pp. 10-21. Holt, Nueva York

Misterska, E., Głowacki, M. & Harasymczuk, J. (2009). Polish adaptation of Bad Sobernheim Stress Questionnaire-Brace and Bad Sobernheim Stress Questionnaire-Deformity. *European Spine Journal,* Vol.18, No.12, (August, 2009), pp.1911-1919.

Nicholson, G. P., Ferguson-Pell, M., Smith, K., Edgar, M. & Morley, T. (2003). The objective measurement of spinal orthosis use for the treatment of adolescent idiopathic scoliosis. *Spine,* Vol. 28, No.19, pp. 2243-2250.

Olafsson, Y., Saraste, H. & Ahlgren, R. M. (1999). Does bracing affect self-image? A prospective study on 54 patients with adolescent idiopathic scoliosis. *European Spine Journal,* Vol.8, No.5, pp.402-405.

Pane, S., Solans, M., Gaite, L., Sera-Sutton, V., Estrada, M. y Rajmil, L. (2006). *Instrumentos de calidad de vida relacionada con la salud en la edad pediátrica. Revisión sistemática de la literatura: actualización,* In: Agencia de Evaluación de Tecnología e Investigación Médicas, 20/3/2011, Available from http://www.gencat.cat

Payne, W., Ogilvie, J., Resnick, M., Kane, R., Transfeldt, E. & Blum, R. (1997). Does scoliosis have a psychological impact and does gender make a difference? *Spine,* Vol.22, No.12 (June 1997), pp.1380-1384.

Planella, J. (2006). *Subjetividad, Disidencia y Discapacidad.* Fundación ONCE, 84-88934-20-3, Madrid

Quiceno, J. & Vinaccia, S. (2008). Calidad de vida relacionada con la salud infantil: una aproximación conceptual. *Psicología y salud,* Vol.18, No.1 (Enero-Junio 2008),pp. 37-44, 1405-1109

Reichel, D. & Schanz, J. (2003). Developmental psychological aspects of scoliosis treatment. *Pediatric rehabilitation,* Vol.6, No. 3-4, pp.221-225.

Roland, M. & Morris, R. (1983). A Study of the Natural History of Back Pain: Part I: Development of a Reliable and Sensitive Measure of Disability in Low-Back Pain. *Spine,* Vol.8, No.2, pp. 141-144.

Rosenberg, M. (1965). *Society and the adolescent self-image.* Princeton University Press, Princeton

Saccomani, L., Vercellino, F., Rizzo, P. & Becchetti, S. (1998). Adolescenti con scoliosi: aspetti psicologici e psicopatologici. *Minerva Pediatrica,* Vol. 50, No.1-2, pp. 9-14.

Salaberria, K., Rodríguez, S. & Cruz, S. (2007). Percepción de la imagen corporal. *Osasunaz,* Vol.8 ,pp. 171-183.

Sanders, J., Polly, D., Cats-Baril, Jones, J., Lenke, L., O'Brien, M., Stephens Richards, B., Sucato, D., AIS Section of the Spinal Deformity Group (2003). Analysis of patient and parent assessment of deformity in idiopathic scoliosis using the Walter Reed Visual Assessment Scale. *Spine,* Vol.28, No.18, pp.2158-2163.

Sapountzi-Krepia, D., Psychogiou, M., Peterson, D., Zafiri, V., Iordanopoulou, E., Michailidou, F. & Chrinodoulou, A. (2006). The experience of brace treatment in children/adolescents with scoliosis. *Scoliosis,* Vol.1, No.8, pp 1-7. URL: www.scoliosisjournal.com

Schilder, P. (1950). *The image and appearance of the human body.* Routledge, 0415-21081-X, Great Britain

Schwartzmann L. (2003). Calidad de vida relacionada con la salud: aspectos conceptuales. *Ciencia y Enfermería,* Vol. 9, No.2 (Diciembre 2003), pp. 9-21, 0717 2079

Seiffege-Krenke, I. & Klessinger, N. (2000). Long-term effects of avoidant coping on adolescents' depressive symptoms. *Journal of Youth and Adolescence,* Vol. 29, pp.617-630.

Selye, H. (1956). *The stress of life.* MCGraw- Hill, Nueva York

Smith, F, Latchford, G., Hall, R. & Dickson, R. (2008). A cross-sectional investigation of eating pathology in adolescent females with scoliosis and diabetes. *Adolescent Health,* Vol. 42, No. 1, (January 2007), pp.58-63

Solano, L. (2001). *Tra mente e corpo.* Raffaello Cortina, 978-88-7078-691-0, Milano

Takemitsu, M., Bowen, J. R., Rahman, T., Glutting, J.J. & Scott, C. B. (2004). Compliance monitoring of brace treatment for patients with idiopathic scoliosis. *Spine,* Vol. 29, No.18, pp.2070-2074.

The World Health Organization Quality of life assessment (WHOQOL), (1995). Position Paper from the World Health Organization. *Social Sciences &. Medicine,* Vol.41, No.10, pp. 1.403-1.409.

Tones, M., Moss, N. & Polly, D. W. (2006). A review of quality of life and psychosocial issues in scoliosis. *Spine,* Vol.31, No. 26, (Dicembre 2006), pp. 3027-3038.

Toro, J. (2010). *El adolescente en su mundo,* Pirámide, 978-84-368-2367-7, Madrid

Torralba, F. (1998). *Antropología del cuidar.* Fundación Mapfre, Madrid

Vandal, S., Rivard, C. H. & Bradet, R. (1999). Measuring the compliacen behavior of adolescents wearing orthopedic braces. *Issues in comprehensive pediatric nursing,* Vol.22, No.2-3, pp. 59-73.

Vasiliadis E, Grivas T. (2008). Quality of life after conservative treatment of adolescent idiopathic scoliosis. In *The Conservative Scoliosis Treatment, Grivas,* pp.409-13, IOS press, 978-1-58603-842-7, Netherlands

Vasiliadis E., Grivas T. & Gkoltsiou, K. (2006). Development and preliminary validation of Brace Questionnaire (BrQ): a new instrument for measuring quality of life of brace treated scoliotics. *Scoliosis,* Vol.1, No. 7, pp.1-8. Available from www.scoliosisjournal.com

Vasiliadis, E., Grivas, TB, Savvidou O, Triantafyllopoulos G.(2006). The influence of brace on quality of life of adolescents with idiopathic scoliosis. Stud Health Technol Inform.,Vol. 123, pp.123:352

Verdugo A., Córdoba, L., Gómez, J. (2006). Adaptación y validación al español de la Escala de Calidad de Vida Familiar (ECVF). *Siglo Cero: Revista Española sobre Discapacidad Intelectual,* Vol.37, No. 218, pp.41-48, 0210-1696

Ware, J. & Sherbourne, C. (1992). The MOS 36-Item Short-Form Health Survey (SF-36): I. Conceptual Framework and Item Selection. *Medical Care,* Vol.30, No.6, pp. 473-483

Weiss, H. (2003). La rehabilitación de la escoliosis. *Control de calidad y tratamiento de los pacientes.* Paidotribo, Barcelona

Weiss, H. & Cherdron, J. (1994). The impact of Schroth's rehabilitation programme on the self concept of patients with scoliosis. *Rehabilitation,* Vol.33, pp.31-36.

Weiss, H., Reichel, D., Schanz, J. & Zimmermann-Gudd, S. (2006). Deformity related stress in adolescents with AIS. *Studies in health technology and informatics,* Vol.123, pp. 347-351.

Weiss, H., Werkmann, M. y Stephan, C. (2007). Brace related stress in scoliosis patients - Comparison of different concepts of bracing. *Scoliosis,* Vol.2, No.1,p.10

World Health Organization (1948). *Basic Documents.* WHO, Ginebra

Yrjönen, T., Ylikoski, M., Schlenzka, D. & Poussa, M. (2007). Results of brace treatment of adolescent idiopathic scoliosis in boys compared with girls: a retrospective study of 102 patients treated with the Boston brace. *European Spine Journal,* Vol.16, No.3, pp.393-397.

17

Psychological Aspects of Scoliosis Treatment in Children

Ryszard Tomaszewski[1] and Magdalena Janowska[2]
[1]*Silesian Medical University, Katowice,*
[2]*Upper Silesian Child Health Centre, Department of Pediatric Orthopedics and Traumatology, Katowice,*
Poland

1. Introduction

Scoliosis in children is a serious therapeutic problem. Generally, scoliosis can be divided into several categories: congenital, neurological idiopathic etc occurring in children, adolescents [1].

In prenatal or after birth case, parents learn about their child's diagnosis soon after his or her birth or even in a prenatal period during fetal ultrasound examination [2] - This information is always difficult for a parent. How they will cope with the problem of their child's illness largely depends on the support they receive and give to each other, their personalities and the way the information is forwarded by their doctor. Information in the prenatal period may allow a child's parents to be better prepared for this situation, seek medical and psychological help.

In the case of idiopathic scoliosis parents experience a shock having learnt about the illness of their child, but a shock of a different kind. They often cannot believe that their children's spine being normal at birth, suddenly began to develop incorrectly. The problem of idiopathic scoliosis also applies to children who, at their teenage years, may mentally suffer from a very strong deformity of their shape. The cause of idiopathic scoliosis is generally unknown. Treatment of scoliosis primarily relies on rehabilitation, but if the curvature reaches a certain angle (about 20 degrees), then the rehabilitation treatment is complemented with brace treatment [3, 4,5]. The aim of treatment of scoliosis with the use of a brace or surgery is to stop the progression and possible correction of the curvature.

Coming to terms with wearing a brace is usually difficult and often a lengthy process As it is known every surgical procedure (including the one associated with scoliosis) is a difficult situation for patients and either their parents. If one wants a child to accept this method of treatment, it needs to be accepted by a child's parents. Due to stress they have the right to feel the negative emotions like anger among others. In some patients' case, anger may be externalized more in a direct manner, for example by shouting, raising voice tone (as it is in the case of external anger), while in others anger may be hidden, repressed, not shown to the object of a situation (internal anger) [6]. A difficult situation, a long-term illness, physical deficiency or hospitalization and surgery can often trigger reactions of anger which can be expressed directly or suppressed. The cause of such reactions is usually fear of the disease itself (respondents described it as a fear of how they will function, what they will be able to do, how they will cope with school situations such as not being able to carry books to school or participate in sports activities) or surgery (with the most frequent question: are you sure I will wake up?, how much will it hurt?). The mere awareness of the fact that a person is ill can create a source of nagging anxiety. A sick child's imagination suggests everything in his or her mind which can be connected with the concept of a disease such as a heart failure, physical disability, being rejected by others. A negative image of the disease, its course and effects may increase a child's anxiety [7]. We must not forget that anger is one of the stages prior to the acceptance of a prolonged illness without the expression of which it is usually impossible to reconcile with the situation and thus to find strength to fight the illness [8].Deciding on the method of treatment patients must know that this is best for them and often the only form of help. It is important that they know the initial treatment plan which will allow them to take a little control over the process. It is vital that both doctors and patients and their parents bear in mind that a positive attitude towards treatment has a huge impact on its results. The very way of information transfer is of the utmost importance. It is important that the information should be received by both parents and the children (Their age, intellectual level and already observed sensitivity must be taken into account. Talking with parents and a child or a teenager about the disease and the proposed method of treatment the principle of finding the positives in difficult situations should be implemented (eg a brace will be worn for a specified time, the operation is to shorten the time of wearing the brace and to accelerate the healing process)[9].

Restrictions to physical capabilities and even functional disturbances of individual organ systems are possible consequences of scoliosis. Following diagnosis, there is a need for a certain amount of adjustment to the new situation. Regular repetition of specific exercises, visits to the family doctor and to specialists, adaptation to a brace and rehabilitation measures all have a lasting impact on the life situation of an adolescent. The initial shock that frequently follows a diagnosis of scoliosis may result in emotional uncertainty; feelings of fear, depression, helplessness or hopelessness need to be overcome. These symptoms are usually most severe at the beginning of the treatment. However, even if a patient comes into terms with it, they may repeatedly re-appear during the long process. Very often does it happen that other difficult life situations make the depressed mood associated with the need to treat by means of a corset and difficulties in reconciling with this fact return. Uncertainty produced by scoliosis about the further progress of the illness may result in changes in the attitude of the patient to himself and his body. Knowing that one will never have a perfect body can lead to doubts about self-worth and a lessening of self-esteem. [10].

The study (Botens-Helmus C, Klein R, Stephan C) using the BSSQ questionnaire (Bad Sobernheim Stress Questionnaire) have shown higher scores in these areas. Patients wearing orthopedic corsets evaluated the following events as being stressful (scale 0-3, 0-most stressful, 3-least stressful):

I feel conspicuous by the appearance of my back

1. I find it hard to show my back public
2. I feel embarrassed in situations, in which other people can see my naked back
3. I don't feel embarrassed showing my back
4. I try not to get too close to other people to avoid that they become aware of my scoliosis
5. When deciding what kind of clothes to wear or how to wear my hair, I take care my back is hidden

6. Scoliosis is a part of me, people have to accept me the way I am
7. Because of the scoliosis I avoid activities/hobbies, which otherwise I would love to do[10].

BRQ is another questionnaire which illustrates the quality of patients' life very well. The questions of the questionnaire were grouped into eight specific domains: general health perception, psychical functioning, emotional functioning, self-esteem and aesthetics, vitality, school activity, bodily pain, social functioning. The subscales of these eight dimensions can be combined to produce a total score. Higher scores mean a better quality of life. In the studies (Vasiliadis E et al) which made use of the BRQ questionnaire, a reduced quality of life of children and adolescents affected by scoliosis were demonstrated . There are minor differences as far as specific domains are concerned among the authors, however, they all stress that patients achieved the lowest results in psychical functioning[11,12,13,].

This problem applies in particular to girls during puberty period. They are ashamed to undress before physical education lessons, go to the pool or even leave the house wearing T-shirts. These difficulties are also very pronounced in male-female relationships which begin to form in that time. Their negative experiences in this area may affect relations with the opposite sex and lead to difficulties in the sphere of intimacy throughout the whole life. Brace wearers may feel unattractive, ugly, unworthy of interest of the opposite sex and this, in consequence, may lead to closing within oneself and to reluctance as far as establishing any new social contacts is concerned, not to mention the emotional and physical intimacy.

Changes in lifestyle and life plans due to giving up particular sporting or leisure interests or limitations to the choice of career represent further burdens for the patient. The relation of the patient to the parental home is affected to the extent that adolescents are usually restricted in their movement towards autonomy by necessary treatment measures. Contact with his own age-group may be hampered by his special role as a scoliosis patient and separations from his social circle by periods in clinics or hospitals are detrimental to the process o orientation towards the peer group[14,15].

Observing people of both sexes with scoliosis would seem that boys will deal with this problem much better. [16].Obinwanne F Ugwonali and the coworkers' study evaluating differences in the functioning of the gender(CHQ domains: Psychical Functioning, Role/Social Limitation, Bodily Pain, Behaviour, Mental Health, Parental Impact - Emotional, Parental Impact-Time, Family Activities, Family Cohesion) have shown that there were no differences between braced boys andgirls, except for Family Activity, which was significantly higher among boys [17]. One can suppose that the boys in question have, in fact, tried not to show inconveniences they experienced.

Teenagers do not want to look different from their peers and, although bracing is not associated with pain, it is distribing for patients. There is evidence that bracing tends to affect them psychologically due to disturbances of their perceptions of self and body image [17,18].

A lot of scientific research and observations [19,20,21,7]point at a lower life quality of children and teenagers being treated due to scoliosis. Although this kind of treatment is not associated with pain, it is a disturbing one for patients and tends to affect them psychologically due to disturbances of the perceptions of self and body image [6]. Adolescence is a difficult psychological period in its own right and, when it is compounded with scoliosis and bracing, can produce immense psychological stress, resulting in altered body image [6]. The study (Parent EC, Hill D, Moreau M, Mahood J, Raso J, Lou E ; Freidel K, Reichel D, Steiner A, Warschburger P, Petermann F, Weiss H, Aulisa A, Guzzanti V, Perisano C) explored differences in perceptions of body image, happiness and satisfaction between adolescence with scoliosis wearing a Boston brace and a control group. The main results obtained is that girls with scoliosis had a statistically significant poorer perception of happiness and satisfaction in comparison to girls in the control group have a better body image perception as well as a better perception of happiness and satisfaction in comparison to the control group . The study shows that adolescence with scoliosis had a poorer body image perception than adolescents in the control group. [6]

However, brace-based treatment significantly interferes with several aspects of patients' life , which may determine high levels of stress and negatively impact on every-day life . In fact, AIS patients, especially those subjected to conservative treatment, may experience social isolation, depression and reduced participation in leisure activities. As a result, the prevalence of psychological disorders may be as high as 19% . Therefore, scoliosis is currently recognized as an important risk factor for psychological discomfort and poor QoL, especially in brace-treated patients [21].

Clinical variables that may affect overall quality of life include severity of the condition, skeletal maturity(Risser Sign), duration of brace treatment and degree of correction (conservative and/or surgical). However, the extent to which all these factors influence a particular patient's ability to benefit from the brace will depend on his/her physical, emotional and social wellbeing [7].High correction bracing has been shown to have favorable outcomes when the patient is compliant . However, bracing is considered to be a traumatic experience which may leave lasting emotional scars. The condition may itself precipitate social problems, with brace treatment further affecting self and body image , interactions with others ,overall quality of life and generally being a stressful experience for patients [7]. L. Rivett, A.Rothenberg and al. explore two patients group.on the basis of their compliance histories. For the purpose of this study, compliance was defined as wearing of the brace for 20–23hours per day and compliance to a prescribed exercise routine, ideally carried out at least four times per week. Non-compliant subjects wore the brace for fewer than 20 hours per day and exercised less than four times per week. Each patients were described using BrQ test concerning 34 question about general health perception, physical functioning, emotional functioning, self esteem and aesthetics, vitality, school activity, bodily pain and social functioning.[7].It is noteworthy that non-compliant subjects do not regard themselves as being in poor general health or experiencing bodily pain (differences between the groups not significant for these two domains), but they clearly lack vitality , have low self esteem , and physical , emotional and social function is at significantly lower level.

Personal observation of children and adolescents wearing orthopedic braces confirm the depressed mood in this group. The group also seemed to cope worse with the difficulties typical for their peers. It had been expected that young people with scoliosis would possess higher levels of neuroticism when compared to healthy children (neuroticism, being neurotic is a personality feature which consists of a strong emotional instability, low resistance to stress, a tendency to feel anxious easily). The opposite of neuroticism is emotional balance. Eysenck was the first to have used this notion in temperament theory

PEN [22, 23,24].A study on a group of 34 children (aged 11-16,5) treated for scoliosis and wearing braces (Open anxiety test by E. M. Choynowski and E. Skrzypek: What are you like? [22] did not confirm the hypothesis that children wearing a brace exhibit a neurotic personality type. Instead, the test did, however, show a different relationship - this group attempted to present themselves in a better way than they really are. It is highly likely that the reason for this was low self-esteem of the subjects. People with a positive self-image evaluate themselves the way they are, along with their advantages and disadvantages, they do not need to worry about being thought of only in positive terms by others. It is worth noting that similar results occurred when testing children suffering from enuresis [25]. Only 1 / 3 of them rated elevated neurotism while 73% of the children in this group showed elevated scores on the lie scale. An important observation seems to be obtained on the basis of Z. Juczyński's KompOs Scale [25] that children wearing a brace showed great persistence in action. This feature is probably very useful in all accomplishments occurring in those children's lives, as well as in treatment by means of a brace. It is therefore a very good predictor in the treatment and rehabilitation of scoliosis.

Our own observations of patients with scoliosis indicate that, very often, do they feel inferior to a group of their healthy peers. Not rarely do such people move away from social life. They do not meet with their peers after school, they do not participate in social events, birthday parties organized by others. Unfortunately, this is the case of the vicious circle principle (eg I'm not going to someone's birthday party despite being repeatedly invited and, in the result, I am not invited any more).

For patients being operated on several times, limited school attendance and its related problems may seem to be a big issue. For this reason, some parents and children decide on an individual course of learning, which in most cases, has a negative effect on self-esteem of hospitalized people. Very often does it deepen the sense of isolation and the feeling of being rejected by peers. A person not involved in daily life of the class ceases to feel as if he/she was treated as a part of it. Not knowing the course of everyday events in the life of the class, they may have trouble finding common topics to talk about with other students.

Aulisa A, Guzzanti V et a,l in their analyses did not show differences in QoL depending on the curve type (data not shown). However, patients with thoraco-lumbar curves were less satisfied with management than those with thoracic curves at the SRS-22 [21].

Teenagers (aged 14.5-18) awaiting scoliosis surgery who were examined by means of Anger Expression Scale (AX) [19] showed, in most cases (except for one person), much greater intensity of internal anger rather than external one. This information would suggest that such people deliberately do not express anger. One can assume that they are afraid to express negative feelings in order not to face disapproval and rejection, especially by their peers, as it was confirmed by the results obtained in the study described above - the lie scale.

Assessing pain control, (Beliefs About Pain Control Questionnaire (BPCQ) by S. Skevington and Z. Juczyński [25] young people from the same research group a month before surgery mostly associated the pain they experienced accidentally which means that neither them nor doctors had influence on the pain. In the second place they pointed their own opportunity to help and then the influence of the doctors. Those who were able to master severity of the pain and trusted their doctors in this respect, found their mood elevated. They felt they could have impact on their own life (or felt cared for by the doctors) which made them feel better. Those, however, who believed that their pain was accidental did not usually do anything to reduce it ("it won't work after all") [26].

Surgical treatment of scoliosis often turns out to be a difficult experience for patients and their families.[24]. Initially, at parents and older patients (teenagers) there usually appears anxiety associated with the operated site. Many times can one hear them frightfully say: What will it be like if it doesn't work? May the spine during surgery be damaged? However, the most frequent second-reaching emotion is the hope that the rigors of rehabilitation, wearing a corset and other related problems will come to an end. Young patients seem to like the fact that the treatment will shorten the time they have to wear the orthopedic corset . It is important that both patients and parents believe that this method of treatment will bring benefits. It is also necessary to keep them informed whether there is going to be one or more surgical procedures because such information will allow patients and their families prepare for this situation. Patients would also like to inquire how much time is expected to make them return to their full efficiency.

Our own experiences [4] indicate that patients' and parents' positive attitude towards operation, feeling influence upon this difficult situation and having confidence in doctors is extremely important. The study showed that patients who believed that they could help themselves endured the pain they experienced after the surgery better and they assessed it as lower when compared to those who declared that they had no influence on the situations in their lives. Such a correlation also applied to having trust in doctors and medical personnel as well as the trust that these people are able to help them. The vast majority of respondents judged that the mood a few weeks before the surgery had an effect on the one assessed several days after. People positively oriented to treatment felt much better after the surgery than those who assessed their mood before the operation as low.

Psychological support should always be provided to AIS patients, through group therapy as well as individual counseling, in order to promote disease and treatment acceptance and minimize psychological discomfort [27].

It is therefore legitimate to provide patients suffering from scoliosis and their families with the contact with a psychologist, especially in difficult stages of the illness (at the time of diagnosis, before operations, immediately after their completion, and in difficult situations). It is particularly worth working on gaining greater control over pain before the surgery which would allow to reduce the pain. Working on expressing one's emotions, especially anger which is a natural part of experiencing the disease as well as working on self-esteem, would also be very helpful [28].

It is concluded that patients with scoliosis and their families need to be provided with psychological support through the whole period of the treatment.[29] Patients and parents should make contact with a psychologist prior to orthopedic treatment in order to gain mutual trust before this difficult and stressful event. It is also important because a psychologist may notice additional family problems earlier (eg a child's emotional situation, family conflicts), or pay attention to the sensitivity of the patient. These are factors which can increase stress and anxiety associated with awaiting treatment.

Particularly important is the contact between the psychologist and the patient who will undergo surgical treatment. Both the patient and parents should be prepared for it. It would be very helpful if the patients were able to help relieve stress and pain by means of capability of positive thinking and relaxation techniques.

In case of very strong fear of the patient, the psychologist could have influence on the shift of operations, recognizing that the patient should be given more time to get familiar with this difficult situation.

Psychological help should be primarily based upon the support of the acceptance of the disease, the ways of its treatment as well as finding positives in this difficult situation. It is also important that patients and their parents should have the opportunity to request a psychologist's help in case of other difficulties that may arise in their lives.

A support group would be extremely beneficial (for people with scoliosis of both sexes), where patients could gain support from other patients, who were faced with similar problems and managed to overcome them.

It is generally discouraged that patients with scoliosis should have an individual course of learning. Such a situation (especially in case of learning from home) may increase the sense of lower self-esteem, and the feeling of isolation from the peer group.

2. References

[1] T, Edgar M, Margulies J. Etiology of Idiopathic Scoliosis: Current Trends in Research, J Bone Joint Surg Am. 2000;82(8):11571-157

[2] Lange J, Steen H ,Brox J. Long-term results after Boston brace treatment in adolescent idiopathic scoliosis, Scoliosis 2009, 4:17

[3] Janowska M, Tomaszewski R, Woś H. Psychologiczne aspekty operacyjnego leczenia skoliozy u młodzieży. Pediatria Polska 2008 ; 83, 4, 96

[4] Hall C., Lindzey G. Teorie osobowości. PWN. Warszawa 2002; :507

[5] Marc A, Lai M, Burton S, Manna D.The Reliability and Concurrent Validity of the Scoliosis Research Society-22 Patient Questionnaire for Idiopathic Scoliosis. 2003;28(1):63-69

[6] Sapountzi-Krepia D. Panteleakis G, Zangana D . Perceptions of body image, happiness and satisfaction in adolescents wearing a Boston brace for scoliosis treatment. Journal of Advanced Nursing,2001, 35(5): 683 690

[7] Rivett L, Rothberg A, Stewart A. The relationship between quality of life and compliance to a brace protocol in adolescents with idiopathic scoliosis: a comparative study. BMC Musculoskelet Disord. 2009; 10: 5.

[8] Misterska E, Glowacki M, Harasymczuk J.Personality characteristics of females with adolescent idiopathic scoliosis after brace or surgical treatment compared to healthy controls.Med Sci Monit. 2010 Dec;16(12): 606-15.

[9] Janowska M, Sobol G, Woś H, Samardakiewicz M, Barsow S, Sposoby przekazywania informacji o chorobie nowotworowej małym pacjentom. Lekarz 2006, 1-2/06

[10] Botens-Helmus C, Klein R, Stephan C. The reliability of the Sobernheim Stress Questionnaire (BSSQbrace) in adolescencts with scoliosis during brace treatment. Scoliosis 2006; 1:22.

[11] Vasiliadis E, Grivas TB, Savvidou O. The influence of Brace on Quality of Life of Adolescents with Idiopatic Scoliosis, Stud Health Technol Inform2006.123: 352-356

[12] Vasiliadis E, Grivas TB, Quality of life after conservative tratment of adolescent idiopatic scoliosis, Stud Health Technol Inform. 2008; 135:409-13

[13] Vasiliadis E, Grivas TB, Gkoltsiou K. Development and preliminary validation of Brace Questionnaire (BrQ):a new instrument for measuring quality of life of brace treated scoliotics.Scoliosis 2006;1:1-8

[14] Reichel D, Schanz J. Developmental psychological aspects of scoliosis treatment. Pediatric Rehabilitation, 2003; 6(3–4): 221–225

[15] Sapountzi-Krepia D, Psychogiou M, Peterson D. The experience of brace tratment in children/adolescents with scoliosis. Scoliosis 2006; 1:8.

[16] Payne W, Ogilvie J .Does Scoliosis Have a Psychological Impact and Does Gender Make a Difference?. Research Education Foundation. 1996;August 21.

[17] Ugwonali O, Lomas G, Choe J at all. Effect of bracing of the quality of life of adolescents with idiopathic scoliosis. The Spine Journal .2004;4: 254-260.

[18] Korovessis P, Zacharatos S, Koureas G.. Comparative multifactorial analysis of the effects of idiopathic adolescent scoliosis and Scheuermann kyphosis on the self-perceived health status of adolescents treated with brace. Eur Spine J. 2007 April; 16(4): 537–546.

[19] Mahood H Raso M, Lou J .Score distribution of the Scoliosis Quality of Life Index questionnaire in different subgroups of patients with adolescent idiopathic scoliosis. Spine ;2007 Jul 15;32(16):1767-77.

[20] Freidel K, Reichel D, Steiner A .Idiopathic scoliosis and quality of life. Stud Health Technol Inform. 2002;88:24

[21] Aulisa A , Guzzanti V,Perisano C .Determination of quality of life in adolescents with idiopathic scoliosis subjected to conservative treatment. Scoliosis. 2010; 5: 21.

[22] Skrzypek E. Tymczasowy podręcznik do testu jawnego niepokoju Jaki jesteś?. Pracownia Psychometryczna PAN. Warszawa 1968

[23] Khetani N, Donaldson S, Wright JG.What do patients and parents know about surgery for adolescent idiopathic scoliosis?: a knowledge questionnaire. Spine 2008 Sep 15;33(20):E754-8.

[24] Janowska M, Zwolińska-Karafioł B, Woś H. Moczenie mimowolne u dzieci a poziom neurotyzmu. Lekarz 2007, nr 4, s. 83-87

[25] Juczyński Z. Narzędzia pomiaru w promocji i psychologii zdrowia. Pracownia Testów Psychologicznych Polskiego Towarzystwa Psychologicznego. Warszawa 2001, s. 103

[26] Salisbury M, LaMontagne L, Hepworth J, Cohen F. Parents' self-identified stressors and coping strategies during adolescents' spinal surgery experiences .Clin Nurs Res. 2007 Aug;16(3):212-30.

[27] Chafetz R, Mulcahey M, Betz R, Impact of Prophylactic Thoracolumbosacral Orthosis Bracing on Functional Activities and Activities of Daily Living in the Pediatric Spinal Cord Injury Population. Spinal Cord Med. 2007; 30(1): 178–S183.

[28] Saccomani L, Vercellino F, Rizzo P, Becchetti S. Adolescents with scoliosis: psychological and psychopathological aspects. Minerva Pediatr. 1998 Jan-Feb;50(1-2):9-14.

[29] Bridwell K, Shufflebarger H, Lenke L, Parents' and Patients' Preferences and Concerns in Idiopathic Adolescent Scoliosis . Spine 25, (18): 2392–2399.

Section 5

The Patient's Perspective

18

Untreated Early Onset Scoliosis - The Natural Progression of a Debilitating and Ultimately Deadly Disease

Janez Mohar
Orthopaedic Hospital Valdoltra
Slovenia

1. Introduction

An early onset idiopathic scoliosis refers to idiopathic deformity that presents itself from birth to ten years of age and includes an infantile type (identified from birth to three years of age) and a juvenile type (identified from three to ten years of age). In contrast to adolescent idiopathic scoliosis (identified from ten years of age to the age of skeletal maturity), the juvenile idiopathic scoliosis patients, especially male, have a much higher risk of large curve development, since deformity occurs at a younger age and thus has a longer growth potential. Males are on average diagnosed earlier and become skeletally mature at a later age than females (Lenke & Dobbs, 2007). While some juvenile curves spontaneously regress, approximately 70% of them progress and ultimately require some form of treatment, either observation, orthotic management or surgical correction, with each treatment form being used at different Cobb angle intervals and progression landmarks. The absence of treatment for progressive early onset scoliosis usually results in severe adult idiopathic scoliosis, a condition that reduces quality of life, endangers general health and may ultimately lead to serious cardiopulmonary complications and premature death.

In the following text, describing and referencing a case of an adult patient with untreated early onset idiopathic scoliosis, I will try to summarise evidence-based facts and data regarding health related issues, natural progression and surgical management of untreated early onset and adolescent idiopathic scoliosis that results in severe adult deformity.

2. Living with spinal deformity - a lonely man's life story

A male was born in 1958 at a maternity ward with normal labour and delivery to a family of five, his father working as a farmer and mother as a housewife. At the age of eight his parents noticed his bad posture with a hump on his back and the referring paediatrician diagnosed him with idiopathic scoliosis. At the time of his first admission to an orthopaedic hospital's paediatric ward in 1966, the records show that his health status and chest radiograph of heart and lung were normal and that skeletal radiographs showed a right thoracic primary curve with a Cobb angle measuring 65° and severe vertebral torsion between the fourth and tenth thoracic vertebrae. The thoracic curve was flexible and corrected under Glisson traction harness to 36°. He was treated with scoliosis exercises and hard bed tractions and extensions daily as was customary at the time. After six months of treatment his thoracic curve Cobb angle measured 60° with curve correction under Glisson traction harness measuring 40°. After eight months of treatment he was discharged from the hospital and further treatment was to be continued after three months, yet records show no acceptance at the planned date. The reason for his non-attendance at follow-up was given by him during a later interview in which he described his mother's decision to stop his treatment due to difficult family circumstances after his father's death during his hospitalisation.

There is little medical history for this patient until the age of 51. He worked full-time as a furniture technologist and lived with his brother in an apartment block. In 2009 he was admitted to a general hospital's gastroenterological department because of three day duration melaena, resulting in hypocalcaemia and haemodynamically relevant normocytic anaemia. During hospitalisation, signs of chronic alcohol abuse with elevated liver enzymes, liver steatosis and predelirant syndrome became apparent. Oesophagogastroduodenoscopy revealed signs of reflux oesophagitis grade B, erosive antral gastritis and erosive bulbar duodenitis with a Forrest III duodenal ulcer, and antibiotic treatment was administered due to signs of acute bronchitis. In 2010 he visited an orthopaedic surgeon for back pain, originating from the left side of the thoracic spine and radiating to the area of posterior left hemithorax and left lumbar. He also had left hip and neck pain, and he complained about a four year duration of shortness of breath when walking short distances. Upon examination we found a short stature with obesity and severe kyphoscoliotic right thoracic deformity with left lumbar compensatory curve and normal neurologic status. His right thoracic rigid primary curve Cobb angle between Th4 and Th11 was 125° with the apex on Th8. There was also a kyphotic angulation with a Cobb angle of 70° between Th2 and Th10 with the apex on Th7 and a left lumbar compensatory scoliotic, slightly flexible curve with a Cobb angle of 75° between Th12 and L4 with the apex on the L2/L3 intervertebral disc. The deformity was classified according to the Lenke Classification System as type 3C+. Physical and radiological examination by a referred internal medicine physician revealed a generalised cyanosis, peripheral oedema, left basal lung wheezes and crackles, diminished right hemithoracic movements and breath sounds over the right lung field. Chest radiograph revealed a left shifted cardiac dilatation with signs of increased pulmonary vascular resistance on bilateral basal areas and the left lung field. Spirometric pulmonary function tests revealed a severe chronic combined obstructive-restrictive ventilatory disturbance, his ECG showed signs of right ventricular hypertrophy and blood laboratory tests revealed secondary polycythaemia with hypoxaemia, hypercapnia and compensated respiratory acidosis. Severe kyphoscoliotic deformity was found to be the cause of chronic respiratory hypoventilatory insufficiency, aggravated by a long-term smoking habit that resulted in right-sided decompensated heart failure. He was prescribed with bronchodilatators, diuretics and home oxygen therapy.

Shortly after he was admitted to our spinal surgery department for further preoperative imaging work-up and respiratory physical therapy. His pulmonary function tests were as follows: forced vital capacity (FVC) 0,71 litres (21%), forced expiratory volume in one second (FEV1) 1,039 litres (14%) and FEV1/FVC index 54% with arterial oxygen saturation of 89%. Echocardiographic examination revealed a right ventricle and atrium hypertrophy with tricuspid regurgitation (Fig. 1.).

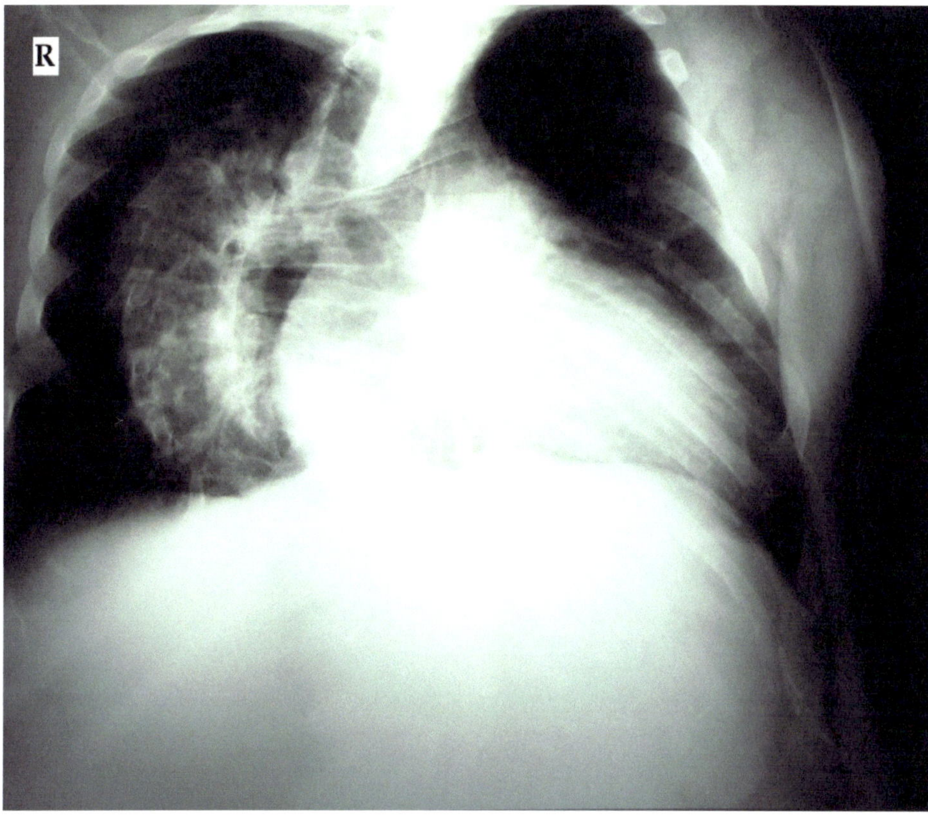

Fig. 1. Anteroposterior chest radiograph showing cardiac enlargement (cardiothoracic index measuring 60%) and severe right thoracic spinal column curvature.

The patient was scheduled for corrective deformity surgery but died at home in his sleep at the age of 52, shortly before his intended admittance to the hospital, due to a cardiorespiratory failure as a consequence of a severe combined obstructive-restrictive respiratory disease and pulmonary heart decompensation. No autopsy was performed.

3. Untreated idiopathic scoliosis - a spine surgeon's perspective

An untreated idiopathic scoliosis after skeletal maturity is one of spine surgeon's greatest challenges, because its three dimensional rigid deformity and patient's often decreased physiological reserve related to cardiopulmonary insufficiency, chronic pain and age present a complex multidisciplinary approach to solving the problem, where doing as little as needed to achieve the best possible overall result often contradicts our way of surgical thinking, accustomed to successfully treating young and generally healthy adolescents (Fig. 2.).

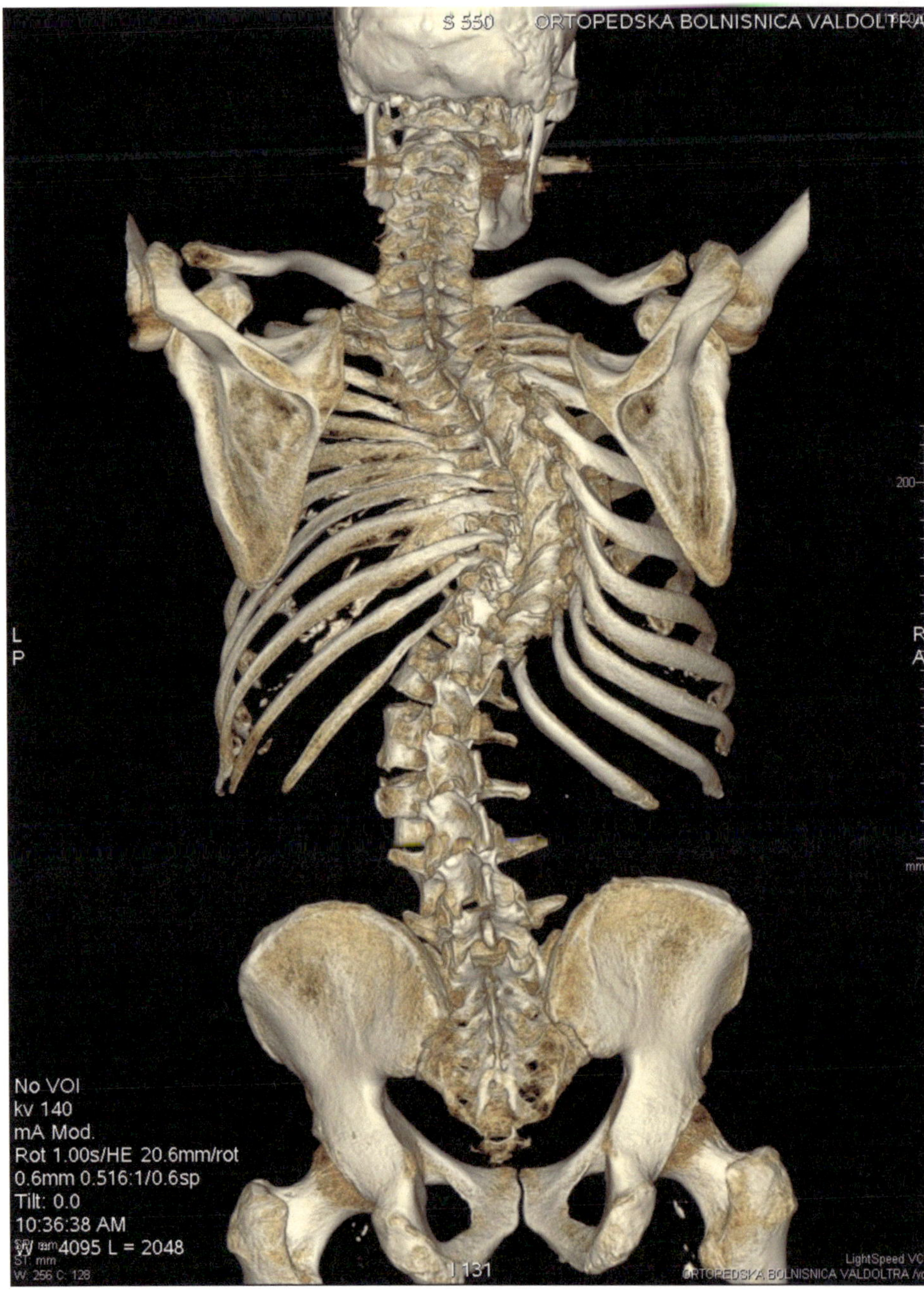

Fig. 2. 3D CT preoperative reconstruction of patient's deformity.

The decision on the proper method of surgical treatment is often based on personal experience with a demanding technique, awareness of conflicting evidence of complications and of short- to long-term results of these relatively rare spinal operations.

4. Mortality

An untreated idiopathic early onset scoliosis has a worse prognosis than late onset adolescent type as concluded in the long-term follow-up study of untreated idiopathic scoliosis patients (Nilsonne & Lundgren, 1968; Pehrsson et al., 1992). Both studies report significantly increased mortality from respiratory failure or cardiovascular diseases compared to the general population with increased risk of death after 40 years of age. Increased mortality was found in patients with infantile and juvenile scoliosis, but not in patients with adolescent scoliosis, although it cannot be said that adolescent type never causes death from cardiopulmonary failure (Asher & Burton, 2006). A mortality of untreated scoliosis is related to the severity of the curve. In a study by Pehrsson et al. from 1991 it was found that respiratory failure occurred only in patients with a predicted vital capacity (VC) of less than 45% and a curve greater than 110°, the findings being consistent with the knowledge of the influence of deformity on immature lung development and function, that is before the termination of growth of the number of alveoli until the age of eight years (Pehrsson et al., 1991). In a study by Rom and Miller, the authors surprisingly encountered ten patients over a four year interval with kyphoscoliotic curves greater than 100° who had survived into the seventh decade without clinically significant cardiorespiratory embarrassment, although they concluded that severe deformity is not compatible with a long and active life (Rom & Miller, 1978).

4.1 Health related issues

There is a number of lifelong health impairment issues related to the untreated adult idiopathic scoliosis. In a long-term follow-up and prognosis study of untreated patients suffering from idiopathic scoliosis, the authors analysed 194 patients who were seen at the University of Iowa between 1932 and 1948. In 69 of those patients pulmonary function studies were done with findings published in 1981 (Weinstein et al., 1981). They reported a significant correlation between reduction in VC and FEV1, and increasing severity of the curve only in patients with thoracic curves, yet a marked reduction and significant limitation of pulmonary function in the non-smokers did not occur until thoracic curve approached a Cobb angle of 100°. In the later follow-up study of the same baseline group of patients the authors concluded that a Cobb angle greater than 50° at skeletal maturity is a significant predictor of decreased pulmonary function (Weinstein et al., 2003). Shortness of breath seems to be the main symptom of decreased pulmonary function in adult idiopathic scoliosis patients, associated with thoracic and large double curves with wheezing being the indicator of a poor prognosis. The new evidence shows that decreased chest wall motion, resulting in decreased pulmonary function, also affects adult patients with relatively small curves and that pulmonary stress testing should be the diagnostic method of choice. The mechanics of breathing in patients with severe thoracic scoliosis is similar to that seen in normal subjects with increased ventilatory drive and in patients with advanced chronic obstructive pulmonary disease with a pattern of respiratory muscle activation being essentially an automatic response of the central respiratory controller (Estenne et al., 1998).

A restrictive ventilatory impairment, a reduction in dynamic pulmonary compliance with breathing against an increased load and an impaired diaphragmatic function in patients with severe thoracic scoliosis, results in a rapid and shallow breathing pattern with increased activation of abdominal muscles during the expiration phase that results in a higher end expiratory gastric pressure, which is associated more frequently with symptoms of a gastroesophageal reflux disease (Fig. 3.).

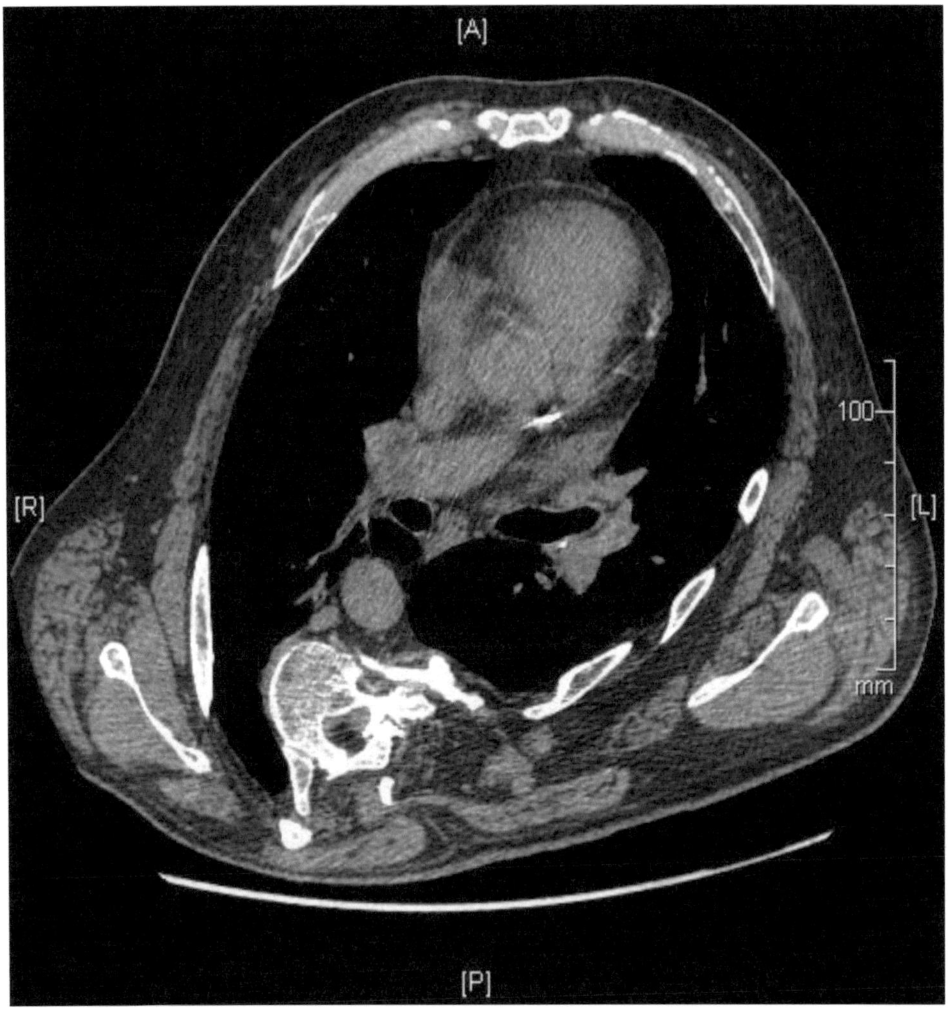

Fig. 3. Transthoracic axial CT image of a patient showing a marked rotation of a dysplastic thoracic vertebra, hypertrophic heart and decreased inflation of lung fields, occupying a reduced thoracic space.

The pathophysiological mechanism of respiratory impairment in spinal deformity follows a specific pattern; chest wall restriction results in a decreased VC and total lung capacity, tidal volume and flow rates are reduced in proportion to the reduction of VC. The ventilation-perfusion mismatch leads to hypoxaemia, resulting in active pulmonary vasoconstriction and hypercapnia secondary to alveolar hypoventilation with renal compensation of respiratory acidosis. Pulmonary vasoconstriction and pulmonary hypertension lead to right ventricular hypertrophy (cor pulmonale), ultimately resulting in right heart failure. An acute respiratory failure that usually follows an acute respiratory infection and right heart failure are thus the two most frequent causes of death in patients with untreated severe kyphoscoliotic deformity.

An increased risk of cardiovascular diseases has been reported among the population of untreated idiopathic scoliosis patients with systemic arterial hypertension being the most commonly overrepresented finding. There seems to be the same pathophysiological mechanism linkage of developing arterial hypertension among patients with obstructive sleep apnoea and night time hypoventilatory episodes with desaturations occurring in patients with severe scoliosis. There is also a higher incidence of congenital heart valve disease among the adult scoliotic population.

The prevalence of both acute and chronic back pain is more common among untreated scoliosis patients than among the general population, with symptoms rarely causing disability. The typical adult scoliotic patient's back pain is rarely severe, usually asymmetrical, often extravertebral and almost always disappears with rest. A long-term pain management programme is rarely needed. There seems to be no correlation between the type and the severity of the curve and back pain, except among patients with thoracolumbar curves, where a translatory shift of the vertebrae has been postulated as the cause, although Kostuik and Bentivoglio found an increasing prevalence and severity of pain with curves greater than 45° (Kostuik & Bentivoglio, 1981, as cited in Hu, 2006). It seems that double curves are least likely to be associated with increased pain. The more frequently reported site of back pain is on the convexity of the curve and in female patients the onset of back pain can be related to the first pregnancy. Lumbar radiculopathy can occur and appears to be confined to the concave side of the compensatory curves but other neurologic impairment is rare (Fig. 4.).

The knowledge of the impact of deformity on quality of life among adult patients with untreated idiopathic scoliosis is somewhat incomplete. Self-image is decreased, but less prevalent than among adolescent patients with idiopathic scoliosis. The frequency of mental health problems does not differ from the general population, although Ascani et al. in their uncontrolled analysis of a group of 187 patients with untreated idiopathic scoliosis and an average follow-up of 33.5 years found real psychological disturbances in 19% of cases, mostly women with thoracic curves greater than 40° (Ascani et al., 1986). Recent studies have showed that marriage and childbearing rates are not affected by adult idiopathic scoliosis to the threshold of relatively larger curves, although the Stockholm series in 1968 found 76% of female patients were unmarried. The authors of an Italian series study from 1986 concluded that the highest percentage of married patients was among those with thoracolumbar curves and the lowest percentage of unmarried patients was among women with thoracic curves. Adult idiopathic scoliosis does not affect employment rate or inability to work, although women with curves greater than 40° and patients with lumbar curves adapt less well to strenuous physical work.

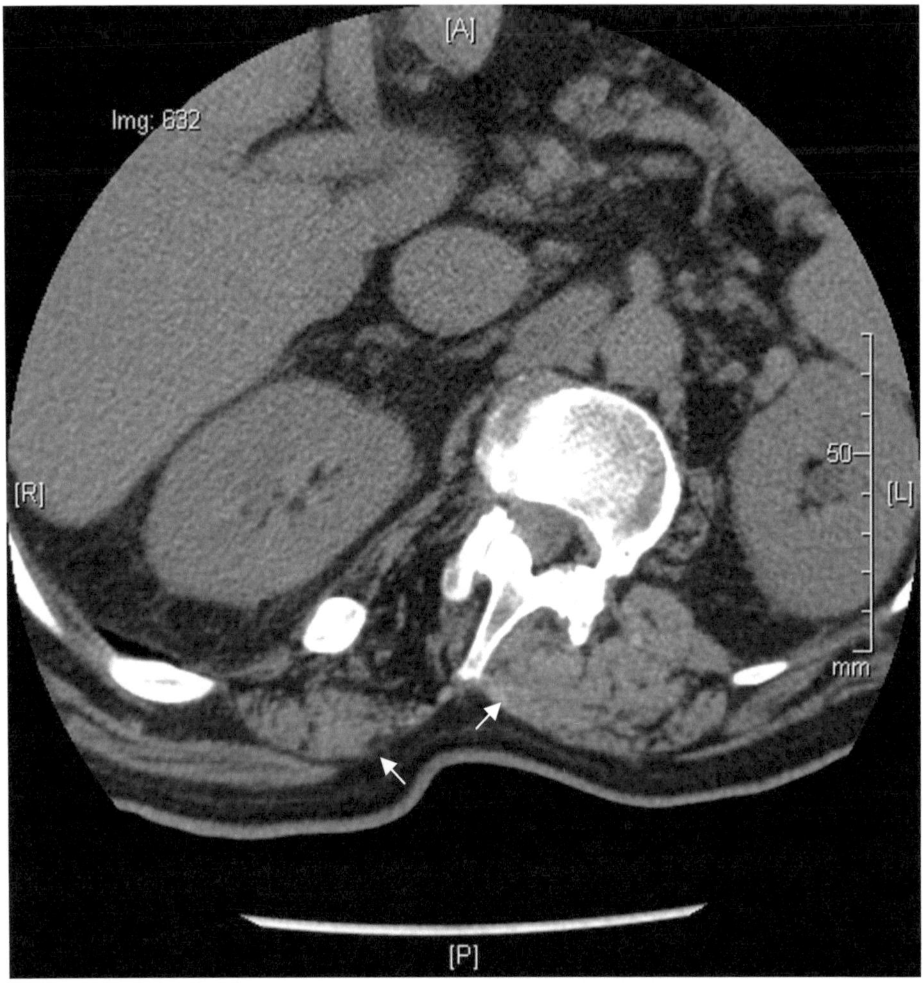

Fig. 4. Transabdominal axial CT image of a patient: notice a shift in abdominal organs due to vertebral rotation and asymmetry of paravertebral muscles (arrows).

4.2 Natural progression of deformity in adult idiopathic scoliosis

The progression of idiopathic scoliotic deformity after skeletal maturity depends on the type and severity of the curve. The threshold for progression seems to be a Cobb angle of 30°. Single thoracic curves between 50° and 80° are most likely to progress at an average of 0.73°/year with an additional risk factor for progression being the apical vertebral rotation of more than 30%. Another risk factor for progression is a translatory shift between two vertebral segments that usually takes place at the lower end of the curve or at the transitional vertebrae, most frequently in the thoracolumbar curves. The lumbar component of double major curves is more likely to progress than the thoracic component and right lumbar apex curves are twice as likely to progress than left apex lumbar curves. The lack of L5 deep seating and greater than 33% apical rotation in lumbar curves are also risk factors for progression. Table 1. shows a comparison between two groups of patients with untreated adult idiopathic scoliosis with regard to curve progression after skeletal maturity based on studies of by Weinstein et al. (2003) and Ascani et al. (1986).

			Iowa study group	Italian study group
No. of patients			117 (79 available for curve progression analysis)	187
Mean age			66 years	43 years, 7 months
Sex	Male		13 (11%)	36 (19.2%)
	Female		104 (89%)	151 (80.8%)
Average follow-up			51 years	33.5 years
Curve type	Thoracic		48 (41%)	74 (39.6%)
	Thoracolumbar		14 (12%)	29 (15.5%)
	Lumbar		32 (27%)	17 (9%)
	Double major		23 (20%)	67 (35.9%)
Average progression of curve by type	Thoracic		0.47° /year	0.47° /year
	Thoracolumbar		0.90° /year	0.40° /year
	Lumbar		0.28° /year	0.56° /year
	Double major	Thoracic component	0.26° /year	0.45° /year
		Lumbar component	0.31° /year	0.47° /year
Average progression of all types of curves combined			0.44° /year	0.47° /year
			0.46° /year	

Table 1. A comparison of demographic and curve progression data between two groups of patients with untreated adult idiopathic scoliosis.

The average progression of all types of curves combined is the same for both groups of patients, regardless of an age difference of approximately 20 years between groups, the conclusion being that the progression of the curve after skeletal maturity shows the same steady increase. Based on relevant literature findings, it is safe to conclude that the progression of any type of curve in idiopathic scoliosis after skeletal maturity rarely exceeds 1°/year, although there may be rare exceptions to this rule. In contrast with the findings shown in Table 1, other relevant literature suggests that thoracic curves tend to increase more than lumbar curves, lumbar curves more than thoracolumbar curves and thoracolumbar curves more than double major curves. Curves in untreated scoliotic women who have had one or more pregnancies progress somewhat more than curves in women with no pregnancies. Patients with discernible body alignment decompensation at the end of growth seem to improve with time.

During the 43 years since his last measurement, the Cobb angle of thoracic curve of the reported patient progressed from 60° to 125°, the average progression being therefore 1.5°/year, although this rate is exaggerated since most of the progression of the curve must have happened whilst growing up. Since we do not have radiographs from 1967, the measurement was taken from the patient's written records - we cannot asses the time of his skeletal maturity and progression of the curve until then.

4.3 The development of early onset idiopathic scoliosis surgery - from Harrington hook and rod instrumentation to modern-day operative techniques

In 1962 Dr. Paul R. Harrington published his results in treating idiopathic scoliosis by introducing a metal hook and rod system, and a major advance in the field of surgical management of spinal deformities was made. The original Harrington rod operated on a ratchet system, attached by hooks to the spine at the top and bottom of the curvature that, when cranked, would distract or straighten the curve. At the time of the reported patient's hospitalisation for his early onset idiopathic scoliosis, the corrective operations of spinal deformities with Harrington instrumentation were common in Slovenia, yet his termination of treatment and the lack of follow-up ruined his chances of leading a relatively healthy life. We can only speculate that the attending physician planned to continue conservative treatment with tractions and bracing until his adolescence, since the knowledge of the impact of spondylodesis on the growing spine (i.e. danger of developing a crankshaft phenomenon and loss of truncal height) was available at the time or that he would have been scheduled for repeated instrumented corrections until the right age for definitive fusion.

Long-term follow-up studies of patients, operated upon with Harrington instrumentation for juvenile and adolescent idiopathic scoliosis, report good general functioning compared with sex and age matched control groups. No significant differences in the single Scoliosis Research Society (SRS) Instrument domain scores between operated patients and control groups, no important impairment of health-related quality of life, no significant correlation between patient's self-reported outcome and preoperative curve magnitude or postoperative rate of correction and an overall high degree of long-term postoperative satisfaction were found (Dickson et al., 1990; Padua et al., 2001; Mariconda et al., 2005). Although Harrington instrumentation was historically a very successful system for treating juvenile and adolescent idiopathic scoliosis, some drawbacks and complications have been reported, namely some loss of correction after time, pseudoarthrosis and broken rods, no improvement of the rib hump with correction being achieved only in coronal plane, flat back syndrome and associated adjacent segment disease at the most caudad levels of fusion that may result in higher incidence of back pain and back fatigue. Despite these complications and the fact that differences in study designs do not allow for a direct comparison of long-term follow-up studies of untreated adult idiopathic scoliosis and studies of patients operated upon with Harrington instrumentation for idiopathic scoliosis, the reported patient would have undoubtedly led a very different life with regards to quality, health issues and life expectancy if he had been operated upon when young.

A preoperative plan for early onset idiopathic scoliosis has to include issues of expected postoperative loss of spinal height and limited growth of the thoracic cage, affecting lung development. The risk of developing a crankshaft phenomenon postoperatively can be prevented by the use of standard anterior and posterior fusion procedures, indicated for older juveniles or growing-rod posterior instrumentation systems, indicated for younger children in whom a diminished chest-wall growth and volume is a concern. The growing-rod posterior instrumentation systems include posterior growing single-rod and Luque trolley systems, dual growing-rod and hook/screw implant systems, McCarhty's Shilla technique of posterior apical growth arrest and fusion construct with proximal and distal non-locking screw to rod fixation and rib-to-rib or ribs-to-spine hybrid constructs, widely known for its use in surgical management of thoracic insufficiency syndromes.

For patients with a scoliotic Cobb angle of more than 80°, with or without thoracic or thoracolumbar kyphosis of more than 70°, a perioperative halo-gravity traction protocol is recommended: a six up to eight-pin halo frame is placed slightly below the equator of the skull just above the eyebrows and the cephalad portion of the earlobes under general anaesthesia with pins tightened to six to eight inch pounds of torque, the axial traction weight is applied in the upright position of the spine through the halo and gradually increased daily for two to twelve weeks with cranial nerve and extremity neurologic examinations performed every eight hours and radiographic improvement of deformity monitored weekly until 32% to 50% of body weight loading is reached (Rinella et al., 2005). The purpose of this protocol, which is particularly useful in patients with previous spine surgeries or intraspinal pathology, is a slow perioperative correction of severe and rigid deformities and improvement of sagittal and coronal alignment while at the same time maximization of cardiopulmonary function and nutritional status before a definitive anterior and/or posterior fusion is performed.

Growth modulation techniques are new procedures utilised for smaller deformities to avoid secondary manifestations of scoliosis. They include a convex intervertebral disc stapling technique, in which continued concave growth maintains or even corrects a deformity over time, and anterior tethering technique, in which a polypropylene tether, attached to the heads of the screws, placed in the vertebral bodies anteriorly, prevents motion of the spine only when bending away from the tether.

4.4 Adult idiopathic scoliosis - rethinking good luck in spinal deformity surgery

Surgical treatment of severe adult idiopathic scoliosis deformity always presents a challenge for spine surgeons, not just because of demands of technically difficult operations, but also because of a high-level mental processing during diagnostic and patient selection stages of treatment, postoperative addressing of frequent complications and a long rehabilitation process. As a rule, a multidisciplinary approach is used and the key to successful treatment outcome is proper patient selection, where the benefits of surgery outweigh the risks. The indications for surgery include: back pain failing conservative care, progressive leg pain or neurologic deficit, muscle fatigue secondary to spinal imbalance, curve progression, progressive pulmonary compromise secondary to deformity and severe deformity resulting in poor body image, with goals of surgery being: a decrease in pain, stability of the curve, cessation of progression of the curve and pulmonary compromise, and improvement of neurologic symptoms (Hu, 2006).

Adult idiopathic scoliosis surgery differs from adolescent idiopathic scoliosis in terms of higher rates of reported mortality and morbidity associated with complications. In its 2011 degenerative lumbar and major adult deformity analysis the SRS queried its morbidity and mortality multicentre, multisurgeon database for the year 2007, associated with 22,957 reported cases, 6,782 of them being adult scoliosis, and stratified it using the American Society of Anesthesiologists' (ASA) physical status classification (Fu et al., 2011). They found a 8.4% overall complication rate and complication rates for ASA Grades 1 through 5 being 5.4%, 9.0%, 14.4%, 20.3% and 50.0%, respectively with mortality rates being 0.03%, 0.1%, 0.3%, 2.2% and 33.3%, respectively. In the subgroup of adult patients with spinal deformity, morbidity and mortality rates for ASA Grades 1 through 4 were 10% and 0%, 16% and 0.2%, 22% and 0.7% and 31% and 4%, respectively. In its 2011 SRS Morbidity and Mortality of

Adult Scoliosis Surgery report, the same database was queried to identify 4,980 submitted cases of adult scoliosis, 2,425 of them being adult idiopathic scoliosis, from 2004 to 2007 in order to asses complication rates on the basis of type of scoliosis, age, use of osteotomy, revision surgery status and surgical approach (Sansur et al., 2011). The overall complication rate was 13.4% with the previously reported adolescent idiopathic scoliosis surgery complication rate being 5.7%, therefore supporting the notion that advanced age leads to increased risk for the development of complications. The most common complications were dural tears (2.9%), implant complications (1.6%), deep wound infections (1.5%), acute neurologic deficits (1.0%), superficial wound infections (0.9%), delayed neurologic deficits (0.5%), wound haematoma (0.4%), epidural haematoma (0.2%), pulmonary embolus (0.2%), deep venous thrombosis (0.2%) and sepsis (0.1%). Significantly higher complication rates were identified in osteotomies (particularly infections), revision surgery and combined anterior-posterior surgery with complication rates not being influenced by scoliosis type (degenerative vs. adult idiopathic scoliosis) or age (less than 60 years vs. greater than 60 years). The mortality rate was 0.3% associated with cardiopulmonary causes, sepsis and excessive blood loss with intraoperative death. The complication rates were greater in patients with higher ASA grades with infections, respiratory complications and haematomas demonstrating a 7-fold, an 8-fold and a 9-fold increase in rate, respectively when comparing ASA Grade 1 patients to ASA Grade 4 patients.

Surgical site infections seem to be one of the most frequent complications in adult spinal deformity surgery associated with long operation times that involve exposure at several levels and increased blood loss, resulting in higher morbidity, mortality and healthcare costs. A retrospective analysis of 830 adult patients with a mean age of 55.4 years who underwent surgery for kyphosis or scoliosis between 1996 and 2005 demonstrated a 5.5% overall surgical site infection rate (2% superficial and 3.5% deep to fascia) with risk factors being obesity and a history of prior surgical site infections warranting a separate drain in a subcutaneous layer and a modification in perioperative antibiotic prophylactic regimens (Pull ter Gunne et al., 2010). The increased subcutaneous fat layer in obesity increases retraction forces to provide exposure, leading to increased tissue necrosis while at the same time increased tissue thickness creates dead space between fascia and skin stitches. For combined anterior-posterior surgeries, staged procedures with exposure to two anaesthetics and a recovery period between two surgeries seem to have a higher infection rate than same-day procedures. Malnourishment in the recovery period is a particular risk factor for developing infections and other complications, therefore a total parenteral hyperalimentation and/or staging procedures over a longer period is warranted, allowing nutritional depletion recovery to baseline.

Other most frequently reported adult scoliosis surgery complications are residual pain (reported rates ranging from 5% to 15%), pseudoarthrosis with or without implant failure (reported rates ranging from 5% to 27 %), progressive spinal decompensation, postoperative non-resolving visual loss, delayed postoperative paraplegia attributed to ischaemia of the spinal cord from postoperative hypovolaemia and mechanical tension of spinal blood vessels on the concavity of the curve, syndrome of inappropriate antidiuretic hormone hypersecretion, pancreatitis, superior mesenteric artery syndrome, ileus, pneumothorax, haemothorax, chylothorax, lung atelectasis, pneumonia, fat embolism and urinary tract infections.

With reported increasing rates of complications with age for adults undergoing scoliosis surgery, the surgeon's and patient's decision for operation must be based on evidence-based reported outcomes. In its 2011 risk-benefit assessment of surgery for adult scoliosis, the SRS retrospectively reviewed its prospective, multicentre spinal deformity database and queried 206 patients, 86% of them having a history of untreated adolescent idiopathic scoliosis, who completed the Oswestry Disability Index (ODI), Short Form-12 (SF-12), Scoliosis Research Society (SRS-22) and Numerical Rating Scale (NRS) for back and leg pain questionnaires at two year follow-up (Smith et al., 2011). Adult scoliotic patients were distributed among age groups of 22 to 44 years, 45 to 64 years and 65 to 85 years, having perioperative complication rates of 17%, 42% and 71%, respectively, with elderly patients having greater disability, worse health status and more severe back and leg pain at baseline than younger patients. Decompression, osteotomy and pelvic fixation were more commonly performed in the surgical treatment of older patients with operating room time, blood loss and length of hospital stay being all significantly greater in the same group. At two year follow-up there were significant improvements in ODI, SRS-22 and NRS for back and leg pain within each age group and significant improvements in SF-12 among those aged 45 to 64 and 65 to 85. The authors concluded that these data demonstrate the potential benefits of surgical treatment for adult scoliosis and suggest that the elderly, despite facing the greatest risk of complications, may stand to gain a disproportionately greater improvement in disability and pain with surgery. They also stressed that occurrence of major complications with adult deformity surgery does result in a modest impact on general health status and that within the confines of appropriate practice and in the absence of significant progressive neurologic deficits, the ultimate management decision should typically be guided by patient choice. The question remains whether this also holds true for patients with progressive cardiopulmonary compromise facing surgery.

With these data in mind a rough preoperative assessment of mortality, complication rate and surgical benefits for the reported patient can be made. The patient was ASA Grade 4, therefore he would have a 4% mortality and a 31% complication probability with a probability for infections, respiratory complications, haematoma and trombembolic events being 8.2%, 3.2%, 0.9% and 1.1%, respectively. When stratified by patient age (≤60 years), type of scoliosis (idiopathic), use of osteotomy (yes), revision status (no revision) and surgical approach (posterior only) the patient would have a complication probability of 9.9%, 13.3%, 9.9% and 10.3%, respectively. Being obese the patient would have a significant probability for postoperative wound infection and by quoting Smith et al., his age group would represent a 42% overall probability for operative complications with probability for minor and major complications being 27% and 15%, respectively, although two years after surgery the expected improvement of disability, back pain and health status would be statistically significant. Based on presented statistical probabilities, an accurate overall probability for mortality, morbidity and improvement cannot be drawn because of the use of different statistical methods in the studies and therefore these values should serve simply as rough guidelines for surgeons, patients and health insurance companies. Major reconstructive surgery of deformities cannot be seen and understood from a strictly mathematical and technical point of view, for the nature of our trade deals with so many dependent and independent factors leading to different circumstances and finally outcomes that "artistic form" in its basic meaning may be a better term when trying to comprehend the unpredictable aspects of complex surgery.

Obtaining a solid fusion by providing rigid internal fixation while at the same time correcting curves and achieving spinal balance in the coronal and sagittal plane are the main goals of adult deformity surgery. Surgical planning in adult idiopathic scoliosis must address technical problems of adjacent segment degeneration and junctional kyphosis at the levels proximal to instrumented fusion, osteopenic bone requiring multiple fixation levels with hybrid systems of transpedicular screws, segmental hooks and/or sublaminar wires, rigidity of the curve requiring release procedures and/or osteotomies with emphasis on priority of achieving and maintaining coronal and sagittal balance to curve correction.

The technical possibilities of modern day spinal surgery allow a surgeon to correct and maintain correction and spinal balance in the most difficult triplanar deformities. It is usually the impact of corrective surgery on possible neurologic deficits and direct or indirect iatrogenous visceral damage that limits the degree of correction, warranting complex anaesthesia with perioperative neurovascular monitoring during the operation and extensive postoperative intensive care management during the recovery period. The danger of poor general health deterioration during and after the extreme physical stresses of prolonged and very invasive surgery is also an issue that demands modification of an otherwise technically feasible surgical plan. The surgical plan must address the issues of approach, levels of fusion, fixation techniques with the use of proper implant and instrumentation selection, spinal column and rib cage release and osteotomy techniques, proper deformity manipulation techniques together with construct manoeuvering and the use of optimal bone grafting methods with efficient bailout and conversion procedures available during every stage of operation in case of complications.

Controversy exists around using combined anterior and posterior approaches or just posterior approaches in correcting rigid spinal deformities, but the current trend is the use of safer posterior approaches that still allow the option of using several different osteotomy techniques. Combined approaches are used when addressing a multiple level rigid deformity requiring anterior release, anterior corpectomy and structural grafting, especially in thoracolumbar kyphoscoliosis for re-establishment of lumbar lordosis. The use of an open anterior approach in a high-risk patient with pulmonary compromise has its drawback in decreasing pulmonary function. In a prospective study on pulmonary function before and after anterior spinal surgery in adult idiopathic scoliosis, the authors found a long-term decrease in mean FVC of 0.21 litres in all patients and a decrease in mean FVC of 0.31 litres in patients who underwent anterior surgery without posterior surgery in spite of mean Cobb angle correction of 31% (Wong et al., 1996). They concluded that a deleterious effect on lung function in a combined approach appears to be more important than a mechanical benefit of correcting a curve, that posterior spinal surgery alone tends to have a beneficial effect on pulmonary function and that an anterior alone or a combined approach should not be undertaken to improve pulmonary function.

When addressing an adult deformity through posterior approach, three different osteotomy techniques; Smith-Petersen osteotomy (SPO), Pedicle Subtraction Osteotomy (PSO) and posterior Vertebral Column Resection (pVCR) are commonly used (Doward & Lenke, 2010). SPO is a posterior column osteotomy that includes a posterior release through facetectomy and re-alignment of the sagittal and/or coronal plane deformity through posterior instrumentation compression with a mobile disc serving as a fulcrum. With SPO, the degree of kyphotic correction is in the range of 9.3° to 10.7° per level or 1°/mm of bone resected and the technique, although providing the least correction of the three, can be used on multiple levels with reduction in operative time, blood loss, and risk of neurologic complications. A PSO or eggshell osteotomy involves a resection of the pedicles, decancellation of a wedge of the vertebral body via a transpedicular corridor and a posterior closing of the wedge through instrumented compression. The corrective power of a single PSO is roughly the amount of three SPOs, yet the average blood loss is nearly twice as much as three SPOs. Indications for a PSO include angular kyphosis, or if performed asymmetrically, angular scoliosis, significant sagittal imbalance and corrections at levels lacking anterior flexibility. The degree of kyphotic correction is on average of 32° at the operated level, making it a powerful single osteotomy technique, but with expected higher technical demands, operative times, blood loss and complication rates, especially neurologic deficits, than SPO. The most powerful and demanding of the three osteotomy techniques is pVCR, where after a posterior resection of the entire spinal level, the proximal and distal limbs are brought together and the curvature of the spine is corrected with the use of an interbody cage, acting as a fulcrum. The corrective power of a single pVCR can be as much as 100° in kyphoscoliotic cases. Indications for pVCR include sharp, angular kyphotic and/or scoliotic deformity in the thoracic and thoracolumbar spine, resection of hemivertebrae and intravertebral spinal tumours and shortening of the spine proximal to a tethered region. The prevalence of complications when using pVCR is significant with longer operative times and increased blood loss.

The aim of treatment in the reported high-risk patient was the retainment or at best improvement of pulmonary function with correction of kyphotic and, to a moderate degree, thoracic scoliotic curve while at the same time enabling a good body balance by correcting the somewhat flexible lumbar scoliotic curve. The preoperative plan consisted of a three week halo traction, respiratory physical therapy and hyperalimentation after which a neurovascular monitored, all posterior approach would be performed with laminar hook placement from Th1 to Th4 and pedicle screw insertion from Th9 to L4 vertebrae. The rib release on the apical concave side of the curve would be performed next, followed by an asymmetrical triple SPO at Th6/7, Th7/8 and Th8/9 motion segment. A concave side distraction, a convex side compression and a derotation manoeuvre over a contoured rod would follow after which a pelvic cancellous and posterior element cancellous and cortical autograft would be placed on decorticated laminae and a standard wound closure would complete the operation. The patient would be mobilised within 24 to 48 hours in an intensive care unit and a custom thoracolumbosacral orthosis would be fitted in the following days. He would receive respiratory and orthopaedic physical therapy once moved to the ward and would be discharged from the hospital when physically independent, with follow-up visits scheduled one, three and six months after discharge, yet the potential success of this kind of treatment plan would sadly never be known.

5. Conclusion

Early and late onset idiopathic scoliosis, although treatable either by observation and exercises, bracing or surgery may become a serious health concern if left untreated. In modern health care systems with proper screening programmes of school age children and adolescents, the probability for missed cases and development of adult idiopathic scoliosis is low. School screening is not only an instrument for early detection and decrease in the number of patients who will eventually experience operative treatment, but it is also an indispensible tool for research on scoliosis aetiology (Grivas et al., 2007). There is great diversity in the policies for scoliosis screening worldwide and between different professional associations, e.g., The American Academy of Orthopedic Surgeons recommends screening girls at ages 11 and 13, and screening boys at 13 or 14 years of age and The American Academy of Pediatrics recommends scoliosis screening with the Adam's forward bending test at routine health visits at 10, 12, 14 and 16 years of age. Still, with rare patients not responding to follow-up visits, as was the case with the reported patient, migration of people from rural to urban areas and immigration of people from developing and underdeveloped countries as a result of globalisation, a spine surgeon must expect to see and treat difficult cases of adult idiopathic deformity.

Early onset idiopathic, compared to late onset scoliosis has a worse prognosis if left untreated because of larger curve development potential and increased mortality risk from cardiopulmonary failure, related to severity of the curve. Patients with untreated adult idiopathic scoliosis have a decreased pulmonary function, especially those with a Cobb angle greater than 50° at skeletal maturity. They have an increased risk of cardiovascular diseases and they have a higher frequency of back pain compared to the general population. Adult idiopathic scoliosis, with the exception of severe curves, does not affect marriage and childbearing, mental health and employment rate or inability to work. The progression of idiopathic scoliotic deformity after skeletal maturity shows a steady increase of less than 1°/year in the majority of cases and single thoracic curves between 50° and 80° are most likely to progress with body alignment decompensation at the end of growth improving with time.

Surgical treatment of severe adult idiopathic scoliosis deformity is technically demanding, has high rates of reported mortality and morbidity and should therefore be reserved only for experienced spine surgeons. The complication rates are strongly correlated to ASA grades, advancing age, osteotomies, revision surgery and combined anterior-posterior approaches, but possible benefits for surgical treatment are great, especially among the elderly. In a modern tertiary health care service setting with the use of multidisciplinary diagnostic and supportive treatment options, intraoperative neurovascular monitoring and safer posterior osteotomy and instrumentation techniques, the possibilities of reducing risk and increasing the success rates of these challenging procedures are improving.

6. Acknowledgement

The author would like to thank F. Bizjak, MD†, B. Pavlin, MD, MSc, N. Hero, MD, MSc, R. Kramar, MD and R. J. Cirman, MD, MSc for their lifelong commitment to treating spinal deformities, without whose efforts the Department of Spinal Surgery and Paediatric Orthopaedics at the Orthopaedic Hospital Valdoltra would not be as it is today.

7. References

Ascani, E., Bartolozzi, P., Logroscino, C.A., Marchetti, P.G., Ponte, A., Savini, R., Travaglini, F., Binazzi, R. & Di Silvestre, M. (1976). Natural history of untreated idiopathic scoliosis after skeletal maturity. *Spine*, Vol.11, No.8, (October 1986), pp. 784-789, ISSN 0362-2436

Asher, M.A. & Burton, D.C. (March 2006). Adolescent idiopathic scoliosis: natural history and long term treatment effects, In: *Scoliosis*, 31.03.2006, Available from http://www.scoliosisjournal.com/content/1/1/2

Dickson, J.H., Erwin, W.D. & Rossi, D. (1889). Harrington instrumentation and arthrodesis for idiopathic scoliosis. A twenty-one-year follow-up. *J Bone Joint Surg Am.*, Vol.72, No.5, (June 1990), pp. 678-683, ISSN 1535-1386

Dorward, I.G. & Lenke, L.G. (1996). Osteotomies in the posterior-only treatment of complex adult spinal deformity: a comparative review. *Neurosurg Focus*, Vol.28, No.3:E4, (March 2010), pp. 1-10, ISSN 1092-0684

Estenne, M., Derom, E. & De Troyer, A. (1987). Neck and abdominal muscle activity in patients with severe thoracic scoliosis. *Am J Respir Crit Care Med.*, Vol.158, No.2, (August 1998), pp. 452-457, ISSN 1073-449X

Fu, K.M., Smith, J.S., Polly, D.W.Jr., Ames, C.P., Berven, S.H., Perra, J.H., McCarthy, R.E., Knapp, D.R.Jr., Shaffrey, C.I. & The Scoliosis Research Society Morbidity and Mortality Committee (1999). Correlation of higher preoperative American Society of Anesthesiology grade and increased morbidity and mortality rates in patients undergoing spine surgery. *J Neurosurg Spine*, Vol.14, No.4, (April 2011), pp. 470-474, ISSN 0022-3085

Grivas, T.B., Wade, M.H., Negrini, S., O'Brien, J.P., Maruyama, T., Hawes, M.C., Rigo, M., Weiss, H.R., Kotwicki, T., Vasiliadis, E.S., Sulam, L.N. & Neuhous, T. (November 2007). SOSORT consensus paper: school screening for scoliosis. Where are we today?, In: *Scoliosis*, 26.11.2007, Available from http://scoliosisjournal.com/content/2/1/17

Hu, SS. (2006). Adult scoliosis, In: *Rothman-Simeone The Spine*, H.N. Herkowitz, S.R. Garfin, F.J. Eismont, G.R. Bell, R.A. Balderston, (Ed.), pp. 1046-1057, Saunders Elsevier, ISBN 978-0-7216-4777-7, Philadelphia, Pennsylvania, USA

Lenke, L.G. & Dobbs, M.B. (1889). Management of juvenile idiopathic scoliosis. *J Bone Joint Surg Am.*, Vol.89, No.1, Suppl.1, (February 2007), pp. 55-63, ISSN 1535-1386

Mariconda, M., Galasso, O., Barca, P. & Milano, C. (1992). Minimum 20-year follow-up results of Harrington rod fusion for idiopathic scoliosis. *Eur Spine J.*, Vol.14, No.9, (November 2005), pp. 854-861, ISSN 0940-6719

Nilsonne, U. & Lundgren, KD. (1930). Long-term prognosis in idiopathic scoliosis. *Acta Orthop Scand.*, Vol.39, No.4, (1968), pp. 456-465, ISSN 0001-6470

Padua, R., Padua, S., Aulisa, L., Ceccarelli, E., Padua, L., Romanini, E., Zanoli, G. & Campi, A. (1976). Patient outcomes after Harrington instrumentation for idiopathic scoliosis: a 15- to 28-year evaluation. *Spine*, Vol.26, No.11, (June 2001), pp. 1268-1273, ISSN 0362-2436

Pehrsson, K., Bake, B., Larsson, S. & Nachemson, A. (1946). Lung function in adult idiopathic scoliosis: a 20 year follow up. *Thorax*, Vol.46, No.7, (July 1991), pp. 474-478, ISSN 0040-6376

Pehrsson, K., Larsson, S., Oden, A. & Nachemson, A. (1976). Long-term follow-up of patients with untreated scoliosis. A study of mortality, causes of death, and symptoms. *Spine*, Vol.17, No.9, (September 1992), pp. 1091-1096, ISSN 0362-2436

Pull ter Gunne, A.F., van Laarhoven, C.J. & Cohen, D.B. (1992). Incidence of surgical site infection following adult spinal deformity surgery: an analysis of patient risk. *Eur Spine J.*, Vol.19, No.6, (June 2010), pp. 982-988, ISSN 0940-6719

Rinella, A., Lenke, L., Whitaker, C., Kim, Y., Park, SS., Peelle, M., Edwards, C. 2nd & Bridwell, K. (1976). Perioperative halo-gravity traction in the treatment of severe scoliosis and kyphosis. *Spine*, Vol.30, No.4, (February 2005), pp. 475-482, ISSN 0362-2436

Rom, W.N. & Miller, A. (1946). Unexpected longevity in patients with severe kyphoscoliosis. *Thorax*, Vol.33, No.1, (February 1978), pp. 106-110, ISSN 0040-6376

Sansur, C.A., Smith, J.S., Coe, J.D., Glassman, S.D., Berven, S.H., Polly, D.W.Jr., Perra, J.H., Boachie-Adjei, O. & Shaffrey, C.I. (1976). Scoliosis research society morbidity and mortality of adult scoliosis surgery. *Spine*, Vol.36, No.9, (April 2011), pp. 593-597, ISSN 0362-2436

Smith, J.S., Shaffrey, C.I., Glassman, S.D., Berven, S.H., Schwab, F.J., Hamill, C.L., Horton, W.C., Ondra, S.L., Sansur, C.A., Bridwell, K.H, & the Spinal Deformity Study Group. (1976). Risk-benefit assessment of surgery for adult scoliosis: an analysis based on patient age. *Spine*, Vol.36, No.10, (May 2011), pp. 817-824, ISSN 0362-2436

Weinstein, S.L., Zavala, D.C. & Ponseti, I.V. (1889). Idiopathic scoliosis: long-term follow-up and prognosis in untreated patients. *J Bone Joint Surg Am.*, Vol.63, No.5, (June 1981), pp. 702-712, ISSN 1535-1386

Weinstein, S.L., Dolan, L.A., Spratt, K.F., Peterson, K.K., Spoonamore, M.J. & Ponseti, I.V. (1883). Health and function of patients with untreated idiopathic scoliosis: a 50-year natural history study. *JAMA*, Vol.289, No.5, (February 2003), pp. 559-567, ISSN 0098-7484

Wong, C.A., Cole, A.A., Watson, L., Webb, J.K., Johnston, I.D. & Kinnear, W.J. (1946). Pulmonary function before and after anterior spinal surgery in adult idiopathic scoliosis. *Thorax*, Vol.51, No.5, (May 1996), pp. 534-536, ISSN 0040-6376

Section 6

Congenital Scoliosis

Congenital Kyphoscoliosis Due to Hemivertebra Treatment Options and Results

Andrés Chahin Ferreyra and Gonzalo Arriagada Ocampo
Spine Center Clinica Las Condes
University of Chile
Chile

1. Introduction

The clinical impact of congenital vertebral malformations is variable and depends mainly on the type of spinal malformation and the location of this (McMaster & Ohtsuka, 1982). Defects of formation, segmentation and combination of these presents different rates of progression and final severity of the deformity.

The natural history of congenital kyphoscoliosis has been well documented and shows that most of untreated patients progress to severe deformities (Winter et al., 1968) (Figure 1), and may even present neurological compromise (McMaster & Singh, 1999).

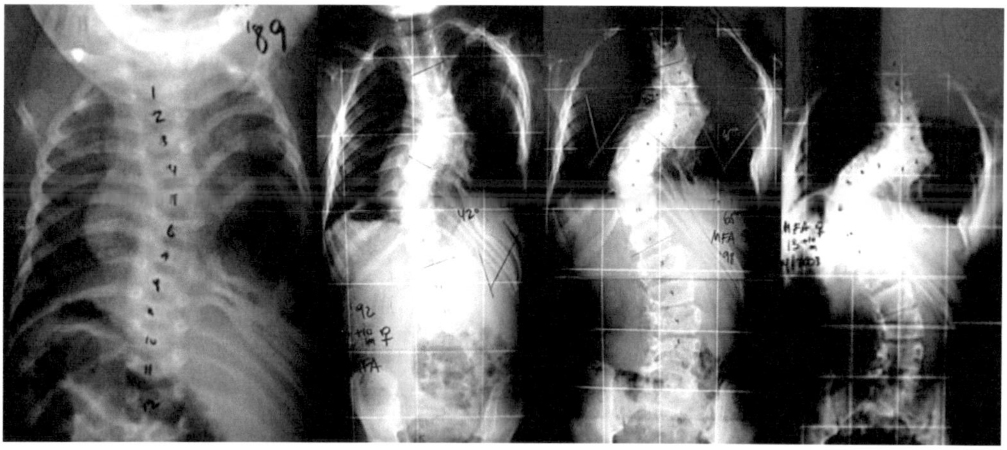

Fig. 1. Natural history of congenital spinal deformity from the newborn period to 13 years of age.

Not been defined the best surgical treatment for hemivertebra deformity. Surgical treatments described include: "in situ" fusion, convex hemiepiphysiodesis and hemiartrhodesis and hemivertebra resection.

The "in situ" fusion and convex hemiepiphysiodesis and hemiartrhodesis have limited effectiveness and unpredictable results in terms of halting the progression and correction of the deformity. Resection of the hemivertebra appears as a surgical alternative that allows to stop the progression of the curve and correct the deformity.

2. Etiology

Congenital kyphoscoliosis is defined as spinal deformity present at birth due to abnormal vertebral development.

Congenital spine malformations are produced by defects in somitogenesis during the embryonic development comprised between 5 and 8 weeks of gestation (Kusumi & Turnpenny, 2007). Are frequently associated with cardiac, urologic and respiratory abnormalities in up to 60% of cases (Basu et al., 2002; Beals et al., 1993), and also to neural axis abnormalities in up to 38% of cases (Basu et al., 2002; Bradford et al., 1991).

The exact cause of congenital vertebral malformations is unknown, however, many experimental studies in animals suggest that maternal exposure to various noxas (carbon monoxide, smoking, alcohol, valproic acid, etc.) during this critical period of embryonic development can lead to defects in the development of the spine (Hensinger, 2009).

There is no hereditary pattern in the development of vertebral malformations, however, has been identified specific genetic abnormalities which are associated with development of spondylothoracic dysplasia and Alagille syndrome (Bulman et al., 2000; Erol et al., 2004).

Current evidence suggests that both environmental and genetic factors were involved in the development of the spinal malformations.

3. Classification

Vertebral congenital anomalies are classified as defects of formation (hemivertebra, wedge vertebra), segmentation defects (bars, block vertebra) and mixed (bar with contralateral hemivertebra).

The hemivertebra is a defect of formation and according to the presence or absence of adjacent intervertebral discs, can be classified as fully segmented, partially segmented or unsegmented (Putti, 1910, as cited in Winter & Lonstein, 2010) (Figures 2 - 3).

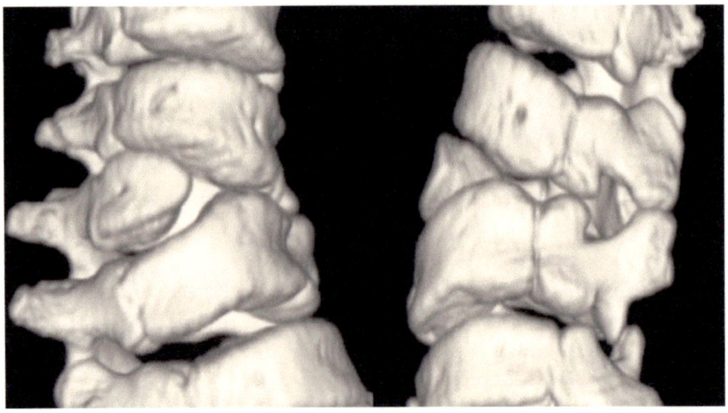

Fig. 2. 3D CT scan reconstruction of fully segmented hemivertebra.

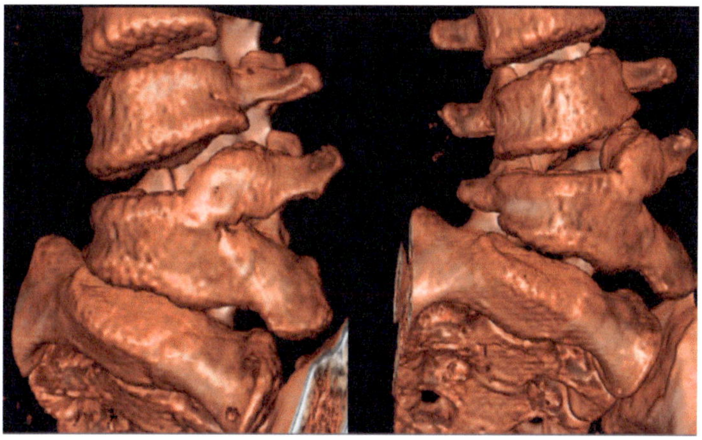

Fig. 3. 3D CT scan reconstruction of partially segmented hemivertebra.

On the other hand, according to its alignment and relationship with the rest of the spine can be classified as "incarcerated", if it maintains the pedicle alignment without protrudes vertebral contour, or as "non incarcerated", if it loses the pedicle alignment and protrudes vertebral contour (McMaster & Ohtsuka, 1982).

4. Epidemiology

The exact prevalence of congenital vertebral malformations is unknown but was estimated at 1 per 1000 live births (Giampietro et al., 2003). The incidence of hemivertebra reaches 0.125% at 12000 antenatal ultrasonography (Freeman et al., 2001).

The deformity secondary to vertebral malformation can alter the sagittal and coronal plane, being congenital kyphosis and lordosis much less common than congenital scoliosis, which includes 80% of cases (McMaster & Ohtsuka, 1982; Winter et al., 1968).

The hemivertebra is the most common spinal malformation present in 35% to 45% of congenital kyphoscoliosis (McMaster & Ohtsuka, 1982; Mohanty & Kumar, 2000).

In relation to the types of hemivertebra, McMaster & David, in their study of 154 hemivertebra found 65% fully segmented hemivertebra, 22% partially segmented and 12% unsegmented (McMaster & David, 1986).

5. Natural history

The natural history of congenital kyphoscoliosis is well known, however, due to the large variability of vertebral malformations present in the congenital kyphoscoliosis is not possible to accurately predict the risk of progression. Several studies conclude that 25% of congenital kyphoscoliosis not progress, 25% presents moderate progress and 50% presents severe progress requiring surgical resolution (McMaster & Ohtsuka, 1982).

The degree of scoliosis produced by hemivertebra depends on following 4 factors (McMaster & David, 1986):

Type of hemivertebra: segmented and non incarcerated hemivertebra progress to most severe deformities.

Location: location of the hemivertebra in transitional zones between mobile segments and less mobile or fixed segments (cervicothoracic, thoracolumbar and lumbosacral) determines a greater trunk imbalance and clinically visible deformities, developing shoulders asymmetry and pelvic obliquity in cases of high thoracic and lumbosacral hemivertebra, respectively (Figure 4).

Number of hemivertebra and its relationship: contralateral hemivertebra in the same area of the spine tend to generate compensatory curves and less severe deformities unlike hemivertebra located in different areas of the spine and hemivertebra located ipsilaterally (Figure 5).

Age of patient: the first 5 years of life and puberty are the 2 periods of rapid growth of the spine where the deformity may progress rapidly (Dimeglio, 2001).

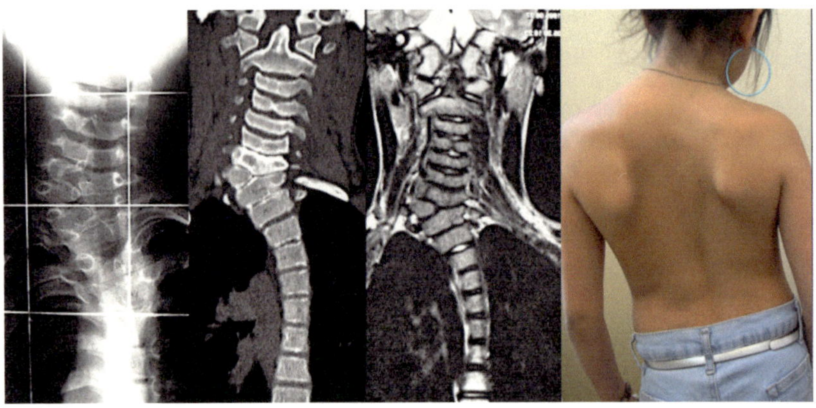

Fig. 4. 12 year old girl with T1 hemivertebra, note the important deformity and trunk imbalance due to his location in cervicothoracic transitional zone.

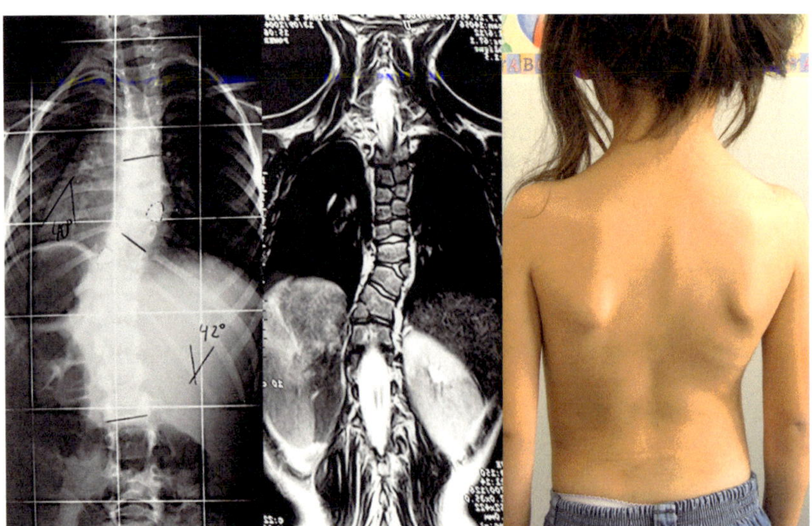

Fig. 5. 5 year old girl with balanced congenital deformity, multiple butterfly vertebra in the upper toracic spine and opposite side hemivertebra in T9 and T11.

The hemivertebra associated with contralateral bar has the worst prognosis of progression (5 to 10 degrees/year) followed by two unilateral hemivertebra (2 to 5 degrees/year), single fully segmented hemivertebra (1 to 3 degrees/year) and wedge vertebra (1 to 2 degrees/year) (McMaster & Ohtsuka, 1982) (Table 1).

Type of formation failiure	Rate of progression
Hemivertebra with contralateral bar	5 to 10 degrees/year
Two unilateral hemivertebra	2 to 5 degrees/year
Single fully segmented hemivertebra	1 to 3 degrees/year
Wedge vertebra	1 to 2 degrees/year

Table 1. Formation defects progression.

In relation to specific types of hemivertebrae and curve magnitude at the end of growth, unsegmented incarcerated hemivertebra never progresses beyond 30 degrees, partially segmented hemivertebra progresses to angular values that do not exceed 40 degrees and fully segmented hemivertebra progresses to values higher than 40 degrees.

Studies about natural history of congenital scoliosis due to hemivertebra confirm the progressive course of the deformity, with curves above 40 degrees at skeletal maturity in 64% to 84% of cases (McMaster & Ohtsuka, 1982; McMaster & David, 1986).

6. Treatment options

Each patient with kyphoscoliosis due to hemivertebra is unique, therefore, the choice of treatment will be based on the risk of curve progression during growth.

Conservative treatment, based on observation and brace has proved ineffective in the control of curve progression, often requiring surgical resolution. As mentioned above, most congenital kyphoscoliosis due to hemivertebra require surgery to prevent the development of severe deformities.

The key is the early detection of the deformity and early surgical management to prevent secondary curves progress and avoid to become structural, preventing the development of severe deformities wich requires complex surgeries and extensive spinal fusion.

Classically it describes three surgical procedures: "in situ" fusion , whose aim is to stop curve progression without correction of this, convex hemiepiphysiodesis and hemiartrhodesis, which aims to halt the progression and achieve gradual correction deformity at the time, and finally, hemivertebra resection which aim is to stop the progression, correction of the curve acutely and prevent the development of secondary curves.

6.1 Conservative treatment

Periodic monitoring is indicated only in patients with clinical and radiographic balanced and non progressive deformities.

Brace has no place in the treatment of congenital kyphoscolisis, only have some utility in the control of secondary curves in selected cases.

6.2 Surgical treatment

The goals of surgical treatment are to achieve a solid fusion to stop the progression of the curve, and reach the end of growth with a spine properly aligned and well balanced.

There are 2 categories of surgical procedures; prophylactic surgery and corrective surgery. Prophylactic surgeries are intended to prevent progression of curve ("in situ" fusion) or gradual correction of curve across the time (hemiepiphyisiodesis). On the other hand, the corrective procedures aim to correct the deformity and prevent the development of secondary curves (hemivertebra resection).

Surgical treatment should be early and ideally should be performed before 5 years of age.

The incorporation and use of instrumentation in young children, especially the use of pedicle screws, is one of the most important advances in recent years. Its proven efficacy and safety, have made the outcomes of different surgical techniques are progressively better and with fewer complications related to the use of implants (Hedequist et al., 2004; Ruf & Harms, 2002).

6.2.1 “In situ” fusion

Cataloged in prophylactic surgical procedures, "in situ" fusion is the oldest surgical strategy for treatment of congenital kyphoscolisis. It corresponds to fusion of a short spinal segment includes vertebral malformation, preserving spinal mobility without significant compromise on the length of the spine at the end of growth.

Patients without or minimal deformity, but with malformations whose progression is virtually assured (fully segmented hemivertebra, hemivertebra with contralateral bar) are the best candidates for this surgery (McMaster & David, 1986; Winter & Moe, 1982).

Classically "in situ" fusion was described by a unique posterior approach without instrumentation associated with the use of corrective brace. Has been described a posterior approach and combined anterior and posterior approach with or without instrumentation

The long-term follow-up showed a high rate of progression attributed to the presence of a flexible callus, present in 39% of patients with remaining growth (Winter & Moe, 1982), and the crankshaft phenomenon, present in 15% of total patients and in 36% of patients younger than 4 years (Kesling et al., 2003).

Patients with anterior growth potential require a anterior or combined approach to prevent the development of the crankshaft phenomenon. In cases of congenital lordosis, anterior fusion is the key to preventing the progression of the deformity, unlike the cases of congenital kyphosis, where the exclusive posterior approach and posterior fusion preserving the anterior spinal growth allow gradual correction of the deformity (Winter et al., 1996).

The use of instrumentation has been shown to improve fusion rates and the degree of curve correction, with a low rate of complications associated with the use of implants (Hedequist et al., 2004), however, this does not result in a significant improvement in long-term clinical outcomes (Farley et al., 2011).

The results of this surgical strategy remain unpredictable with incidence rates of progression after surgery ranging from 11% to 42% of cases. Goldberg et al. indicate that of 43 patients underwent fusion "in situ", 25.6% required reoperation for unacceptable progression of curve (Goldberg et al., 2002), a rate that does not differ from the rate of surgeries presented in natural history studies of Mc Master (McMaster & Ohtsuka, 1982; McMaster & David, 1986), and suggests that this procedure would be ineffective in the management of congenital kyphoscoliosis, and it does not modify the natural history of the disease.

Today this technique is practically abandoned because of the inability to control the progression of the curve, the high rate of reoperations and poor clinical outcomes in the long-term follow-up.

6.2.2 Convex hemiepiphysiodesis and hemiartrhodesis

Considered in prophylactic surgery, the goal is to halt the growth of the convexity of the curve and maintain growth of the concavity achieving theoretically the gradual correction of the deformity. It is imperative that the patient have growth potential in the concavity of curve, therefore that surgery is reserved for formation vertebral defects and should be performed early, before 5 years of age.

Is recommended with curves under 50 degrees, because curves greater than 50 degrees have higher incidence of fusion.

The classic indication is patient with fully segmented hemivertebra without other spinal malformation.

Requires combined anterior and posterior approaches to prevent development of deformities in the sagittal plane. The anterior hemiepiphysiodesis involves removing 1/3 of the intervertebral disc and its corresponding vertebral endplates and fuse them, and the posterior hemiarthrodesis involves the exclusive convex side exposure and its fusion with or without instrumentation (Shen, F. & Arlet, V 2008)

The anterior hemiepiphysiodesis may be made by classic combined open anterior and posterior approaches, endoscopic or transpedicular posterior approach.

We do not recommend this technique when deformity have a major kyphotic component, because the growth of the posterior elements of the concavity may generate significant progression of the deformity in the sagittal plane in 36% of cases (Cil et al., 2004).

Uzumcugil et al. in a review of different series of patients treated with convex hemiepiphysiodesis and hemiarthrodesis notes that the hemiepiphisiodesis effect is achieved in 20% to 77% of cases, fusion effect in 17% to 70% and progression in the 0% to 21%, demonstrating that this technique results are unpredictable (Uzumcugil et al., 2004). In cases where hemiepiphisiodesis effect is achieved, the average curve correction does not exceed 15 to 20 degrees (Winter & Lonstein, 1988).

The overall results of this technique are variable and unpredictable, however, this technique has a low complication rate, virtually only related to anterior approaches.

6.2.3 Hemivertebra resection

The first report of resection of hemivertebra was made by Royle in 1928. Despite the high rate of complications and initial technical difficulties, has gradually incorporated as a valid surgical alternative.

The aim is to remove the source of the deformity, correction of the curve and prevent the development of secondary curves.

Currently considered the method of choice for the treatment of congenital kyphoscoliosis secondary to isolated hemivertebra.

The best indication of hemivertebra resection is: patients younger than 5 years with thoracolumbar, lumbar or lumbosacral hemivertebra associated to initial trunk imbalance.

Classically hemivertebra resection was described by combined anterior and posterior approach in 1 or 2 stages. Also have been reported simultaneous anterior/posterior approaches.

Posterior exclusive approaches have become popular. Traditional or classic vertebral resection or eggshell techinque are the surgical options described for the posterior vertebral excision (Figure 6 - 7).

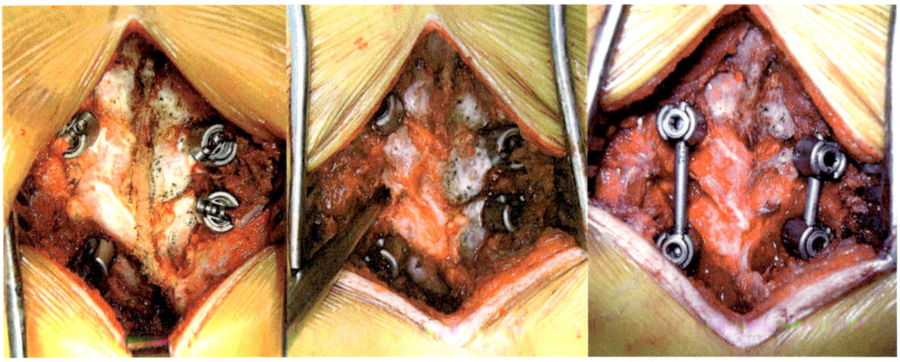

Fig. 6. Eggshell technique.

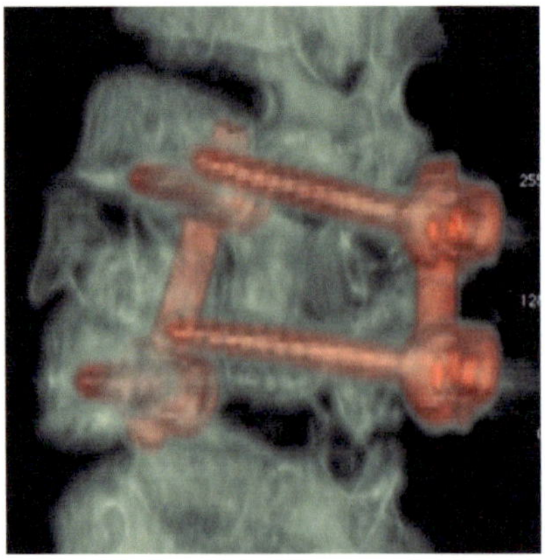

Fig. 7. 3D CT scan reconstruction of hemivertebra resection with eggshell procedure.

Initially, to close the gap left by the resected hemivertebra were applied corrective casts and brace for a 6 months period. Then posterior instrumentation was introduced, which allowed the compression of the convexity using wires, hooks and rods. Finally, the incorporation and use of pedicle screws in young children has made more rigid and shorter fixations, allowing monosegmental pedicular instrumentation with good outcomes at medium-term follow-up. (Ruf & Harms, 2003; Ruf et al., 2009).

There are also some reports of series where anterior instrumentation was used with good results in the short-term follow-up (Elsebaie et al., 2010; Garrido et al., 2008).

The operating time of anterior and posterior combined approach that goes from 280 to 435 minutes, slightly above the average operating time exclusive posterior approach, ranging from 225 to 380 minutes (Arriagada et al., 2009).

Holte et al. in a series of hemivertebra resection by combined approach showed overall complication rate of 65% with 21% of neurological complications (Holte et al., 1995). Over time, the overall complication rate decreased to values from 0% to 30%, with 5% to 10% of neurological complications, particularly transient neurological injury.

Recent research indicates that complication rates associated to the exclusive posterior approach (14%) is slightly higher than the combined approach (9%), without significant differences in relation to neurological complications (Jalanko et al., 2010).

Combined approaches are mainly associated with medical complications derived from anterior approaches (thoracotomy) and posterior approaches are mainly associated with complications derived from implant failure and the need for reoperations.

The global analysis of hemivertebra resections, regardless of approach, shows average correction of 35% to 81% in the coronal plane and 8% to 79% in the sagittal plane, with a minimum follow-up of 2 years.

In the short and medium-term follow-up, surgeries perfomed through combined approach allow corrections of scoliosis from 35% to 77%, without significant differences with respect to the exclusive posterior approach, which allows correction of 27% to 81% (Table 2).

Approach	Instrument.	Correction (%)		Operative time (min)	EBL (ml)	Complic. (%)
		Scoliosis	Kyphosis			
Posterior	Posterior	27 - 81	33 - 80	225 -380	114 - 885	8 - 40
Combined	Anterior	56 - 64	31 - 49	120 -133	150 - 169	8 - 13
	Posterior	35 - 77	32 - 42	280 - 435	280 - 2767	8 - 38

Table 2. Results of hemivertebra resection strategies.

The use instrumentation in the exclusive posterior approach with unilateral or bilateral monosegmental fixation is associated with frequent implant failures and the need for additional surgeries. The use of a third bar or the use of postoperative brace allows to reduce that risk.

The traditional or classic vertebral resection by exclusive posterior approach, regardless instrumentation was used, achieved corrections above 40% with minimal loss of correction during long-term follow-up. By contrast, vertebral resection with eggshell technique shown corrections of 27% in the medium-term follow-up, with a loss of scoliosis correction of 25% (Table 3).

Posterior Approach	Correction (%)		Operative time (min)	Complic. (%)	
	Scoliosis	Kyphosis		Total	Neuro
Classic	54 - 81	50 - 80	225 - 380	8 - 40	0 - 10
Eggshell	27	28	225	29	0

Table 3. Results posterior approach: classic and eggshell technique.

The growth potential of patients and the use of monosegmental fixations preserving unfused levels makes the progression and loss of correction is an expected and predictable phenomenon. Apparently eggshell resection would not allow such accurate and complete removal of adjacent intervertebral discs as well not proper preparation of adjacent vertebral plates to provide adequate anterior fusion. Furthermore, pedicle instrumentation monosegmental not be able to slow the growth of the hemivertebra above, allowing the progression of the curves.

With the eggshell technique produces better results than the "in situ" fusion and convex hemiepiphysiodesis in terms of correction and control the progression of the curve, with a similar complication rates, so that this technique appears as an intermediate alternative between these 2 strategies and complete resection of the hemivertebra, achieving acceptable and predictable angular correction, avoiding the potentially serious complications of complete vertebral resection.

For all these reasons we believe that, although the eggshell technique allows minor corrections that technique of complete resection of hemivertebra, remains a safe and less invasive alternative that can be used in a special group of patients who require surgery with low risk and predictable results, even when the magnitude of these results is less than those obtained with the complex vertebral resection by combined or single posterior approach.

7. Conclusion

The spinal malformations arise from defects in very early stages of embryonic development, due to this presents a wide variety of vertebral anomalies and their frequent association with malformations in other systems (cardiac, urologic, respiratory and neural axis).

Numerous studies of the natural history of congenital spinal deformities due to hemivertebra are categorical in the progressive nature of these deformities. It is therefore important to define accurately the type of malformation detected in the patient and determine the potential risk of progression. The most common spinal defect is the hemivertebra, which causes about 50% of cases of congenital kyphoscoliosis.

The ideal treatment for hemivertebra deformity should be able to correct the deformity, stop curve progression and prevent the development of structured secondary curves, with low complication rate.

It is demonstrated that the conservative treatment and use of brace has no place in the management of congenital kyphoscoliosis, therefore the treatment is mainly surgical.

Strict controls of patients, to objectify the evolution of the deformity is vital to define a possible surgical treatment at the right time.

Young children with deformities which have a guaranteed progression and demonstrate a curve progression with clinical repercussion are candidates for surgery. To achieve the best results, we recommend surgical treatment within 5 years of age.

Has been described three surgical options for management of kyphoscoliosis due to hemivertebra: "in situ" fusion, convex hemiepiphysiodesis and hemiartrhodesis and hemivertebra resection.

The literature review shows us that the in situ fusion is a procedure incapable to correct and control the progression of the curve, without changing the natural course of disease, for this reason its use has been virtually abandoned today.

On the other hand, the convex hemiepiphysiodesis and hemiarthrodesis is a safe procedure that shows some effectiveness in terms of correction and control of the progression, but the results are completely unpredictable in time.

Finally, resection of hemivertebra enables setting an adequate and predictable correction of the curve and stop progression, but is associated with a considerable number of complications inherent to surgery or related to use of implants, which can be potentially severe.

For all the above, there is no ideal treatment for this condition, each individual case must be analyzed, carefully assessing the condition of patient, potential risks and expected outcomes.

8. Acknowledgment

To our families, friends and colleagues.

9. References

Arriagada, G., Chahin, A., Pantoja, S & Chamorro, M. (2009). Hemivertebrae Resection with Eggshell Procedure for Congenital Kyphoscoliosis: Results in Children Aged From One to Seven Years. *Coluna/Columna*. Vol.8, No.3, (July/September 2009), pp. 337-343, ISSN 1808-1851

Basu, P., Elsebaie, H. & Noordeen, M. (2002). Congenital spinal deformity: a comprehensive assessment at presentation. *Spine*. Vol.27, No.20, (October 2002), pp. 2255–2259, ISSN 1528-1159

Beals, R., Robbins, J. & Rolfe, B. (1993). Anomalies associated with vertebral malformations. *Spine*. Vol.18, No.10, (August 1993), pp. 1329-1332, ISSN 1528-1159

Bradford, D., Heithoff, K. & Cohen M. (1991). Intraspinal abnormalities and congenital spine deformities: A radiographic and MRI study. *Journal of Pediatric Orthopaedics*. Vol.11, No.1, (January/February 1991), pp. 36-41, ISSN 1539-2570

Bulman, M., Kusumi, K. & Frayling, T. (2000). Mutations in the human delta homologue, DLL3, cause axial skeletal defects in spondylocostal dysostosis. *Nature Genetics*. Vol.24, No.4, (April 2000), pp. 438-441, ISSN 1546-1718

Cil, A., Yazici, M., Alanay, M., Acaroglu, E., Uzumcugil, A, Surat, A. (2004). The Course of Sagittal Plane Abnormality in the Patients With Congenital Scoliosis Managed With Convex Growth Arrest. *Spine*. Vol.29, No.5, (March 2004), pp. 547-553, ISSN 1528-1159

Dimeglio, A. (2001). Growth in pediatric orthopedics. *Journal of Pediatric Orthopaedics*. Vol.21, No.4, (July/August 2001), pp. 549-555, ISSN 1539-2570

Erol, B., Tracy, M., Dormans, J., Zackai, E., Maisenbacher, M., O'Brien, M., Turnpenny, P. & Kusumi, K. (2004). Congenital scoliosis and vertebral malformations: characterization of segmental defects for genetic analysis. *Journal of Pediatric Orthopaedics*. Vol.24, No.6, (November/December 2004), pp. 674-682, ISSN 1539-2570

Farley, F., Have, K., Hensinger, R., Streit, J., Zhang, L. & Caird, M. (2011). Outcomes After Spinal Fusion for Congenital Scoliosis Instrumented Versus Uninstrumented Spinal Fusion. *Spine*. Vol.36, No.2, (January 2011), pp. E112-E122, ISSN 1528-1159

Freeman, B., Ouellet, J., Twining, P. & Webb, J. (2001). *Antenatal diagnosis and ultimate outcome of fetal hemivertebrae.* Scoliosis Research Society annual meeting 2001; http://www.spineuniverse.com/professional/research/srs/2001/antenatal-diagnosis-ultimate-outcome-fetal

Giampietro PF, Blank RD, Raggio CL, et al. (2003). Congenital and idiopathic scoliosis: clinical and genetic aspects. *Clinincal Medicine & Research*. Vol.1, No.2, (April 2003), pp. 125-136, ISSN 1554-6179

Goldberg, C., Moore, D., Fogarty, E. & Dowling, F. (2002). Long-term results from in situ fusion for congenital vertebral deformity. *Spine*. Vol.27, No.6, (March 2002), pp. 619-628, ISSN 1528-1159

Hedequist, D., Hall, J. & Emans, J. (2004). The safety and efficacy of spinal instrumentation in children with congenital spine deformities. *Spine*. Vol.29, No.18, (September 2002), pp. 2081-2086, ISSN 1528-1159

Hedequist, D., Emans, J., Proctor, M. (2009). Three rod technique facilitates hemivertebra wedge resection in young children through a posterior only approach. *Spine*. Vol.34, No.6, (March 2009), pp. E225-E229, ISSN 1528-1159

Hensinger, R. (2009). Congenital scoliosis: etiology and associations. *Spine*. Vol.34, No.17, (August 2009), pp. 1745-1750, ISSN 1528-1159

Holte, D., Winter, R., Lonstein, J. & Denis, F. (1995). Excision of hemivertebrae and wedge resection in the treatment of congenital scoliosis. *The Journal of Bone and Joint Surgery Am*. Vol.77, No. 2, (February 1995), pp. 159-171, ISSN 1535-1386

Kesling, K., Lonstein, J., Denis, F., Perra, J., Schwender, J. Transfeldt, E. & Winter, R. (2003). The crankshaft phenomenon after posterior spinal arthrodesis for congenital scoliosis: a review of 54 patients. *Spine*. Vol.28, No.3, (February 2003), pp. 267-271, ISSN 1528-1159

Kusumi, K. & Turnpenny, P. (2007). Formation errors of the vertebral column. *The Journal of Bone and Joint Surgery Am.* Vol.89, Supplement 1, (February 2007), pp. 64-71, ISSN 1535-1386

McMaster, M. & Ohtsuka, K. (1982). The natural history of congenital scoliosis: A study of two hundred and fifty-one patients. *The Journal of Bone and Joint Surgery Am.* Vol.64, No.8, (October1982), pp. 1128-1147, ISSN 1535-1386

McMaster, M. & David C. (1986). Hemivertebra as a cause of scoliosis: a study of 104 patients. *The Journal of Bone and Joint Surgery Br.* Vol.68-B, No.4, (August 1986), pp. 588-595, ISSN 0301-620X

McMaster, M. & Singh, H. (1999). Natural history of congenital kyphosis and kyphoscoliosis. A study of one hundred and twelve patients. *The Journal of Bone and Joint Surgery Am.* Vol.81, No.10, (October1982), pp. 1367-1383, ISSN 1535-1386

Mohanty, S. & Kumar, N. (2000). Patterns of presentation of congenital scoliosis. *Journal of Orthopeadic Surgery.* Vol.8, No.2, (December 2000), pp. 33-37, ISSN 1022-5536

Nasca, R., Stelling, F. & Steel, H. (1975). Progression of congenital scoliosis due to hemivertebrae and hemivertebrae with bars. *The Journal of Bone and Joint Surgery Am.* Vol.57, No.4, (June 1975), pp. 456-466, ISSN 1535-1386

Ruf, M. & Harms, J. (2002). Pedicle screws in one and two year old children: Technique, complications, and effect on further growth. *Spine.* Vol.27, No.21, (November 2002), pp. E460-E466, ISSN 1528-1159

Ruf, M. & Harms, J. (2003). Posterior hemivertebra resection with transpedicular instrumentation: early correction in children aged 1 to 6 years. *Spine.* Vol.28, No.18, (September 2003), pp. 2132-2138, ISSN 1528-1159

Ruf, M., Jensen, R., Letko, L. & Harms, J. (2009). Hemivertebra resection and osteotomies in congenital spine deformity. *Spine.* Vol.34, No.17, (August 2009), pp. 1791-1799, ISSN 1528-1159

Shen, F. & Arlet, V. (2008). Congenital Scoliosis, In: *Spinal Disorders. Fundamentals of Diagnosis and Treatment,* Boos, N. & Aebi (Ed.), M., pp. 693-711, Springer, ISBN 978-3-540-40511-5, Germany

Uzumcugil, A., Cil, A., Yazici, M., Acaroglu, E., Alanay, A., Aksoy, C. & Surat, A. (2004). Convex growth arrest in the treatment of congenital spinal deformities, revisited. *Journal of Pediatric Orthopaedics.* Vol.24, No.6, (November/December 2004), pp. 658-666, ISSN 1539-2570

Winter, R., Moe, J. & Eilers, V. (1968). Congenital scoliosis: A study of 234 patients treated and untreated: Part I. Natural history. *The Journal of Bone and Joint Surgery Am.* Vol.50 , No. 1, (January 1968), pp. 1-15, ISSN 1535-1386

Winter, R. & Moe, J. (1982). The results of spinal arthrodesis for congenital spinal deformity in patients younger than five years old. *The Journal of Bone and Joint Surgery Am.* Vol.64 , No. 3, (March 1982), pp. 419-432, ISSN 1535-1386

Winter, R., Lonstein, J. Denis, F. & de la Rosa, H. (1988). Convex growth arrest for progressive congenital scoliosis due to hemivertebrae. *Journal of Pediatric Orthopaedics.* Vol.8, No.6, (November 1988), pp. 633-638, ISSN 1539-2570

Winter, R., Lonstein, J. & Boachie-Adjei, O. (1996). Instructional Course Lectures, The American Academy of Orthopaedic Surgeons: Congenital Spinal Deformity. *The Journal of Bone and Joint Surgery Am*. Vol.78-A, No. 2, (February 1996), pp. 300-311, ISSN 1535-1386

Winter, R. & Lonstein, J. (2010). Scoliosis Secondary to a Hemivertebra. Seven Patients With Gradual Improvement Without Treatment. *Spine*. Vol.35, No.2, (January 2010), pp. E49-E52, ISSN 1528-1159